The Clinical Relevance of Kindling

The Clinical Relevance of Kindling

Edited by

Tom G. Bolwig
Professor of Psychiatry, Department of Psychiatry, Rigshospitalet,
University of Copenhagen, Denmark

and

Michael R. Trimble
Consultant Physician in Psychological Medicine, National Hospital
for Nervous Diseases, Queen Square, and Senior Lecturer in
Behavioural Neurology, Department of Neurology, Institute of
Neurology, Queen Square, London, UK

JOHN WILEY & SONS
Chichester · New York · Brisbane · Toronto · Singapore

Other Wiley Editorial Offices

John Wiley & Sons, Inc., 605 Third Avenue,
New York, NY 10158-0012, USA

Jacaranda Wiley Ltd, G.P.O. Box 859, Brisbane,
Queensland 4001, Australia

John Wiley & Sons (Canada) Ltd, 22 Worcester Road,
Rexdale, Ontario M9W 1L1, Canada

John Wiley & Sons (SEA) Pte Ltd, 37 Jalan Pemimpin 05-04,
Block B, Union Industrial Building, Singapore 2057

Library of Congress Cataloging-in-Publication Data:

The Clinical relevance of kindling/edited by Thomas G. Bolwig and
    Michael R. Trimble.
        p. cm.
    Based on a symposium held in Helsingør, Denmark, Nov. 2–11, 1988.
    Includes bibliographies and index.
    ISBN 0 471 92449 0
    1. Kindling (Neurology)—Congresses. 2. Epilepsy—
Pathophysiology—Congresses. 3. Neuropsychiatry—Congresses.
I. Bolwig, Tom G. II. Trimble, Michael R.
    [DNLM: 1. Kindling (Neurology)—congresses.   WL 102 C6414 1988]
RC322.5.C58   1989
616.8'5307—dc20
DNLM/DLC
for Library of Congress   89-14757
                                                                CIP

British Library Cataloguing in Publication Data

The clinical relevance of kindling.
    1. Man. Nervous system. Diseases
    I. Bolwig, Tom G. II. Trimble, Michael R.
    616.8
    ISBN 0 471 92449 0

Phototypeset by Input Typesetting Ltd, London
Printed and bound by Courier International, Tiptree, Colchester

Contents

Contributors vii

Preface ix

Acknowledgements xi

1 Do kindling-like phenomena unify hypotheses of psychopathology?
   Tom G. Bolwig 1

2 Kindling: clinical relevance and anatomical substrate
   R. J. Racine, G. O. Ivy and N. W. Milgram 15

3 Chemical kindling
   *Claude G. Wasterlain, Anne M. Morin, Denson G. Fujikawa and
   Jeff M. Bronstein* 35

4 Kindling and antiepileptic drugs
   M. Schmutz and K. Klebs 55

Discussion — Session 1 69

5 Kindling and neurotransmitter systems: seizure suppression by
   intracerebral grafting of fetal neurons
   David I. Barry, Jørn Kragh and Benedikte Wanscher 75

6 Kindling and memory
   Jerzy Majkowski. 87

7 Kindling, behaviour and memory
   J. Mellanby and L. Sundstrom 103

Discussion — Session 2 113

8 Kindling, anxiety and personality
   Robert E. Adamec. 117

9 Kindling, psychopathology and cerebral mechanisms in ethanol
   withdrawal
   Ralf Hemmingsen 137

Discussion — Session 3 147

10 The process of epilepsy: is kindling relevant?
    E. H. Reynolds 149

11 The prognosis of epilepsy
    Mogens Dam and Anne Sabers 161

12 Kindling, epilepsy and behaviour
    M. R. Trimble. 177

Discussion — Session 4 191

13 Convulsive therapy and kindling
    Max Fink 195

14 Kindling and manic-depressive illness
    Robert M. Post and S. R. B. Weiss 209

15 Addictive behavior and kindling: relationship to alcohol
    withdrawal and cocaine
    James C. Ballenger and Robert M. Post. 231

Discussion — Session 5 259

16 Kindling and panic disorder
    Raben Rosenberg 263

17 Kindling, drug holidays and disorders of movement
    R. Fog and H. Pakkenberg. 275

Discussion — Session 6 281

Subject index 287

Contributors

R. E. Adamec, *Departments of Psychology and Basic Medical Science, Memorial University, St John's, Newfoundland, Canada*

J. C. Ballenger, *Department of Psychiatry and Behavioral Sciences, Medical University of South Carolina, USA*

D. I. Barry, *Neurobiology Research Group, Department of Psychiatry, Rigshospitalet, University of Copenhagen, Denmark*

T. G. Bolwig, *Department of Psychiatry, Rigshospitalet, University of Copenhagen, Denmark*

J. M. Bronstein, *Epilepsy Research Laboratory, VA Medical Center, Sepulveda, California, USA*

M. Dam, *University Clinic of Neurology, Hvidovre Hospital, Hvidovre, Denmark*

M. Fink, *Department of Psychiatry and Behavioral Science, State University of New York at Stony Brook, New York, USA and International Association of Psychiatric Research, St James, New York, USA*

R. Fog, *Laboratory of Psychopharmacology, St Hans Hospital, Roskilde, Denmark*

D. G. Fujikawa, *Epilepsy Research Laboratory, VA Medical Center, Sepulveda, California, USA*

R. Hemmingsen, *Department of Psychiatry, Bispebjerg Hospital, Copenhagen, Denmark*

G. O. Ivy, *Department of Psychology, Scarborough College, University of Toronto, Scarborough, Ontario, Canada*

K. Klebs, *Research and Development Department, Pharmaceuticals Division, Ciba-Geigy Ltd, Basel, Switzerland*

J. Kragh, *Neurobiology Research Group, Department of Psychiatry, Rigshospitalet, University of Copenhagen, Denmark*

J. Majkowski, *Department of Neurology and Epileptology, Medical Center for Postgraduate Education, Warszawa, Poland*

J. Mellanby, *Department of Experimental Psychology, University of Oxford, UK*

N. W. Milgram, *Department of Psychology, Scarborough College, University of Toronto, Scarborough, Ontario, Canada*

A. M. Morin, *Epilepsy Research Laboratory, VA Medical Center, Sepulveda, California, USA*

H. Pakkenberg, *Department of Neurology, Hvidovre Hospital, Hvidovre, Denmark*

R. M. Post, *Biological Psychiatry Branch, National Institute of Mental Health, Bethesda, Maryland, USA*

R. Racine, *Department of Psychology, McMaster University, Hamilton, Ontario, Canada*

E. H. Reynolds, *Maudsley and King's College Hospitals, London, UK*

R. Rosenberg, *Department of Psychiatry, Rigshospitalet, University of Copenhagen, Denmark*

A. Sabers, *University Clinic of Neurology, Hvidovre Hospital, Hvidovre, Denmark*

M. Schmutz, *Research and Development Department, Pharmaceuticals Division, Ciba-Geigy Ltd, Basel, Switzerland*

L. Sundstrom, *Department of Experimental Psychology, University of Oxford, UK*

M. R. Trimble, *Department of Psychological Medicine, National Hospitals for Nervous Diseases and Institute of Neurology, London, UK*

B. Wanscher, *Neurobiology Research Group, Department of Psychiatry, Rigshospitalet, University of Copenhagen, Denmark*

C. G. Wasterlain, *Epilepsy Research Laboratory, VA Medical Center, Sepulveda, California, USA*

S. R. B. Weiss, *Biological Psychiatry Branch, National Institute of Mental Health, Bethesda, Maryland, USA*

Preface

Since the discovery by Graham Goddard of the kindling phenomenon in 1967 this new concept in the neurosciences has been the subject of a steadily increasing number of research reports as well as three books. From being originally an area of experimental neurophysiology, kindling gradually has become a vital area of interest in the search for pathophysiological explanations of neurological and psychiatric disorders in man. Bringing together a group of authors, we have wished to shed more light on some of the controversial and more or less well-documented aspects of this whole intriguing area of research.

The first chapter by Bolwig lays the groundwork for the rest of the book by discussing certain areas of psychopathology where kindling may have relevance.

The second chapter by Racine reviews the present knowledge of basic characteristics of the kindling phenomenon and points to a possible use of the concept in understanding human epileptogenesis. Wasterlain then discusses differences and similarities between electrically and chemically induced kindling in animals, and Schmutz tackles the problems of the differential action of various antiepileptic drugs on kindling development and on the kindled state. The importance of the ascending noradrenergic projection system for a suppressive action on the development of kindling is described by Barry who discusses the modulation of excitability of epileptic brain regions in the rat following grafting of fetal neurons.

An area of controversy is the relation between kindling and memory formation. Majkowski reviews current hypotheses, and based on cat experiments points to differences in spatio-temporal distribution of impulses being responsible for events at the interface between epileptogenesis and memory consolidation. Following this some studies by Mellanby describe impairment of memory and behaviour in rats not fully kindled and with reversible EEG-changes. Further implications of limbic kindling on behaviour are reviewed by Adamec who finds that repeated spread of seizures into the amygdala of the cat leads to behavioural changes which serve as a model for the interictal

ix

phenomena seen in certain epileptic patients. The last chapter on behaviour and kindling in laboratory animals by Hemmingsen has the suggestion that repeated episodes of alcohol withdrawal and not the intoxication as such are the background for the severe consequences of heavy drinking such as delirium tremens and epileptic convulsions.

The following chapters are clinical studies. Reynolds discusses the process of epilepsy and carefully sifts the evidence for kindling and for other candidates being responsible for chronicity in epilepsy. Dam likewise, on the basis of the different prognosis of different forms of epilepsy, discusses kindling alongside with neurological, psychological and social factors. Trimble looks at psychopathology associated with epilepsy, and discusses the possibility that kindling may play a role in the psychoses associated with localization-related temporal lobe epilepsy.

Fink reviews the literature concerning ECT and kindling and compares these two forms of repeated electrical stimulation of the brain. He points out the many differences of these processes and discusses the antidepressant and antimanic effect of ECT in relation to the kindling hypothesis. Based on the study of a pharmacological preclinical kindling model Post considers the longitudinal aspects of manic-depressive illness and suggests that the frequency of cycling occurring over time may be best understood in the light of a kindling-like hypothesis.

Studies of well-tested preclinical models as well as clinical experience pointing to a kindling-like pathophysiological background for cocaine intoxication and for alcohol withdrawal are presented by Ballenger.

Finally, the clinical and pathophysiological features characterizing the still controversial clinical entity panic disorder are discussed by Rosenberg, and Fog reviews the different hypotheses for the pathogenesis of tardive dyskinesia with special reference to 'drug holidays'.

We have chosen to include in the text certain sections from the very lively discussion which occurred during our meeting. We hope that in editing this we have retained some of the more important points which were brought out by the discussants.

It is our hope that this book will help clarify some of the many unresolved issues of kindling and its relation to neuropsychiatric illness, and will be an inspiration for further investigations in this important field of research.

TOM G. BOLWIG
Copenhagen

MICHAEL R. TRIMBLE
London

Acknowledgements

The editors gratefully acknowledge the support of Ciba-Geigy of the Nordic Countries, and in particular the enthusiasm of Lars Christian Andersen, Denmark, who participated in the work of planning and coordination of the symposium on the background of which this book has been composed. They also wish to thank all the speakers for providing manuscripts for the book and for their contributions to valuable discussions throughout the meeting.

The Clinical Relevance of Kindling
Edited by T. G. Bolwig and M. R. Trimble
© 1989 John Wiley & Sons Ltd

1

Do kindling-like phenomena unify hypotheses of psychopathology?

TOM G. BOLWIG
Department of Psychiatry, Rigshospitalet, University of Copenhagen, DK-2100 Copenhagen, Denmark

INTRODUCTION

Since the first description of the kindling phenomenon by Goddard (Goddard, 1967; Goddard, McIntyre and Leech, 1969), who demonstrated how repeated administration of an initially subconvulsive electrical stimulus leads to a progressive intensification of seizure activity culminating in a generalized seizure, the number of research reports dealing with aspects of this neurophysiological phenomenon have been steadily increasing (Wada, 1986). In rats stimulated in the amygdala the initial stimulus often elicits focal electrical seizure activity (after-discharge measured on EEG) without clinical seizures. Subsequent stimulation will induce the development of seizures evolving through five stages from facial clonus to rearing and falling (Racine, 1977). Through this development there is reduced responsiveness to sensory stimuli as compared to the normal waking state. When fully kindled, the animals for months will have full strength responses after one or two stimulations (Wada and Sato, 1974). If the animal is stimulated beyond the fully kindled state, spontaneous convulsions will often occur, and interictal spikes are frequent. Kindling can be induced by stimulation of many but not all sites in the brains of different species of animals, including primates. The limbic system and related structures such as the olfactory bulb, the pyriform cortex and the amygdala require relatively few stimulations, whereas hippocampus has a higher kindling rate.

The above-mentioned features, carefully described in laboratory studies, have challenged and inspired many clinicians for whom a precise description of progressive and sequential changes in psychopathology is crucial for their understanding of the relationship of the development of clinical phenomena to underlying neurobiological mechanisms. This has led to speculations and formation of hypotheses concerning a number of previously completely unrelated conditions, all of which, however, with the background that, as in the laboratory studies, repetition of critical stimuli and a time factor are unifying themes.

DOES THE KINDLING MODEL HAVE CLINICAL RELEVANCE?

Kindling in the strictest sense of the model is impossible to intentionally demonstrate in man, and very little evidence exists pointing to proper kindling in patients. In certain forms of epilepsy, however, the kindling model can be applied easily since in such conditions it is possible to measure spontaneous and evoked EEG-changes related to cortical as well as subcortical structures and also to concomitant psychopathological phenomena present before, during, after, and not least important, between epileptic fits. Epilepsy and epilepsy-related conditions are discussed thoroughly in Chapters 10 (Reynolds), 11 (Dam and Sabers) and 12 (Trimble).

In the study of drug abuse and alcoholism we face clinical problems in which the underlying pathological mechanism may be viewed in the light of the kindling model, since in the course of constant abuse, especially of psychomotor stimulants such as cocaine and amphetamine, as well as in heavy alcoholism, there will be both gross psychopathology and often seizures. These aspects are discussed in Chapter 9 by Hemmingsen and Chapter 15 by Ballenger and Post.

While the above-mentioned conditions with frequent and demonstrable epilepsy-like properties have been much studied in relation to kindling for obvious reasons, other conditions such as functional psychosis, especially affective disorder and to a lesser degree schizophrenia, have also been considered. Finally, tardive dyskinesia found after long periods of neuroleptic medication is under discussion (for review, see Glenthøj, Hemmingsen and Bolwig, 1988 and Fog and Pakkenberg, Chapter 17), especially because intermittent treatment as compared to constant medication seems to represent over time a stimulus that may bear some resemblance to kindling.

THE FUNCTIONAL PSYCHOSES

Manic-depressive disorder

Post and Ballenger (1981) were the first to suggest that affective illness in certain forms may bear some resemblance to the progression of behavioral changes observed during kindling experiments. They referred to a review by Grof, Angst and Haines (1974) describing a patient population sample of 594 with recurrent unipolar depression, in which group each episode of illness tended to occur with shorter intervals between successive episodes. This phenomenon of apparent sensitization seemed more evident in the older age ranges. The observation is in good accordance with the purely clinical description given in the textbook of Bleuler (1916), who states that with recurrent episodes of mania and depression shorter intervals between episodes becomes a characteristic, and a condition of chronicity gradually develops.

The idea that the course of manic-depressive illness may be considered a kindling-like process is based on the studies of pharmacological kindling (Post and Kopanda, 1976 and Post and Weiss, Chapter 14), and it was the observation of the different changes of affect ranging from elevation of mood to depression-like conditions that further inspired cocaine use in man to be viewed as a parallel to certain affective disorders. Post and co-workers (1987) showed that there was an environmental context dependent effect, and this further has led to speculations linking pharmacological kindling and other forms of stimuli inducing a sensitization process. The idea that certain life events after one or more episodes of illness will exert an increasing influence in the limbic system and make way for new episodes represents a stress diathesis model (Post et al., 1981).

There is thus a theoretical link between pharmacological kindling, behavioural sensitization and occurrence of mood swings following psycho-social stresses. However, it is not proven that all phases in manic-depressive disorder are precipitated by stressful events, and further manic-depressive illness has very little similarity with the other conditions considered in the light of the kindling model. It is important to reinforce the point that the illness is not a seizure disorder and neither positron emission tomography (PET) nor single photon emission computerized tomography (SPECT) studies have pointed to localized pathology associated with limbic structures in affective disorder.

It is interesting, however, that at least two principles that are efficacious in blocking the development of kindling, namely electroconvulsive therapy (ECT) and carbamazepine, are highly valuable in the therapy of manic-depressive illness, especially of the bipolar type; but the anticonvulsant effects of these two treatment modalities do not explain their efficacy in a non-convulsive disorder. Further, both ECT and carbamazepine have robust effects in diseases completely unrelated to affective disorder such as certain epileptic conditions and delirious conditions and can not, therefore, be immediately used in the argument for manic-depressive psychosis having a kindling-like background.

Schizophrenia

There is not much clinical evidence that makes it reasonable to explain any of the various forms of schizophrenia as a kindling-like phenomenon. Although in manic-depressive illness the course of illness bears some resemblance to the behavioural sensitization seen in the laboratory, this is not the case with schizophrenia. However, theoretically there is a possibility that a kindling-like mechanism could be at work at least in certain forms of schizophrenia. One might speculate for instance, as has been done by Weinberger (1986, 1987), that the brain structures in which neuroleptic drugs are highly efficacious in the treatment of psychotic symptoms might be the site of a dysfunction responsible for the development of the disease. This has been generally related to the high density of dopaminergic nerve connections in the basal ganglia. However, the intriguing finding by Ingvar and Franzén (1973) that there is a decreased blood flow in the frontal regions of schizophrenic patients — a finding which has been confirmed in independent studies — points to an involvement of cortical regions which does not find an explanation in the prevailing subcortical dopamine theory for schizophrenia.

The idea that schizophrenia basically is a brain disease rather than the result of psycho-social problems is not new, and the finding of the above-mentioned metabolic 'hypofrontality', and in certain patients of enlarged cerebral ventricles has given neurobiological explanations an increasing momentum in the past two decades.

In spite of a number of sophisticated studies of brain function *in vivo* and post-mortem investigations, so far no finely circumscribed lesion has been described. It would also be unreasonable to imagine a single nucleus, a cortical region, or a major pathway being implicated by itself. It is more appropriate to think of an involvement of a system of anatomically and neurochemically related cortical and subcortical regions. These would include various periventricular, limbic and diencephalic nuclei such as nucleus accumbens, hypothalamus, medial pallidum and amygdala as well as the so-called limbic cortex, the hippocampal formation and the dorso-lateral prefrontal cortex. These cortical and subcortical components are linked functionally and anatomically. Distortions in perception or hallucinations may reflect a dysfunction of the periventricular, limbic, and diencephalic nuclei, whereas the decreased motivation, social ineffectiveness and flat affect characteristic in many schizophrenics point to a dysfunction of the dorsolateral prefrontal cortex (Weinberger, 1986, 1987).

In favour of the idea that the so-called positive psychotic symptoms represent a dysfunction in the subcortical sites, are findings from depth electrode studies showing that psychotic experiences and perceptual distortions can result from electrical discharges in hippocampus, amygdala or temporal cortex (Gloor *et al.*, 1982) as well as the schizophrenia-like symptomatology following organic diseases such as tumours, trauma, epilepsy and infections involving the limbic system and diencephalon (Davison and Bagley, 1969; Trimble in Chapter 12).

The theory suggested by Weinberger is that the dopamine hyperactivity which has been demonstrated also in receptor studies in man using the PET-technique (Gjedde and Wong, 1988) is secondary to a functional disinhibition between the prefrontal cortex and the deep structures. The efficacy of the neuroleptics in reducing positive symptoms is thus thought to be related to a reduction of dopamine activity in the system described here. The theory seems to gain support from monkey experiments showing that there is impairment of cognitive functions when selective ablation of ascending dopamine afferents to the dorsolateral prefrontal cortex is made (Brozoski et al., 1979).

One of the important features characterizing schizophrenia is the very high probability that the disease will become clinically apparent in late adolescence. Much speculation can be made concerning the role of brain maturation if one accepts the Weinberger concept of a 'lesion' in the connection between subcortical and prefrontal cortical structures.

The possibility of a kindling-like process in the development over time from early childhood to adolescence of a 'lesion' with a secondary, compensatory hyperfunction of dopaminergic areas must be considered speculative, but is a probability seen in the light of the frequent finding of EEG-abnormalities in children hospitalized with a variety of psychiatric disorders, some of which turn out to be early stages of a psychotic disorder. The problem of explaining schizophrenia and manic-depressive disorder as diseases with a neurophysiological background in a kindling-like action is the same: these diseases do not display seizures in their phenomenology. Further, patients with schizophrenia, in contrast to those with affective illness, do not seem to respond to the anticonvulsants ECT and carbamazepine. On the other hand, there seems to be a close relationship between the development of tardive dyskinesia, the antipsychotic effect of neuroleptics and psychopathology. Dopamine, either alone or in co-operation with other transmitter systems, seems to mediate the reinforcing effect of brain stimulation (Crow and Deakin, 1985), and kindling stimulation of the central tegmental area of the cat (Stevens and Livermore, 1978) speaks in favour of the hypothesis suggested insofar as the animals developed progressive fearfulness and loss of social behaviour instead of seizures.

ALCOHOLISM

In their retrospective study Ballenger and Post (1978) showed that it takes more than 10 years for an alcoholic patient to develop severe clinical phenomena such as delirium tremens and convulsions, while milder physical abstinence symptoms begin sooner in the course of a drinking career. The authors suggested that a kindling-like mechanism was the pathophysiological background for the clinical picture (see Chapter 15).

The idea that abstinence more than the toxic influence of alcohol is a critical variable in the predisposition to alcohol withdrawal seizures in patients seems confirmed by the recent findings of Brown *et al.* (1988).

Elucidation of these problems has been attempted through experimental studies such as those briefly described below, and in more details by Hemmingsen (Chapter 9). In an animal model for the study of successive episodes of ethanol intoxication and withdrawal in the rat developed by Clemmesen and Hemmingsen (1984), it was shown that after a number of episodes, i.e. cycles of intoxication followed by withdrawal, an increasing number of animals developed spontaneous seizures, strongly resembling the stage 3–5 kindling response described in studies of electrical amygdala kindling in the rat (Racine, 1977). Experiments have shown that previous alcohol withdrawal facilitates electrical kindling (Carrington, Ellinwood and Kristiansen, 1984) and that amygdala kindling will provoke and increase in the severity of subsequent withdrawal reactions (Pinel, 1980). This clear experimental evidence of cross-sensitization between the two categories of CNS excitation further finds clinical support in the study of Brown *et al.* (1988). In suppport of the idea that kindling is the underlying mechanism for the development of behavioral abnormalities during the course of alcoholism is a recent study by Clemmesen *et al.* (1988). This group, using the 2-deoxyglucose method, showed that spontaneous withdrawal seizures during cycles of intoxication and withdrawal had significantly more pronounced suppression of glucose metabolism in the amygdala as compared to other regions of the brain, and with audiogenic seizures the suppression was most pronounced in the auditory cortex. This points to a certain specificity in the neuropathology of behaviour, stressing the role of the amygdala for the development of seizures following repetition of initially subconvulsive biological events. Further there are not only similarities between electrical kindling and the repeated intoxication–withdrawal episodes, but there are also suggestions that cross-sensitization between the two categories of CNS excitation exists (Brown *et al.*, 1988).

A hyperexcitability of the CNS in delirium tremens and related conditions was recently demonstrated in a study of cerebral blood flow using SPECT by Hemmingsen *et al.* (1988). They studied 12 patients with severe alcohol withdrawal reactions; it was found that a significant correlation existed between increased flow and the occurrence of visual hallucinations and agitation during the acute reaction.

Taken together, clinical observations and animal experiments rather strongly point to the withdrawal phenomenon being of crucial importance for the progressive development of severe behavioural abnormality in connection with repetition of alcohol ingestion, and especially that a kindling-like phenomenon may be at play.

A link between alcoholism, epilepsy with complex partial seizures (CPS) and kindling could be suggested on the background of a study of alcoholics with a 15–20 year drinking career, who developed personality features somewhat similar to those described by Bear and Fedio (1977) in a syndrome characterizing some, but definitely not all, patients with temporal lobe epilepsy (TLE) (Jellinck, 1952; Gross et al., 1976).

ABUSE OF PSYCHOMOTOR STIMULANTS

There is a wealth of observations suggesting a connection between long-term abuse of certain stimulants such as cocaine and amphetamine and severe psychopathology. In review articles (Post and Kopanda, 1976; Post and Ballenger, 1981 and Chapter 15) some of the clinical and especially the pharmacological evidence pointing to a kindling-like effect are discussed. The authors here operate with the concept of pharmacological kindling. Cocaine and lidocaine are shown to have potent effects on the limbic system, in an experimental setting causing localized spindles, after-discharges and seizure activity before the cortical EEG is influenced. These neurophysiological phenomena seem to increase in severity after repeated doses, resulting in increasing effects on behaviour which may eventually become manifest in convulsions very much similar to those seen following electrical amygdala kindling (Post, 1975).

Thus, the time course and quality of physiological focus of the effects of cocaine and lidocaine seem suggestive of a pharmacological kindling mechanism within the limbic system, the stimulant effects of cocaine probably being due to its ability to enhance catecholamines, particularly dopamine (Kelly and Iversen, 1975).

The clinical effects of these two stimulants, which seem to exert increasing social problems, especially on the American continent, lead to arousal, alerting and euphoria. They are substances which can easily been studied in the laboratory where studies with intracerebral administration have shown strong rewarding effects. This may well explain why the abuse of such drugs is very difficult to treat.

Further preclinical studies are necessary before firmer conclusions can be drawn, but undoubtedly the study of pharmacological kindling seems to be a fruitful way to understand the mechanism behind the abuse of stimulants and not least to explore the mechanism of action at a transmitter level in the search for drugs that may effectively block the development of sensitization.

There are some similarities in the clinical picture of cocaine and amphetamine abuse, but there are also differences. While an effect on catecholamines seems to be a common denominator, it is more difficult to see amphetamine psychosis, with its schizophrenia-like features, especially auditory hallucinations and stereotypies, as a result of a kindling process in contrast to cocaine-induced disturbances which may often lead to epileptic seizures.

PSYCHIATRIC MANIFESTATIONS OF EPILEPSY

The clinical relevance for the kindling model in epilepsy is obvious. The kindling concept is derived from laboratory studies of animals rendered epileptic. One of the more important clinical observations suggesting that kindling-like phenomena may contribute to epileptogenesis in humans is that of the 'mirror focus'. It has been observed that epilepsy with complex partial seizures arising from one temporal lobe may progress so that both temporal lobes eventually trigger complex partial seizures. The notion of a mirror focus seems supported by the observation that patients with brain tumours apparently confined to one temporal lobe seem to develop seizure activity generated independently by both temporal lobes (Morrel *et al.*, 1983). It is thus a possible interpretation that repeated seizure activity from one abnormal temporal lobe can itself induce epileptic activity in an originally normal temporal lobe.

The *psychotic manifestations* present in some, but not all, epileptic patients have been thoroughly reviewed by Toone (1981) and Trimble (1988, Chapter 12). Based on these reports it seems evident that patients with epilepsy display an increased incidence of psychopathology both with respect to psychosis such as schizophrenia-like syndromes (Slater and Beard, 1963), and affective disorder (Flor-Henry, 1969) as well as personality disorders. Concerning the question of laterality, a left-sided temporal lobe focus probably is more likely to be associated with a schizophrenia-like psychosis in contrast to the development of affective disorder linked with right-sided non-dominant abnormality. Trimble (1988) emphasizes that in the case of schizophrenia-like psychoses especially, British investigators have used Schneider's criteria for diagnosis, and that a lack of deterioration and negative features are remarkable in these patients. However, the relevance of limbic system dysfunction to the development of psychopathology in epilepsy has been generally agreed upon, also by investigators using different diagnostic criteria (Kristensen and Sindrup, 1978).

Whether the development of the psychoses, which for the schizophrenia-like syndromes may take 12 to 16 years after the start of seizures (Slater and Beard, 1963), are epileptic in origin, i.e. the result of recurrent seizure phenomena, or whether they are the result of unspecific organic changes is still a matter of dispute. Flor-Henry (1969) has advocated for the concept that a link between seizure frequency and psychosis exists, whereas Slater and Beard (1963) represent the opinion that a defined organic damage is the background of psychotic phenomena.

In favour of the idea of a connection between epileptic activity and psychosis are the studies by Heath (1962, 1977) who recorded abnormal EEG-discharges from mesolimbic structures in patients with psychotic symptomatology regardless of the co-existence of epilepsy. He found that such subcortical activity seems inversely related to cortical electrophysiological phenomena in epileptic patients with psychosis. It is interesting that, while norepinephrine is clearly inhibitory to the development of amygdaloid kindling (Adamec and Stark-Adamec, 1983; Barry et al., 1987), an increase in dopamine activity following kindling seems probable. Kindling of the central tegmental area in the cat leads to both increased dopamine activity and development of progressive fearfulness and loss of social behaviour instead of seizures (Stevens and Livermore, 1978). Adamec and Stark-Adamec (1983) suggest that the behavioural changes developing during the kindling process and the epileptogenicity may be independent events, and that the changes in behaviour do not require the development of motor seizures. They propose that long-lasting synaptic potentiation and an increased susceptibility to failure under high drive of neurotransmitter systems antagonistic to seizure expressions (including dopamine) have explanatory value in understanding the persisting interictal changes in the behaviour of patients suffering from epilepsy with complex partial symptomatology.

The *personality changes* of interictal nature likewise are still a matter of great controversy. A large number of studies have been published, and recently reviewed by Sørensen and Bolwig (1987). Survey of the literature, including studies with Minnesota Multiphasic Personality Inventory (MMPI), the Bear–Fedio Inventory, and psychiatric clinical assessments, points to an increased prevalence of emotional and psychological problems in patients with epilepsy in general and temporal lobe epilepsy specifically. However, no consistent picture of the phenomenlogy of personality changes in epilepsy finds support from these studies, while several case reports suggest an interesting relationship between temporal lobe epilepsy and a pronounced interest in philosophical and religious matters, hypergraphia and changes in sexuality, often hyposexuality (Bear and Fedio, 1977). The majority of these studies have been made in patients in hospital settings, some patients undergoing temporal lobectomy, and are thus hardly representative for an 'average' epileptic population. Since the influence of a number of other factors, such as medication, heredity, social factors, age at onset and duration of illness, also seem not to be fully determined, the question of a kindling mechanism behind personality changes in epilepsy is difficult to determine. Further, some of the disturbed partial personality functions in epilepsy in a recent study using Bellak's semi-structured interview (Sørensen et al., 1988) did not point to a difference on adaptive level of ego-functioning between primary generalized epilepsy and epilepsy with complex partial symptomatology. Patients with a temporal lobe focus had the same adapative level regardless of the side localization of the EEG-changes. Taken together, however, it was found that compared with a group of healthy volunteers and patients with a non-neurological, relapsing disorder (psoriasis), the epilepsy groups showed a decrease in the adaptive level of ego-functioning. One of the areas most affected was 'regulation and control of drives' which to a certain extent points to the involvement of the limbic system in the epilepsy groups.

CONCLUSIONS

Kindling, such as it was described originally by Goddard (1967) and subsequently by a number of laboratory researchers, is a concept based on stimulation of certain, especially central brain structures, leading to abnomal behaviour including motor seizures. In the study of certain forms of epilepsy which can be reasonably replicated in the laboratory animal with intracerebral EEG-measurements it is reasonable to assume that kindling may be an important underlying mechanism, just as is the case for other conditions leading to seizure activity, for instance the effect of repeated intake of certain psychomotor stimulants and the alcohol-withdrawal phenomenon.

The well-established paramount importance of the limbic system for the development of psychopathology (Trimble, 1981), together with some of the characteristics of electrical kindling, namely (1) that the primary stimulus is below the seizure threshold, (2) that it is necessary to stimulate with certain intervals, (3) that the fully kindled state remains permanent and (4) that interictal EEG-abnormalities persist, all make it tempting to speculate that diseases such as the functional psychoses may also have a kindling-like background in spite of the fact that these diseases are not seizure disorders. On the background of our present knowledge it is, however, too early to judge whether this is the case. The suggestions, however, are of great interest, and when the neurochemistry of kindling, especially regarding the neurotransmitters, becomes clarified, it will be possible to judge the relative importance of the repetition of the electrical stimulus and that of stress and fear.

It may by then turn out that repeated episodes of psychosocial stress and the kindling phenomenon proper have considerable neurobiological similarities. But only when such a similarity has been made more plausible, will the ideas of a kindling-like effect as an explanation for the development of the functional psychoses be more than speculations.

REFERENCES

Adamec, R. E. and Stark-Adamec, C. (1983). Limbic kindling and animal behaviour — implications for human psychopathology associated with complex partial seizures. *Biol. Psychiat.*, **18**, 269–293.

Bear, D. and Fedio, P. (1977). Quantitative analysis of interictal behavior in temporal lobe epilepsy. *Arch. Neurol.*, **34**, 454–467.

Ballenger, J. C. and Post, R. M. (1978). Kindling as a model for alcohol withdrawal syndromes. *Br. J. Psychiat.*, **133**, 1–14.

Barry, D. I., Kikvadze, I., Brundin, P., Bolwig, T. G., Björklund, A. and Lindvall, O. (1987). Grafted noradrenergic neurons suppress seizure development in kindling-induced epilepsy. *Proc. Natl. Acad. Sci.*, USA, **84**, 8712–8715.

Bleuler, E. (1916). Lehrbuch der Psychiatrie. Springer, Berlin.

Brown, M. E., Anton, R. F., Malcolm, R. and Ballenger, J. C. (1988). Alcohol detoxification and withdrawal seizures: clinical support for a kindling hypothesis. *Biol. Psychiat.*, **23**, 507–514.

Brozoski, T. J., Brown, R. M., Rosvold, H. E. and Goldman, P. S. (1979). Cognitive deficit caused by regional depletion of dopamine in prefrontal cortex of rhesus monkey. *Science*, **205**, 929–931.

Carrington, C. D., Ellinwood, E. H. and Kristiansen, R. R. (1984). Effects of single and repeated alcohol withdrawal on kindling. *Biol. Psychiat.*, **19(4)**, 525–537.

Clemmesen, L. and Hemmingsen, R. (1984). Physical dependence on ethanol during multiple intoxication and withdrawal episodes in the rat: evidence of potentiation. *Acta Pharmacol. Toxicol.*, **55**, 345–350.

Clemmesen, L., Ingvar, M., Hemmingsen, R. and Bolwig, T. G. (1988). Local cerebral glucose consumption during ethanol withrawal in the rat: Effects of single and multiple episodes and previous convulsive seizures. *Brain Res.*, **453**, 204–214.

Crow, T. J. and Deakin, J. F. W. (1988). Neurochemical transmission, behaviour and mental disorder. In: *Handbook of Psychiatry*, Vol. 5. *The Scientific Foundations of Psychiatry* (ed. M. Shepherd), pp. 137–186. Cambridge University Press, Cambridge.

Davison, K. and Bagley, C. R. (1969). Schizophrenia-like psychoses associated with organic disorders of the central nervous system. In: *Curent Problems in Neuropsychiatry* (ed. R. N. Herrington), pp. 113–184.

Flor-Henry, P. (1969). Psychosis and temporal lobe epilepsy. *Epilepsia*, **10**, 363–395.

Gjedde, A. and Wong, D. F. (1987). Positron tomographic quantitation of neuroreceptors in human brain in vivo with special reference to the D2 dopamine receptors in caudate nucleus. *Neurosurg. Rev.*, **10**, 9–18.

Glenthøj, B., Hemmingsen, R. and Bolwig, T. G. (1988). Kindling: a model for the development of tardive dyskinesia? *Behav. Neurol.*, **1**, 29–40.

Gloor, P., Olivier, A., Quesnay, L. F., Anderman, F. and Horowitz, S. (1982). The role of the limbic system in experimental phenomena of temporal lobe epilepsy. *Ann. Neurol.*, **12**, 129–138.

Goddard, G. V. (1967). Development of epileptic seizures through brain stimulation at low intensity. *Nature*, **214**, 1020–1021.

Goddard, G. V., McIntyre, D. C. and Leech, C. K. (1969). A permanent change in brain function resulting from daily electrical stimulation. *Exp. Neurol.*, **25**, 295–330.

Grof, P., Angst, J. and Haines, T. (1974). The clinical course of depression. Practical issues. In: *Classification and Prediction of Outcome of Depression* (ed. F. K. Schattauer), pp. 141–148. Schattauer Verlag, New York.

Gross, M. M., Kierszenbaum, H. S., Lewis, E. and Lee, Y. (1976). Desire to drink: relation to age, blood alcohol concentration, and severity of withdrawal on admission for detoxification. *Ann. N.Y. Acad. Sci.*, **273**, 360–363.

Heath, R. G. (1962). Common characteristics of epilepsy and schizophrenia. *Am. J. Psychiat.*, **118**, 1013–1026.

Heath, R. G. (1977). Subcortical brain function correlates to psychopathology in epilepsy. In: *Psychopathology and Brain Dysfunction* (eds C. Shagass, S. Gershon and A. J. Friedhoff). New York, Raven Press.

Hemmingsen, R., Vorstrup, S., Clemmesen, L., Holm, S., Tfelt-Hansen, P., Sørensen, A. S., Hansen, C., Sommer, W. and Bolwig, T. G. (1988). Cerebral blood flow during delirium tremens and related clinical states studied with Xenon–133 inhalation tomography. *Am. J. Psychiat.*, **145(11)**, 1384–1390.

Ingvar, D. H. and Franzén, G. (1973). Abnormalities of cerebral blood flow distribution in patients with chronic schizophrenia. *Acta Psychiat. Scand.*, **50**, 425–462.

Jellinek, E. M. (1952). Phases of alcohol addiction. *Q.J. Stud. Alcohol*, **13**, 673–684.

Kelly, P. H. and Iversen, S. D. (1975). Selective 6-OHDA-induced destruction of mesolimbic dopamine neurons: abolition of psychostimulant-induced psychomotor activity in rats. *Eur. J. Pharmacol.*, **40**, 45–56.

Kristensen, O. and Sindrup, E. (1978). Personality correlates of sphenoidal EEG foci in temporal lobe epilepsy. *Acta Neurol. Scand.*, **64**, 289–300.

Morrel, F., Rasmussen, T., Gloor, P. and de Toledo-Morrell, L. (1983). Secondary epileptogenic foci in patients with verified temporal lobe tumors. *Electroencephalogr. Clin. Neurophysiol.*, **54**, 26–48.

Pinel, J. P. J. (1980). Alcohol withdrawal seizures: implications of kindling. *Pharmacol. Biochem. Behav.*, **13(1)**, 225–231.

Post, R. M. (1975). Cocaine psychoses: a continuum model. *Am. J. Psychiat.*, **132**, 225–231.

Post, R. M. and Ballenger, J. C. (1981). Kindling models for the progressive development of psychopathology. Sensitization to electrical, pharmacological and psychological stimuli. In: *Handbook of Biological Psychiatry*, Part IV, *Brain Mechanisms and Abnormal Behavior-Chemistry* (eds H. Van Praag, M. H. Lader, O. J. Rafaelsen and E. J. Sachar), pp. 609–651. Marcel Dekker, New York.

Post, R. M. and Kopanda, R. T. (1976). Cocaine, kindling and psychosis. *Am. J. Psychiat.*, **133**, 627–634.

Post, R. M., Ballenger, J. C., Ray, A. C. and Bunney, W. E. Jr. (1981). Slow and rapid onset of manic episodes: Implications of underlying biology. *Psychiat. Res.*, **4**, 229–237.

Post, R. M., Weiss, S. R. B., Pert, A. and Uhde, T. W. (1987). Chronic cocaine administration: sensitization and kindling effects. In: *Cocaine: Clinical and Biobehavioral Aspects* (eds A. Raskin and S. Fischer), pp. 109–173. Oxford University Press, New York.

Racine, R. J. (1977). Modification of seizure activity by electrical stimulation: cortical areas. *Electroencephalogr. Clin. Neurophysiol.*, **35**, 553–556.

Slater, E. and Beard, A. W. (1963). The schizophrenia-like psychosis of epilepsy. *Br. J. Psychiat.*, **109**, 95–112.

Stevens, J. R. and Livermore, A. (1978). Kindling in the mesolimbic dopamine system: animal model of psychosis. *Neurology*, **28**, 36–46.

Sørensen, A. S. and Bolwig, T. G. (1987). Personality and epilepsy: new evidence for a relationship? A review. *Compr. Psychiat.*, **28**, 369–383.

Sørensen, A. S., Hansen, H., Høgenhaven, H. and Bolwig, T. G. (1988). Ego functions in epilepsy. *Acta Psychiat. Scand.*, **78**, 211–221.

Toone, B. (1981). Psychoses of epilepsy. In: *Epilepsy and Psychiatry* (eds E. H. Reynolds and M. R. Trimble), pp. 113–137. Churchill Livingstone, Edinburgh.

Trimble, M. R. (1981). Visual and auditory hallucinations. *Trends Neurosci.*, **4**, 110–112.

Trimble, M. R. (1988). *Biological Psychiatry*. Wiley, Chichester.

Wada, J. A. (ed.) (1986). *Kindling 3*, Raven Press, New York.

Wada, J. A. and Sato, M. (1974). Generalized convulsive seizures induced by daily electrical stimulation of the amygdala in cats: correlative electrographic and behavioral features. *Neurology*, **24**, 565–574.

Weinberger, D. R. (1986). The pathogenesis of schizophrenia: a neurodevelopmental theory. In: *Handbook of Schizophrenia*, Vol. 1, *The Neurology of Schizophrenia* (eds H. A. Nasrallah and D. R. Weinberger), pp. 397–406. Elsevier, Amsterdam.

Weinberger, D. R. (1987). Implications of normal brain development for the pathogenesis of schizophrenia. *Arch. Gen. Psychiat.*, **44**, 660–670.

The Clinical Relevance of Kindling
Edited by T. G. Bolwig and M. R. Trimble
© 1989 John Wiley & Sons Ltd

2

Kindling: clinical relevance and anatomical substrate

R. J. Racine, G. O. Ivy[1] and N. W. Milgram[1]
Department of Psychology, McMaster University, Hamilton, Ontario, L8S 4K1 and [1]Department of Psychology, Scarborough College, University of Toronto, Scarborough, Ontario, Canada

A DESCRIPTION AND DEFINITION OF THE KINDLING PHENOMENON

The phenomenon of kindling was first described in detail by the late Graham Goddard (Goddard, 1967; Goddard, McIntyre and Leech, 1969). Goddard found that repeated electrical stimulation of forebrain sites could eventually lead to the appearance of convulsive activity in rats that had been initially unresponsive to the stimulation. This change in response appeared to involve a long lasting change in brain function. Once the stimulation began to trigger motor seizures, it would continue to produce these responses even after delays of several months. Kindling is now used to investigate the cellular mechanisms of epilepsy in many laboratories around the world.

Electrographic measures — evoked

Most kindling data have been obtained from animals with stimulating electrodes implanted into either the amygdala or hippocampus. In general, limbic system structures are more reactive than other brain sites, with the amygdala and pyriform cortex being the most reactive. Kindling requires the triggering of epileptiform discharge, although appropriate patterns of non-epileptogenic stimulation can facilitate subsequent kindling (Racine, Newberry and Burnham, 1975; Sutula and Steward, 1987). The first epileptiform afterdischarge (AD) triggered by amygdala stimulation is typically about 10 s in duration with relatively weak propagation to anatomically related sites. With repeated stimulation, the discharge increases in duration and amplitude, and these changes are permanent. Animals that have been left for very long periods of time will show strong to full strength electrographic responses on retest. For an overview of recent kindling research, see Wada (1986).

Electrographic measures — spontaneous

The changes described above apply to evoked electrographic responses, but kindling also includes the development of spontaneously occurring epileptiform events. The first of these to appear are interictal spikes that originate from the more reactive limbic sites (including the pyriform cortex and the amygdala — Kairiss, Racine and Smith, 1984). Interictal spikes often appear after as few as two or three ADs have been evoked, and, once the animal is fully kindled, they last for at least several weeks. If the animals continue to receive kindling stimulation after they reach the standard response criterion (a clonic convulsion involving forelimbs and trunk, see below), they will eventually begin to show spontaneous ictal events as well (Pinel, 1981).

Behavioural measures

The typical behavioural response accompanying the initial evoked discharge is an arrest followed by investigatory behaviour. Additional convulsive behaviours appear as kindling progresses until the animal has developed a strong clonic convulsion involving forelimb clonus and a clonic rearing. A 5-stage scale is often used to describe the sequence of behaviours (Racine, 1972). Stage 1 includes mouth movements, stage 2 clonic head movements, stage 3 forelimb clonus, stage 4 clonic rearing and stage 5 rearing and loss of postural control. Stages 4–5 are generally used as criteria for completion of kindling. Stage 1 often appears at a relatively early stage of kindling, while stages 3–5 tend to appear in rapid succession at the later stages of kindling. These responses, like the electrographic ones, are manifestations of permanent changes in brain function. If the animals are retested after a rest period of many months, they will show full strength responses after as few as one or two stimulations (Wada and Sato, 1974).

If stimulation is continued beyond the point at which the animal reaches criterion for the evoked convulsion, spontaneous convulsions will begin to appear. These accompany the spontaneous ictal discharges and include running fits (Pinel, 1981).

Although most of the measurements taken during experiments on the kindling phenomenon have been directed towards seizures and related motor and electrographic events, there is also considerable evidence that kindling can alter the animal's behaviour in other ways. Partial kindling of the ventral hippocampus, for example, enhances the defensive or withdrawal responses of cats exposed to rats (Adamec and Stark-Adamec, 1983). Similarly, Pinel, Treit and Rovner (1977) reported that kindled rats were more reactive to certain stimuli (e.g. a tap to the base of the tail) when compared with non-kindled rats.

The experiments described above were done with electrical stimulation, but it is now clear that kindling can be produced by any procedure that involves the triggering of forebrain epileptiform discharge. Therefore, a reasonable definition of kindling would describe it as the progressive and long-term increase in the strength of epileptiform responses produced by repetition of the epileptiform event.

CLINICAL RELEVANCE I: WHAT DOES THE KINDLING PHENOMENON REPRESENT?

The kindling phenomenon is used to study epilepsy, but epilepsy is a complex and not always clearly defined set of clinical syndromes. A common expectation is that an epilepsy model should mimic the clinical condition that it is supposed to model. Kindling experiments have shown limbic system structures to be the most reactive, so it is not surprising that kindling is often cited as a model of temporal lobe epilepsy. Nevertheless, this may not be the most productive way to think about the relationship between kindling and epilepsy. It leads us to anticipate surface similarities that may not exist because of the different ways in which the epileptogenic conditions were initially invoked. If temporal lobe epilepsy typically starts with hippocampal ischaemia, we might expect a number of differences between the resulting condition and that seen in an animal kindled via electrodes implanted into the amygdala *or* the hippocampus. Nevertheless, the critical neuronal changes that support the epileptic condition may be the same in both cases. Perhaps a better way to view the kindling phenomenon is as a model of chronic epileptogenesis which renders the underlying neuronal mechanisms amenable to experimental investigation. In this respect, the kindling model has many advantages over other epilepsy models. It allows us to study cellular and synaptic mechanisms under tightly controlled conditions, without the gross damage produced by most other chronic models. Unlike clinical conditions, most of the measured events are evoked rather than spontaneous, but it is this very feature that makes the phenomenon amenable to experimental analysis.

When we *do* consider the surface features of kindling (the developing AD and the convulsive responses), we should recognize the complexity of the behaviour. It consists of a number of components that may be relevant when considering the nature of kindling as an epilepsy model. We will now outline some of the dimensions along which the kindling phenomenon varies.

Acute vs chronic

Kindling combines features of both acute and chronic models. In an acute model such as the penicillin/hippocampal slice model, in which epileptiform responses are triggered in a slice preparation by exposure to penicillin, the epileptic responses are rapidly induced, readily reproducible and easily controlled (e.g. Schwartzkroin and Prince 1977). The major drawback of models of this type is that they are not chronic, so the mechanisms involved might be very different from those in the clinical conditions. In a chronic model, such as the alumina focus model (Wyler and Ward, 1984), the epileptogenic agent is applied and the experimenter monitors events as the chronic epileptic condition develops (if and when it does). The effects are not as readily reproducible, and the resulting tissue damage leads to many secondary correlates and makes neurophysiological analysis difficult.

The kindling phenomenon possesses most of the advantages and few of the disadvantages of both categories. It enables the tight control characteristic of the acute models, but it leads to a chronic condition that is free of the gross damage accompanying the lesion models.

Evoked vs spontaneous

There are two different categories of measures related to the developing chronic state that are commonly taken from the kindling preparation. The first are the evoked electrographic and behavioural responses. As described above, the increases in strength of these responses is permanent. Consequently, they reflect the development of the chronic state. The second category are the spontaneous events that provide another source of information about the nature of the epileptic state.

The spontaneous events provide information about which brain areas are becoming epileptogenic in their own right. These areas serve as generators for epileptiform activity. It is much more difficult and time consuming to monitor and analyse spontaneous interictal events, but the data thus far indicate that the pyriform cortex may be the most sensitive area in the brain for the development of a chronic epileptogenic condition (the hippocampus continues to show the lowest threshold for acute activation). The amygdala, entorhinal cortex and ventral hippocampus are somewhat less sensitive, in that order, and the dorsal hippocampus appears to be relatively resistant (Kairiss, Racine and Smith, 1984; Racine, Mosher and Kairiss, 1988). These differences in sensitivity are reflected in evoked measures as well. Kindling rates follow the same order, with the pyriform cortex showing the most rapid kindling and the dorsal hippocampus the least rapid (among the limbic sites tested).

If we wish to draw comparisons between kindling, as an epilepsy model, and the clinical condition, then we should probably focus on the *spontaneous* events. Comparing evoked responses in the kindled preparation with spontaneous responses in the human is likely to yield a number of superficial differences that may be misleading (e.g. see Engel and Cahan, 1986).

Cortical vs subcortial

Although there are some differences in the way in which various limbic sites respond to the kindling treatment, the progression of events is basically similar. The ADs increase in strength, and the animals develop the typical clonic convulsion. Neocortical sites, however, respond quite differently. The ADs initially show much smaller increases in duration and the convulsion approaches a tonic rather than a clonic form. The animal often shows some convulsive activity during the first evoked AD if motor cortical sites are activated. This response often takes the form of a turning of the head and body. As the response increases in strength, the animal may turn and drop or twist into a prone position. Little clonic activity is present during this stage. If kindling is continued, a clonic limbic type seizure begins to develop at the same time that limbic sites become recruited. At this point, the AD begins to show the typical growth seen with limbic kindling (Burnham, 1978; Racine, Burnham and Livingston, 1979).

It is not surprising that neocortical and limbic areas show different forms of development in response to the kindling trains. The circuitry supporting the tonic and clonic forms of discharge have different properties as confirmed by their different response to anticonvulsants. Neocortical ADs are very effectively blocked by phenytoin and procaine, while these drugs serve as activators within limbic sites. Further, limbic ADs are strongly affected by diazepam, which is relatively ineffective on cortical responses (Racine, Livingston and Joaquin, 1975).

Focal vs generalized

During the early stages of kindling, the evoked AD is relatively circumscribed. Amygdala stimulation, for example, will give rise to an AD which is clearly generated from within the stimulated area. Some propagation of this response can be detected in proximal sites (e.g. pyriform and entorhinal cortices), but those responses are generally of lower amplitude and clearly evoked. At this stage the response is focal. As kindling proceeds, more structures become recruited into the discharge in the sense that their cells, once activated, enter a bursting mode independent of input from the stimulated site. Workers in this area typically describe this process as 'generalization'. The generalized response is more sensitive to blockade by certain drugs (e.g. diazepam) than is the focal response (Racine, Livingston and

Joaquin, 1975). Again, this is not too surprising. No modifications are required in the local circuitry to support the *focal* response, while the generalized response requires kindling-induced alterations at a number of sites and a progressive recruitment of these sites into the forebrain discharge. There are many more links in the critical chain of events. A major disrupion at any link, or a uniform weakening of response across many links, could serve to block the discharge.

Responses with or without motor convulsion

It is not unusual for the epileptiform discharge to show dramatic changes in strength before the appearance of convulsive activity (other than mouth movements). In some cases, the longest recorded ADs are evoked just *prior* to the appearance of this convulsive activity. This presumably reflects a stage where the forebrain discharge is showing near maximal levels of propagation but before the stage where the motor systems that drive the skeletal response are recruited into the discharge. These two stages show somewhat different properties. The convulsions can be blocked by pharmacological treatments which do not appear to affect the forebrain discharge (Albright, Burnham and Livingston, 1986). It is not unreasonable to expect that recruitment of motor nuclei might be blocked without interfering with forebrain circuitry. Among many other possibilities, the transmitter systems may differ.

All of these characteristics of the kindling phenomenon should be kept in mind when attempting to determine what the kindling phenomenon is modelling. Racine and Burnham (1984) have argued that kindling should be viewed as a procedure which can elicit a number of different types of epileptiform response, each of which may have its counterpart in a clinical condition. The limbic and neocortical kindled responses, for example, may share certain characteristics with those found in human temporal lobe and neocortical epilepsies. The progression of focal to generalized response may model similar stages in human epilepsy (i.e. the process of secondary generalization).

CLINICAL RELEVANCE II: DO HUMANS SHOW A KINDLING EFFECT?

Kindling is ubiquitous across species

Thus far, it appears that any epileptogenic agent that can trigger an epileptiform discharge in the forebrain can, if repeatedly administered, produce a kindling effect (see Cain, 1986). Human relevance is suggested more strongly, however, by the fact that every vertebrate species tested, from frog to baboon, has shown a kindling effect, although different species may respond somewhat differently. For example, rhesus monkeys kindle relatively slowly (Goddard, McIntyre and Leech, 1969). Whereas baboons kindle rapidly (Wada and Osawa, 1976). Even different rat strains, however, can show large differences in kindling rates (Racine et al., 1973), so we need more information before we can make valid cross-species comparisons. Also, the expression of spontaneous activity may be a more relevant clinical correlate, and there have been few cross-species comparisons of kindling-induced spontaneous events.

The progression of clinical epilepsy may reflect a kindling effect

It is clear that epilepsy can be a progressive disease. For example, the appearance of spontaneous seizures after traumatic injury generally has a delayed onset. Even after its symptoms become severe enough to require medical attention, there is often a continued deterioration. At least some of this time-dependent increase in severity of the epileptic symptoms may be due to a kindling effect. Whatever has caused the initial focal disturbance, lesion, metabolic imbalance, etc., the further development of epileptogenic activity may be dependent upon the frequent appearance of the epileptiform activity itself. The temporal lobe appears to be particularly sensitive to the development of the epileptogenic condition (Hughes, 1985).

Secondary epileptogenesis

It is well established that mirror and secondary foci can develop in experimental preparations. Although there has been some controversy about whether similar phenomena occur in humans, it now seems clear that they do. The arguments have been made that these various foci are simply developing independently as a result of the same initial perturbation (e.g. ischaemias). Morrell (1985), however, has monitored a group of patients in which the seizure activity appears to be induced by a developing tumour. It is extremely unlikely that an identical tumour will develop in the homologous region of the contralateral hemisphere, so these subjects provide a strong test for a secondary epileptogenetic effect. Morrell found clear evidence of secondary foci in many of these subjects. The presence of secondary foci in animal models as well as human epileptics provides another argument for a contribution of kindling to human epilepsy (Morrell, 1973; Morrell, Wada and Engel, 1987).

Demonstrations of kindling in humans

Although kindling procedures cannot be intentionally applied to humans, kindling-like procedures have occurred for other reasons. Sramka, Sedlack and Nadvornik (1977) observed an apparent kindling effect in a patient treated for chronic pain by stimulation of the thalamus. Naoi (1959) and Devinsky and Duchowny (1983) reported a greater than normal incidence of spontaneous seizures in patients treated with electroconvulsive therapy. Other groups (e.g. Small *et al.*, 1981) have failed to detect a kindling effect following electroconvulsive therapy (ECT) in humans. It is clear from animal work, however, that the kindling effect of electroconvulsive shock is dependent upon the spacing of the stimulation trains and whether or not the animal has been treated with an anticonvulsant drug (Ramer and Pinel, 1976; Racine, unpublished observations). The lack of effect in some human studies could be due to either non-optimal (for kindling) spacing of the ECT treatments or to sedation of the subjects during the treatments.

ANATOMICAL SUBSTRATES

Whether comparing the kindling phenomenon, as seen in laboratory animals, with clinical epilepsies, or using kindling to study cellular mechanisms of epilepsy, it is useful to start with a consideration of the circuitry involved. Also, the possibility remains that kindling might be accompanied by structural changes at the cellular level, which might be detected with histological techniques. Progress is being made at both levels of analysis.

Kindling from different sites

Different sites kindle at different rates. Among limbic system and related structures, the olfactory bulb and pyriform cortex kindle with the smallest number of stimulations, while the dorsal hippocampus requires the greatest number of stimulations. There appears to be an anterior/posterior axis along the pyriform lobe (including the olfactory bulb) with anterior sites showing faster kindling rates than posterior sites (Goddard, McIntyre and Leech, 1969; Racine, 1972).

Electrographic correlates

If *spontaneous* epileptiform events are monitored as an index of the sensitivity of a structure for development of a chronic epileptogenic condition, they appear to follow the same order as the kindling rates (Kairiss, Racine and Smith, 1984; Racine, Mosher and Kairiss, 1988). The first spontaneous events often appear from the pyriform cortex (even if another site has received the kindling stimulation). The most resistant site appears to be the dorsal hippocampus. It is also clear, however, that all limbic sites so far tested can participate in the generation of spontaneous events.

Gross histological measures

One of the attractions of the kindling model is that it is free of much of the gross focal damage that is produced by the chemical lesion techniques. There are no obvious sites of damage in the kindled preparation (Goddard, McIntyre and Leech, 1969; Racine, 1972). It should be pointed out, however, that a number of important histological measures have yet to be taken. Cell counts among specific cell types (particularly those believed to provide local inhibition), for example, might even reveal changes not yet detected.

Cell morphology

The data here remain ambiguous. Racine, Tuff and Zaide (1976) found no changes in dendritic structure of neocortical pyramidal cells in cortically kindled animals. Goddard and Douglas (1975) ran an electron microscopic analysis of tissue around the stimulation site in an amygdala-kindled animal. They found evidence for increased terminal volume, but, unfortunately, the placement of the kindling electrode (and, consequently, the marker lesions made via those electrodes) differed between control and experimental groups. Racine and Zaide (1978) reported similar changes in the neocortex of cortically kindled animals, but failed to replicate this result in a more tightly controlled follow-up study (although a trend in the same direction was found). Due to cost and time limitations, this work has not been followed to a successful conclusion and the questions raised in those studies remain unanswered.

Relevance of status models

Local or systemic injection of the neurotoxin kainic acid (KA) can induce a state of status epilepticus (Schwob et al., 1980; Ben-Ari, 1985). There are a number of reasons to believe that this model has relevance for kindling. The progression of seizure development is similar, although it develops rapidly (within 2 h — Lothman and Collins, 1981). The epileptiform discharges start out with a short duration and become longer. The lower frequency spiking between ictal episodes and the convulsive responses are also at least superficially similar to those seen during kindling. Finally, these developments, including status epilepticus, can be induced by electrical stimulation. The status is most easily induced in animals that have already been electrically kindled (McIntyre, Nathanson and Edson, 1982).

Unlike kindling, the induction of status epilepticus by KA *does* lead to gross tissue damage (Schwob et al., 1980; Ben-Ari et al., 1981). If the seizure activity is sufficiently severe and prolonged, there will be massive neural damage found in a number of sites. It is interesting that the pyriform cortex is, again, one of the most sensitive sites. Other sites sustaining damage are the medial dorsal thalamus, nucleus reuniens, and the central amygdaloid nuclei. Damage also appears in the hippocampal formation, but here it is more variable (Buterbaugh *et al.*, 1987; Milgram *et al.*, 1985; Milgram, unpublished observations).

These results raise some interesting possibilities. For example, the first indication of the cell damage produced by induction of status may be quite subtle. If so, these changes might also be induced during kindling. If such changes *are* found in kindling, they might play a role in the developing epileptogenesis.

Status and kindling-induced sprouting

At least one such change common to both the status and kindling models has now been described in the literature. Nadler, Perry and Cotman (1980) reported that exposure to KA led to a sprouting of collaterals from the mossy fibres that originate from dentate gyrus cells. Most of this sprouting appeared to be located close to the cells of origin themselves. Sutula *et al.* (1988) found a similar sprouting effect induced by kindling. It has been argued that this sprouting could lead to an increase in the excitability of the hippocampus.

Astrocyte activation

We have recently discovered another parallel between the effects of status-inducing treatments and kindling. When KA is applied systemically (subcutaneously or intraperitoneally), the first sites to show spontaneous spiking are the pyriform cortex (Milgram, in preparation), the entorhinal cortex (Ben-Ari *et al.*, 1981), or the ventral hippocampus (Lothman and Collins, 1981). O'Shaughnessy and Gerber (1986) compared damage in animals in which status was induced with damage in animals showing only partial seizures, and found that only the animals in status showed sustained damage. The amount of seizure activity can be further controlled by several applications of a barbiturate anaesthetic (sodium pentobarbital) at varying times after the induction of status. As might be expected, more or less damage is produced depending upon how much seizure activity is allowed to occur.

Among the more sensitive techniques for measurement of status-induced neural disruption is the labelling of activated astrocytes. Astrocytes are stellate-shaped glial cells which are involved in the regulation of the neuronal microenvironment and in the repair of neural tissue and phagocytosing of neural debris following trauma. In response to disturbances in the local environment, astrocytes synthesize glial fibrillary acidic protein (GFAP), an intermediate filament protein found only in astrocytes (see review by Eng, 1988). The increased production of GFAP causes hypertrophy of astrocytic processes and perikarya (Figure 1), which dramatically alters their morphology and, possibly, their physiology. The hypertrophy of a population of astrocytes is referred to as reactive gliosis. Reactive gliosis can be initiated by abnormally heightened levels of neuronal activity and is a prominent feature of the brains of humans with epilepsy as well as animals in which epileptogenic activity has been induced by alumina, iron or cobalt (see review by Tiffany-Castiglioni and Catiglioni, 1986).

We (Ivy and Milgram, 1987; Moore *et al.*, 1988) have utilized immunocytochemical procedures to localize astrocyte hypertrophy in the brains of rats in which seizure activity induced by kainic acid was controlled by the administration of barbiturates. Astrocyte hypertrophy varied in proportion to the duration of status epilepticus. Figure 2B shows slight reactive gliosis in the pyriform cortex and amygdaloid areas of a rat injected with KA but prevented from developing motor seizures with barbiturate. With increasing duration of seizure activity, there was a corresponding increase in immunostaining (Figure 2C, D). The structures most severely affected include the pyriform cortex, amygdaloid nuclei, endopyriform nucleus and the dorsomedial, reuniens, and laterodorsal nucleus of the thalamus. The hippocampus and the

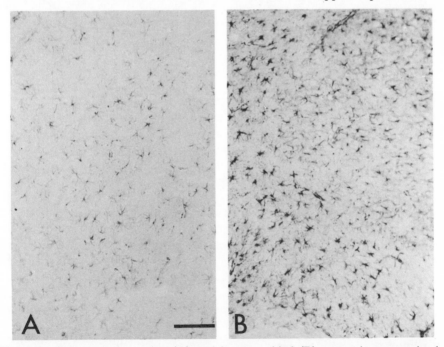

Figure 1. Astrocytes, in resting (A) and hypertrophied (B) states, immunostained with antibodies to GFAP. The astrocytes produce large quantities of this protein in response to abnormal levels of neural activity, as well as to other forms of brain trauma

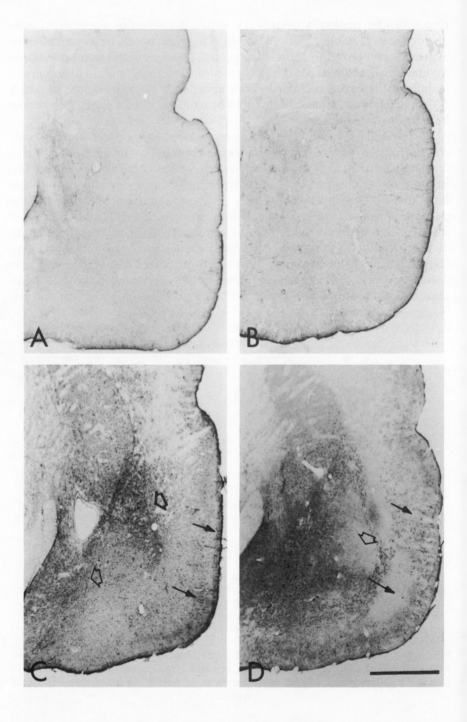

neocortex are generally less heavily affected, although notable astrocyte hypertophy often appears in the CA3 region and in the hilus of the fascia dentata as well as in layer Va of the parietal and temporal neocortex and in layer I throughout the neocortex.

The development of hypertrophy and cell death depend on survival time as well as seizure duration. Increased hypertrophy is reliably evoked after 5 h of status epilepticus. While no cell death is apparent at 24 h after the status, as determined by Nissl stains (Figure 3A), a dramatic necrosis is evident in both the pyriform cortex and the amydala after a survival period of 4 months (Figure 3C). Astrogliosis is still present in the region, as well, forming a glial scar which may persist for the life of the animal (Figure 3D).

In our most recent investigations, we are using the same procedures to monitor these cells in kindled animals (Ivy, Racine and Milgram, in progress). Thus far, we have found reliable activation of astrocytes within the ipsilateral amygdala and pyriform cortex of amygdala kindled animals at 24 h (Figure 4B) and 1 week (Figure 4D) after completion of kindling. Control tissue is shown in Figure 4A, C. The astrogliosis can also be seen in the contralateral hemisphere, particularly after 1 week survival (Figure 4F). In ongoing experiments, astrocytes will be monitored at 1 and 2 months after completion of kindling and after kindling of other brain sites. Although this effect appears to be quite reliable, it remains to be seen whether it reflects cell death. On the other hand, elevation of extracellular potassium *per se* has not been shown to produce activated astrocytes (Tiffany-Castiglioni and Castiglioni, 1986).

MECHANISMS

Work pertaining to mechanisms has been thoroughly reviewed in the literature (e.g. Racine, 1978; Racine and Burnham, 1984; Racine *et al.*, 1986; Burnham, Racine and Okazaki, 1986; McIntyre and Racine, 1986) and there is not much new that can be added, other than the points covered above. We have monitored measures of inhibition and synaptic potentiation and

Figure 2. Sections of pyriform cortex and amygdaloid areas of a non-injected control rat (A) and rats treated systemically with 10 μg/kg of KA (B–D). (B) No seizures. (C) One hour of status epilepticus. (D) Five hours of status epilepticus. The rats were sacrificed 1 week following injections and their brains immunostained with antibodies to GFAP to demonstrate regions of astrocyte hypertrophy. Note the generally increased darkening of the sections from A to D, indicating increased immunoreactivity. Note also the dramatic increase in immunoreactivity in the amygdala (open arrows) and pyriform cortex (solid arrows) after 1 h of seizure activity and the clear neuronal degeneration (see adjacent Nissl stained sections) after 5 h of status. Over time, these regions shrink and become composed largely of glial scar tissue (as shown in the next figure)

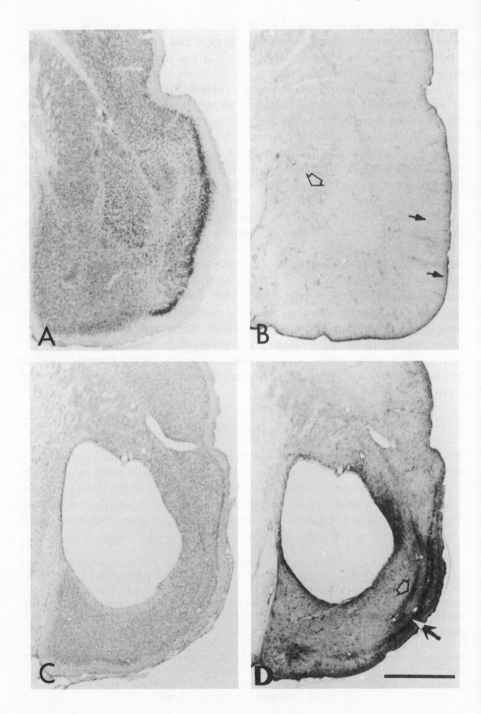

have concluded that there are changes in these measures produced by kindling but that these changes probably do not reflect primary kindling mechanisms (see Racine *et al.*, 1986a, for a thorough presentation of the arguments). Still to be tested is the possibility that the response characteristics of reactive cells have been altered during kindling. Preliminary evidence indicates that this might be the case. Kairiss (1985), for example, found that hippocampal cells from kindled animals were more responsive to intracellular application of depolarizing currents than were cells from control hippocampi (also see Racine *et al.*, 1986a). McIntyre and Wong (1986) reported even more dramatic changes in pyriform cortex cells from kindled animals. Martin *et al.* (1988) found that magnesium gating of NMDA receptor-linked ion channels was reduced in kindled animals. NMDA receptor binding, however, was not affected (Okazaki, McNamara and Nadler, 1988). There are definitely some interesting developments, but it is too early to tell where they will lead.

FUTURE DIRECTIONS

There are some clear gaps in kindling research in terms of the areas of expertise committed to the problem. More work needs to be done at the membrane level in physiology, the ultrastructural level in anatomy, and the ion flux level in both physiology and neurochemistry. There has been a heavy focus on the hippocampus in recent kindling research. There are sound reasons for this, and some of them pertain to clinical relevance, but the area might be better served if there were more comparisons made between structures.

One of the problems with the kindling model may be that the kindled preparation remains in a state of flux for some period of time after completion of kindling. Lewis, Westerberg and Corcoran (1987), for example, measured transmitter levels and metabolites in several transmitter systems and found quite different results at 2 weeks compared to 4 weeks after completion of kindling. Also, Bragdon, Taylor, McNamara and Wilson (in preparation) found that an increase in burst responses in the hippocampus that was present at 4 weeks post-kindling was no longer present at 3 months post-kindling. It

Figure 3. Sections of pyriform cortex and amygdaloid areas of two rats injected with kainic acid and allowed to survive for 24 h (A and B) or 4 months (C and D) following 5 h of status epilepticus. (A) Nissl stain showing normal cell density and pattern. (B) Section immunostained for GFAP. Note the slightly increased immunoreactivity in the amygdala (open arrow) and the pyriform cortex (solid arrows) as compared to the non-injected rat shown in Figure 3A. (C) Nissl stain showing gross shrinkage of amygdala and pyriform cortical regions with concomitant enlargement of the lateral ventricles. (D) Section immunostained for GFAP. Note the glial scars which are especially prominent in the deep layers of the pyriform cortex (solid arrow) and in the presumed remnants of the amygdala (open arrow)

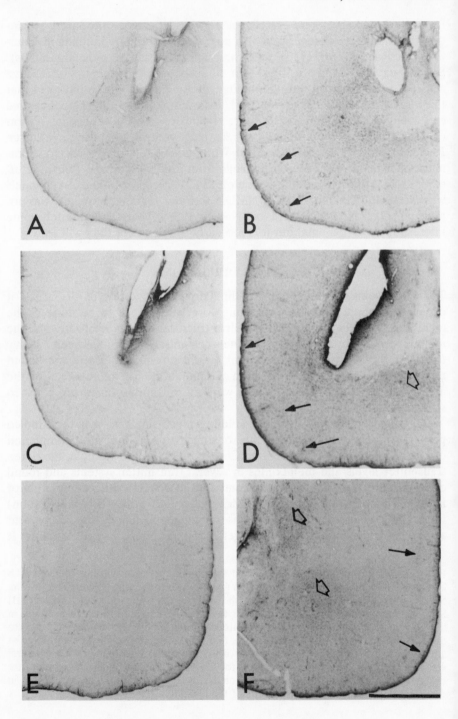

may be necessary to take some measures at delays of 2–3 months after completion of kindling until we have some confidence about the nature of the permanent changes in brain function that support the continued increase in epileptogenesis.

As in most areas, progress sometimes seems painfully slow. We have been able to exclude at least a critical role for many potential mechanisms, but we have not been able to isolate the mechanism(s) that *are* critical. Nevertheless, some of the recent developments (e.g. the kindling-induced sprouting, the activation of astrocytes and the increased response of kindled cells to depolarizing pulses) are encouraging, and most of the controversies (e.g. the relative involvement of the various limbic structures) are resolvable. Consequently, we look forward to the next few years with some optimism.

REFERENCES

Adamec, R. E. and Stark-Adamec, C. (1983). Partial kindling and emotional bias in the cat: Lasting after effects of partial kindling of the ventral hippocampus. I. Behavioral changes. *Behav. Neur. Biol.*, **38**, 205–222.

Albright, P. S., Burnham, W. M. and Livingston, K. E. (1986). Seizure patterns and pharmacological responses in the kindling model. In: Doane, B. K. and Livingston, K. E. *The Limbic System: Functional Organization and Clinical Disorders* (eds B. K. Doane and K. E. Livingston), pp. 147–157. Raven Press, New York.

Ben-Ari, Y. (1985). Limbic seizure and brain damage produced by kainic acid: mechanisms and relevance to human temporal lobe epilepsy. *Neuroscience*, **14**, 375–403.

Ben-Ari, Y., Trenblay, E., Riche, D., Ghilini, G. and Naquet, R. (1981). Electrographic, clinical and pathological alterations following systemic administration of kainic acid, bicuculline or pentetrazole: metabolic mapping using the deoxyglucose method with special reference to the pathology of epilepsy. *Neuroscience*, **6**, 1361–1391.

Burnham, W. M. (1978). Cortical and limbic kindling: similarities and differences. In: *Limbic Mechanisms: The Continuing Evolution of the Limbic System Concept* (K. E. Livingston and O. Hornykiewicz), pp. 507–519. Plenum Press, New York.

Burnham, W. M., Racine, R. J. and Okazaki, M. O. (1986). Kindling mechanisms.

Figure 4. Sections of pyriform cortex and amygdaloid region of rats sacrificed 24 h or 1 week following kindling or stimulation control treatment. Sections were immunostained for GFAP. (A) Section taken through the site of electrode placement in a control rat. (B) Electrode site in kindled rat with 24 h survival. Note the increased immunoreactivity indicating astrocyte hypertrophy both immediately surrounding the lesion and in more distal pyriform cortex (arrows) as compared to A. (C) Electrode site in control animal after 1 week survival. (D) Electrode site in kindled rat with 1 week survival. Note the increased immunoreactivity in the amygdala (open arrow) and pyriform cortex (solid arrows). (E) Site contralateral to that shown in C. (F) Site contralateral to that shown in D. Note the increased astrocyte hypertrophy in amygdala (open arrows) and pyriform cortex (solid arrows)

II. Biochemical studies. In: *Kindling 3* (ed. J. A. Wada), pp. 283–299. Raven Press, New York.

Buterbaugh, G. C., Michelson, H. B., Keyser, D. O. and Jones, B. R. (1987). Pathology and 2-deoxy-D-glucose uptake associated with early and late status epilepticus in kindled rats. *Neurosci. Abstr.*, **13**, 948.

Cain, D. P. (1986). The transfer phenomenon in kindling. In: *Kindling 3* (ed. J. A. Wada), pp. 231–248. Raven Press, New York.

Devinsky, O. and Duchowny, M. S. (1983). Seizures after convulsive therapy: A retrospective case survey. *Neurology*, **33**, 921–925.

Eng, L. F. (1988). Regulation of glial intermediate filaments in astrogliosis. In: *The Biochemical Pathology of Astrocytes* (eds M. D. Norenberg, L. Hertz and A. Schousboe), pp. 79–90. Alan R. Liss, New York.

Engel, J. and Cahan, L. (1986). Potential relevance of kindling to human partial epilepsy. In: *Kindling 3* (ed. J. A. Wada), pp. 37–54. Raven Press, New York.

Goddard, G. V. (1967). Development of epileptic seizures through brain stimulation at low intensity. *Nature*, **214**, 1020–1021.

Goddard, G. V. and Douglas, R. M. (1975). Does the engram of kindling model the engram of normal long term memory? *Can. J. Neurol. Sci.*, **2**, 385–394.

Goddard, G. V., McIntyre, D. C. and Leech, C. K. (1969). A permanent change in brain function resulting from daily electrical stimulation. *Exp. Neurol.*, **25**, 295–330.

Hughes, J. R. (1985). Long-term clinical and EEG changes in patients with epilepsy. *Arch. Neurol.*, **42**, 213–233,

Ivy, G. O. and Milgram, N. W. (1987). A technique for visualizing the neural systems involved in activity related brain damage. *Neurosci. Abstr.*, **13**, 1265.

Kairiss, E. W. (1985). Hippocampal slice studies of kindling-induced epilepsy. Ph.D. thesis, McMaster University, Hamilton, Ontario.

Kairiss, E. W., Racine, R. J. and Smith, G. K. (1984). The development of the interictal spike during kindling in the rat. *Brain Res.*, **322**, 101–110.

Lewis, J., Westerberg, V. and Corcoran, M. E. (1987). Monoaminergic correlates of kindling. *Brain Res.*, **403**, 205–212.

Lothman, E. W. and Collins, R. C. (1981). Kainic acid induced limbic seizures: metabolic, behavioral, electroencephalographic and neuropathological correlates. *Brain Res.*, **218**, 299–318.

Martin, D., Bowe, M. A., McNamara, J. O. and Nadler, J. V. (1988). Kindling depresses magnesium regulation of depolarizing responses to amino acid excitants. *Neurosci. Abstr.*, **14**, 865.

McIntyre, D. C. and Racine, R. J. (1986). Kindling mechanisms. *Prog. Neurobiol.*, **21**, 1–21.

McIntyre, D. C. and Wong, R. K. S. (1986). Cellular and synaptic properties of amygdala-kindled pyriform cortex in vitro. *J. Neurophysiol.*, **55**, 1295–1307.

McIntyre, D. C., Nathanson, D. and Edson, N. (1982). A new model of partial status epilepticus based on kindling. *Brain Res.*, **250**, 53–63.

Milgram, N. W., Green, I., Liberman, M., Riexinger, K. and Petit, T. L. (1985). Establishment of status epilepticus by limbic system stimulation in previously unstimulated rats. *Exp. Neurol.*, **88**, 253–264.

Moore, W., Milgram, N. W., Khurgel, M. and Ivy, G. O. (1988). Time course and brain distribution of seizure-induced astrocyte hypertrophy in rats. *Neurosci. Abstr.*, **14**, 881.

Morrell, F. (1973). Goddard's kindling phenomenon: A new model of the 'mirror focus'. In: *Chemical Modulation of Brain Function* (ed. H. C. Sabelli), pp. 207–223. Raven Press, New York.

Morrell, F. (1985). Secondary epileptogenesis in man. *Arch. Neurol.*, **42**, 318–335.

Morrell, F., Wada, J. and Engel Jr., J. (1987). Appendix III: Potential relevance of kindling and secondary epileptogenesis to the consideration of surgical treatment for epilepsy. In: *Surgical Treatment of the Epilepsies* (ed. J. Engel Jr), pp. 701–707. Raven Press, New York.

Nadler, J. V., Perry, B. W. and Cotman, C. W. (1980). Selective reinnervation of hippocampal CA1 and the fascia dentata after destruction of CA3-CA4 afferents with kainic acid. *Brain Res.*, **182**, 1–9.

Naoi, T. (1959). EEG assessment of electroconvulsive treatment. *Folia Psychiatr. Neurol. Jpn.*, **61**, 871–881.

Okazaki, M. M., McNamara, J. O. and Nadler, J. V. (1988). Regionally-specific reductions in kainate and NMDA receptor binding after angular bundle kindling. *Neurosci. Abstr.*, **14**, 865.

O'Shaughnessy, D. and Gerber, G. J. (1986). Damage induced by systemic kainic acid in rats is dependent upon seizure activity — a behavioral and morphological study. *Neurotoxicology*, **7**, 187–202.

Pinel, J. P. (1981). Spontaneous kindled motor seizures in rats. In: *Kindling 2* (ed. J. A. Wada), pp. 179–192, Raven Press, New York.

Pinel, J. P. J., Treit, D. and Rovner, L. I. (1977). Temporal lobe agression in rats. *Science*, **197**, 1088–1089.

Racine, R. J. (1972). Modification of seizure activity by electrical stimulation. II. Motor seizure. *Electroencephalogr. Clin. Neurophysiol.*, **32**, 281–294.

Racine, R. J. (1978). Kindling: The first decade. *Neurosurgery*, **3**, 234–252.

Racine, R. J. and Burnham, W. M. (1984). The kindling model: In: *Electrophysiology of Epilepsy* (eds P. A. Schwartzkroin and H. Wheal), pp. 153–171. Raven Press, New York.

Racine, R. J. and Zaide, J. (1978). A further investigation into the mechanisms of the kindling phenomenon: In: *Limbic Mechanisms: The Continuing Evolution of the Limbic System Concept* (eds K. E. Livingston and O. Hornykiewicz), pp. 457–493. Plenum Press, New York.

Racine, R., Burnham, W. M. and Livingston, K. (1979). The effect of procaine hydrochloride and diazepam, separately or in combination, on cortico-generalized kindled seizures. *Electroencephalogr. Clin. Neurophysiol.*, **47**, 204–212.

Racine, R. J., Livingston, K. and Joaquin, A. (1975). Effects of procaine hydrochloride, diazepam and diphenylhydantoin on seizure development in cortical and subcortical structures in rats. *Electroencephalogr. Clin. Neurophysiol.*, **38**, 355–365.

Racine, R. J., Mosher, M. and Kairiss, E. W. (1988). The role of the pyriform cortex in the generation of interictal spikes in the kindled preparation. *Brain Res.*, **454**, 251–263.

Racine, R., Newberry, F. and Burnham, W. M. (1975). Post-activation potentiation and the kindling phenomenon. *Electroencephalogr. Clin. Neurophysiol.*, **39**, 261–271.

Racine, R. J., Tuff, L. and Zaide, J. (1975). Kindling, unit discharge patterns and neural plasticity. *Can. J. Neurol. Sci.*, **2**, 395–405.

Racine, R. J., Burnham, W., Gartner, J. and Levitan, D. (1973). Rates of motor seizure development in rats subjected to electrical brain stimulation: strain and interstimulation interval effects. *Electroencephalogr. Clin. Neurophysiol.*, **35**, 553–556.

Racine, R. J., Burnham, W. M., Gilbert, M. and Kairiss, E. W. (1986). Kindling mechanisms: I. Electrophysiological studies. In: *Kindling 3* (ed. J. A. Wada), pp. 263–282. Raven Press, New York.

Ramer, D. and Pinel, J. P. J. (1976). Progressive intensification of motor seizures produced by periodic electroconvulsive shock. *Exp. Neurol.*, **51**, 421–433.

Schwartzkroin, P. A. and Prince, D. A. (1977). Penicillin-induced epileptiform activity in the hippocampal in vitro preparation. *Ann. Neurol.*, **1**, 463–469.

Schwob, J. E., Fuller, T., Price, J. L. and Olney, J. W. (1980). Widespread patterns of neuronal damage following systemic or intracerebral injections of kainic acid: a histological study. *Neuroscience*, **5**, 991–1014.

Small, J., Milstein, V., Small, I. F. and Sharpley, P. H. (1981). Does ECT produce kindling? *Biol. Psychiat.*, **16**, 773–778.

Sramka, M., Sedlack, P. and Nadvornik, P. (1977). Observation of the kindling phenomenon in treatment of pain by stimulation in the thalamus. In: *Neurosurgical Treatment in Psychiatry, Pain and Epilepsy* (eds W. H. Sweet, S. Obrador and J. G. Martin-Rodriguez), pp. 651–654. University Park Press, Baltimore.

Sutula, T. and Steward, O. (1987). Facilitation of kindling by prior induction of long-term potentiation in the perforant path. *Brain Res.*, **420**, 109–117.

Sutula, T., He, X., Cavazos, J. and Scott, G. (1988). Synaptic reorganization induced in the hippocampus by abnormal functional activity. *Science*, **239**, 1147–1150.

Tiffany-Castiglioni, E. and Castiglioni Jr, A. J. (1986). Astrocytes in epilepsy. In Fedoroff, S. and Vernadakis, A. (Eds.), *Astrocytes*, Vol. III, pp. 401–424, Academic Press, New York.

Wada, J. A. (ed.) (1986). *Kindling 3*. Raven Press, New York.

Wada, J. A. and Osawa, T. (1976). Spontaneous recurrent seizure state induced by daily electric amygdaloid stimulation in Senegalese baboons (*Papio papio*). *Neurology*, **26**, 273–286.

Wada, J. A. and Sato, M. (1974). Generalized convulsive seizures induced by daily electrical stimulation of the amygdala in cats: correlative electrographic and behavioral features. *Neurology*, **24**, 565–574.

Wyler, A. R. and Ward, A. A. (1984). The alumina monkey model. In *Electrophysiology of Epilepsy* (eds P. A. Schwartzkroin and H. Wheal), pp. 31–49. Academic Press, New York.

The Clinical Relevance of Kindling
Edited by T. G. Bolwig and M. R. Trimble
© 1989 John Wiley & Sons Ltd

3

Chemical kindling

CLAUDE G. WASTERLAIN, ANNE M. MORIN, DENSON G.
FUJIKAWA and JEFF M. BRONSTEIN
*Epilepsy Research Laboratory, VA Medical Center, Sepulveda, CA 91343,
and Department of Neurology and Brain Research Institute, UCLA School
of Medicine, Los Angeles, CA 90024, USA*

PROLOGUE

Kindling can be induced by intracerebral injection of minute amounts of neurotransmitter receptor ligands, in selective brain locations, providing an adequate interval separates repeated injections. Nanomolar quantities of carbamylcholine and other muscarinic agonists injected into the amygdala produce kindling with an optimal interstimulus interval of 3 days. Carbachol kindling shows full transfer between muscarinic agonists, blockage by picomolar amounts of muscarinic antagonists, and stereospecificity which favors agonists with a high affinity for the muscarinic receptor. Potentiation by cholinesterase inhibitors is also observed. The complex interaction between chemical and anatomical specificity is demonstrated by the ability of muscarinic agonists to kindle amygdala but not cortex, while gamma-aminobutyric acid (GABA) antagonists kindle cortex but not amygdala. This phenomenon of chemical kindling provides strong evidence that kindled epilepsy is the pathological expression of the activation of physiological adaptive synaptic cerebral mechanisms at multiple levels of the central nervous system.

Chemical kindling can be induced by agonists of excitatory neurotransmitters such as acetylcholine and possibly aspartate-glutamate. Other excitatory amino acid analogs generally failed to produce kindling. Antagonists of GABA, benzodiazepines and chloride channel ligands produced chemical kindling, as did some agents which alter catecholamine metabolism, while other antagonists of inhibitory neurotransmitters failed. Transfer of kindling from one chemical type to another and from one anatomical site to another showed an extreme degree of chemical and anatomical specificity. Cellular changes in kindled brains occurred at many levels, suggesting that it is a complex phenomenon resulting from adaptive changes in both synaptic and cellular excitability in multiple but specific neuronal networks. Human epilepsy is frequently associated with extensive destruction of the structures most intimately involved in the mechanism of kindling in animals. This paradox may reflect the important role of the resistant burst-prone area CA2 in lesioned hippocampi. The biochemical mechanism of kindling is unknown, but calcium channels and calcium-dependent enzymes seem to play a significant role in its genesis.

INTRODUCTION

Many investigators working on self stimulation of chronic stimulation of the brain had noted that repeated low-level stimulation sometimes produced epileptic seizures, and that once acquired this behavior was very persistent (Delgado and Sevillano, 1961). Stimulated by Frank Morrel's (1960, 1979) hypothesis of independent mirror foci, Goddard recognized that these acquired seizures represented an important change in brain excitability induced by experience (Goddard, McIntyre and Leech, 1969). At the same time, Goddard (1969) showed that the appearance of seizures in response to repetitive subconvulsive stimulation of specific brain regions could be induced not only by electrical stimulation but also by microinjections of carbamylcholine, an agonist of the excitatory transmitter acetylcholine. Detailed studies of this phenomenon have now described its pharmacology, anatomy, and time course (Vosu and Wise, 1975; Wasterlain and Jonec, 1983). The phenomenon of chemical kindling has provided the strongest evidence to date that epilepsy can be the pathological expression of physiological adaptations in synaptic and cellular excitability. It has been clearly demonstrated that this phenomenon can be induced transynaptically in the absence of any brain lesion. Yet it is not at all clear why chemical kindling with a specific agent works in some brain locations but not in others. We do not understand why some types of kindling show positive transfers while others do not. The possible relationship of kindling to human epilepsy also remains an enigma.

MUSCARINIC KINDLING

In a series of experiments which extended Goddard's original observations, we injected 2.7 nmol of carbachol or of other muscarinic agonists dissolved in a volume of 0.2–1 µl of sterile isotonic artificial spinal fluid into the basolateral amygdala of rats (Wasterlain and Jonec, 1983). The initial injection produced no behavioral response. However, electrographically many animals showed mild spiking from the injection site. When this injection was repeated once a day, seizures gradually appeared over a period of 2–3 weeks and were clinically very similar to those induced by electrical stimulation of the amygdala (Racine, 1972b) (Figure 1). Daily injections of a similar volume of saline or other control solutions did not induce seizures. Mixing the carbachol with blockers of nicotinic synapses such as D-tubocurarine (100 nmol) did not modify the seizures, but addition to carbachol of muscarinic blockers such as atropine or scopolamine blocked them in a dose-dependent fashion. Kindled seizures could be induced by other muscarinic agonists such as muscarine or acetylbetamethylcholine. When stereoisomers of muscarinic agonists were used, only the isomer with high affinity for muscarinic receptors was effective. Inhibitors of cholinesterase potentiated kindling. Finally, the rank order of potency in inducing kindling closely resembled that of affinity for muscarinic receptors. Spontaneous seizures were common (Figure 2), showing that some chemically kindled animals had truly become epileptic. These results indicate that the generation of a kindled focus in this model is entirely dependent on the activation of excitatory muscarinic receptors and completely independent of any cerebral lesions. In other words, it appears to be the pathological expression of physiological synaptic adaptive mechanisms.

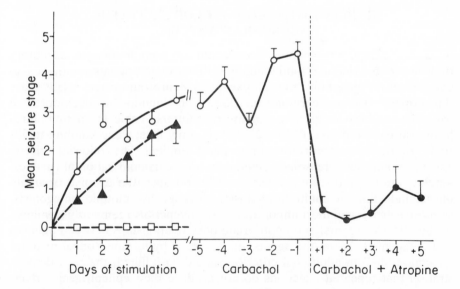

Figure 1. Response to daily intra-amygdaloid injection of carbachol during the first 5 days (1–5) of stimulation, the last 5 days before full kindling (–5 to –1), and the first 5 days of injection of carbachol mixed with equimolar atropine, a blocker of muscarinic receptors (+1 to +5). □, saline; ▲, carbachol 2.7 nmol; ○, carbachol 27 nmol; ●, carbachol 27 nmol + atropine 27 nmol

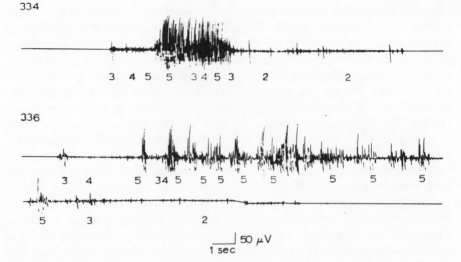

Figure 2. Electrographical recording of spontaneous seizures recorded through bipolar amygdaloid electrodes in two carbachol kindled rats. Numbers indicate the seizures stage at that particular time according to the classification of Racine

KINDLING WITH AGONISTS OF EXCITATORY NEUROTRANSMITTERS

At central muscarinic synapses, acetylcholine is a predominantly excitatory transmitter, and the successful kindling with muscarinic agonists in the amygdala raised the possibility that all excitatory neurotransmitters might share this property. This is clearly not the case. While kindling has been obtained with some agonists of excitatory neurotransmitters (Table 1), many failures have also been reported (Table 2). In fact, only muscarinic kindling fulfills strict criteria for demonstration of chemical kindling. The following criteria appear to represent a reasonable minimum for the demonstration of chemical kindling through intracranial injection of neurotransmitter agonists or antagonists: induction by multiple agonists, blockage by multiple antagonists, stereospecificity, and most importantly, effectiveness of reasonably low doses of the effective agents, and appropriate dose relationships between agonists and antagonists. When the agents are delivered by intraperitoneal or other systemic route, an additional criterion should be fulfilled, that is a demonstration that repeated injections do not produce their epileptogenic effects as a result of a change in the metabolic rate of the agent that would deliver it in epileptogenic concentrations to the brain.

Excitatory neurotransmitters seem intimately involved in electrical kindling of the amygdala, as evidenced by the demonstration that, in the dentate gyrus, NMDA receptors participate in synaptic transmission in kindled ani-

Table 1. Chemical kindling with neurotransmitter agonists or antagonists

	Reference
Glutamate + aspartate	Mori and Wada (1987)
Muscarinic:	
Carbachol, muscarine, ABM	Wasterlain and Jonec (1983)
Pilocarpine	Butebaugh, Michelson and Keyser (1986)
DFP	Girgis (1981)
Peptides:	
met-Enkephalin	Cain and Corcoran (1985)
beta-Endorphin	Cain and Corcoran (1985)
Gaba:	
Bicuculline Am	Wasterlain, Morin and Jonec (1982)
Benzodiazepines:	
Betacarboline	Morin, Watson and Wasterlain (1983)
Metrazol	Gilbert and Cain (1985)
FG 7142	Little, Null and Taylor (1987)
Penicillin	Collins (1978)
Chloride channel:	
Picrotoxin	Cain (1987)
Catecholamines:	
Lidocaine	Post (1981)
Cocaine	Sato and Okamoto (1981)

Am, amygdala; ABM, acetyl-beta-methylcholine.

Table 2. Chemical kindling failures

	Reference
CRF	Weiss et al. (1986)
Morphine	Cain and Corcoran (1985)
L-Enkephalin	Wasterlain et al. (1986)
Bicuculline—Am	Wasterlain, Morin and Jonec (1982a)
Carbachol—cortex	Wasterlain, Farber and Fairchild (1986)

Am, amygdala.

mals but not in controls (Mody and Heinemann, 1987). Chemical kindling with glutamate, aspartate or their agonists has failed in several laboratories (Morin, personal communication; Wasterlain, in preparation). However, a number of arguments suggest that these failures result from technical and practical problems, and do not preclude involvement of excitatory amino acid synapses in kindling. First, glutamate, asparatate and their agonists have excitotoxic properties (Solviter and Dempsey, 1985), so that they are toxic to neurons at a dose only slightly higher than that which includes their physiological effects. Since it is very difficult to control precisely the concentrations of intracerebrally delivered agents, excitotoxic effects might eliminate the most responsive cells and present the appearance of failure. Second, success has been reported using a mixture of aspartate and glutamate (3/1), in the amygdala (Mori and Wada, 1987), and this type of kindling transferred to and from electrical kindling of the same region. Third, noncompetitive blockers of NMDA synapses are quite effective at blocking electrical kindling (Peterson, Collins and Bradford, 1984), and in fact are more effective at preventing epileptogenesis than at inhibiting the expression of well established kindled seizures (Figure 3).

Limited successes have also been obtained in generating chemical kindling by local systemic injection of peptides which have a predominantly excitatory role as neurotransmitters on neuromodulators in brain (Table 1), such as enkephalins or endorphins (Cain, 1981a; Frenk *et al.*, 1982; Corcoran *et al.*, 1984; Cain and Corcoran, 1985). Habituation has been observed using different methods with closely related agents such as morphine (Cain and Corcoran, 1985; Wasterlain *et al.*, 1986). The apparent discrepancy between results using different peptides is not surprising given their complex role in synaptic physiology and our limited understanding of their function.

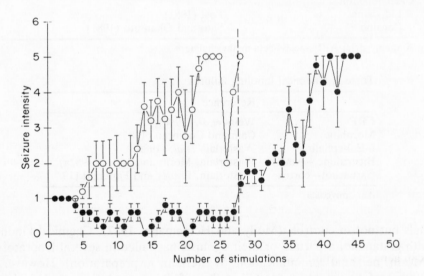

Figure 3. Effect of MK–801, a noncompetitive glutamate antagonist, on entorhinal kindling. Five rats (○) were injected with vehicle 15 min before each stimulation, and 5 paired animals (●) were injected with MK–801 (10 mg/kg i.p.) 15 min before each stimulation. After the first group was fully kindled, we stopped MK–801 (dashed line) but continued once daily stimulation (400 A, 60 Hz, 1 s, AC). MK–801 blocks the ionic channel associated with NMDA receptors. It was very effective in blocking kindled epileptogenesis, but only mildly effective as an anticonvulsant in kindled animals (data not shown)

KINDLING WITH ANTAGONISTS OF INHIBITORY
NEUROTRANSMITTERS

Kindling has been obtained by action at several levels of the GABA–benzodi-azepine receptor complex (Table 1); partial success has been reported with direct GABA blockers such as bicuculline, with agents which bind to the chloride channel sites such as picrotoxin, and with antagonists of benzodi-azepines (Morin, Watson and Wasterlain, 1983). Successful kindling has been reported with repeated systemic injections of metrazol, picrotoxin, bicuculline and other agents (Cain, 1980, 1982; Pinel and Van Oot, 1975; Ito et al., 1977; Pinel and Cheung, 1977; Nutt et al., 1982; Diehl, Smialowski and Totwo, 1984; Fabisiak and Schwark, 1982) (Table 1). Success has been much more limited with intracerebral injections. Bicuculline, picrotoxin and penicillin (Collins, 1978; Nutt et al., 1982; Cain, 1987) can all produce seizures when injected intracortically. However, the spread of those seizures remains local, and generalized kindled seizures are never obtained (Figure 4). This is surprising in view of the success of systemic injections and of the similarity between the clinical manifestations of seizures kindled using these agents systemically or using muscarinic or electrical stimulation. If behavioral analogy of kindled progression implies the use of common circuitry, the failure of seizure spread after intracortical bicuculline injection is difficult to understand. Again, technical factors might account for this failure, since gliosis might limit the effects of repeated injections. The very large number of local stimulations needed for spread of cortical electrical kindling to the limbic system might not be achievable by chemical kindling because of gliosis at the site of injection.

Agents which bind to benzodiazepine receptors come closest to a full demonstration of chemical kindling since the phenomenon was induced by inverse agonists such as betacarboline; could be blocked by multiple agonists such as diazepam and clonazepam; and could also be blocked by antagonists which displace inverse agonists without having any action of their own, such as RO 15–1788 (Morin, Watson and Wasterlain, 1983; Morin, 1984). Thus it appears that many agents which weaken GABAergic recurrent inhibition can generate a kindling-like phenomenon. Conversely, agents which increase inhibition by acting on various components of the GABA–benzodiazepine receptor complex, such as muscimol, gamma-vinyl GABA, benzodiazepines and barbiturates, are inhibitors of many types of kindling (Wasterlain, Morin and Jonec, 1982a; Racine, 1978).

Agents which interact with other inhibitory neurotransmitters, such as catecholamines, have also been reported to induce chemical kindling and their role in electrical kindling of the amygdala is well established (Downs and Eddy, 1932a; Corcoran et al., 1976; McIntyre and Wong, 1986). For example, lidocaine and cocaine have been used in successful kindling experi-

SEIZURES INDUCED BY INTRACORTICAL BICUCULLINE

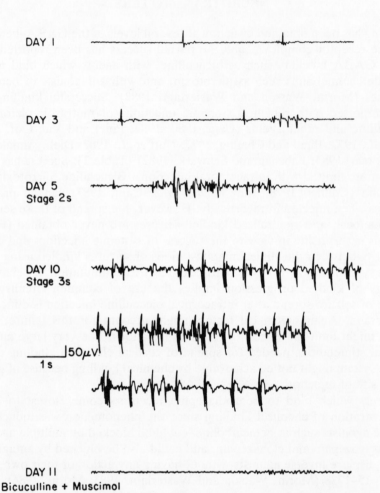

Figure 4. Electrographic response to daily intracortical injection of the GABA receptor blocker bicuculline. Seizures were blocked when bicuculline was mixed with the GABA agonist muscimol. Upon repeated bicuculline injections, we observed limited behaviorial and electrographic seizure progression, but these seizures remained unilateral and full kindling was never reached in any animal even after over 100 injections

ments (Post and Kopanda, 1975, 1976; Post, Kopanda and Lee, 1975; Kopanda and Black, 1976; Wagman, deJong and Prince, 1967). However, the pharmacology of their kindling action has not been explored in detail, and its precise site of action and relation to the catecholaminergic effects have not been defined.

ANATOMICAL SPECIFICITY OF KINDLING CIRCUITS

Seizures induced by many types of kindling are strikingly similar. For example, stage 2 through 5 seizures are nearly identical in electrical kindling of the amygdala, the pyriform cortex, entorhinal cortex, medial septum and the hippocampus, and in chemical kindling of the amygdala or hippocampus with carbachol, or by systemic injection of metrazol, bicuculline, and many other types of kindling. The metabolic anatomy of chemically kindled seizures is very similar to that of electrically caused seizures (Figures 5, 6). The initial injection of carbachol results in enhanced metabolic activity at the site of injection, which disappears as seizures start spreading. Stage 3–5 seizures, which are generalized, with clonic activity of many muscle groups on both sides, are characterized by enhanced glucose metabolism in the hippocampus, entorhinal cortex, substantia nigra, and disappearance of the hypermetabolism at the site of injection. A similar evolution has been described in electrical kindling of the amygdala (Engel, Wofson and Brown, 1978). This similarity of behavioral seizures, electrographic spread and metabolic anatomy suggests that the final common pathway of generalized seizures of many types may involve a common circuitry. If this is true, we should observe transfer of kindling between the late stages of many kindling subtypes, be they electrical

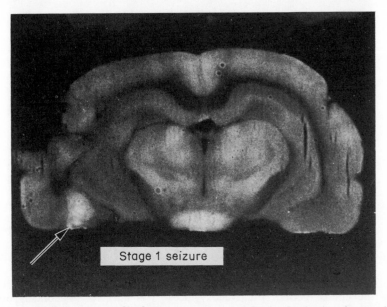

Figure 5. Autoradiogram of [^{14}C]2-deoxyglucose uptake in the brain of a rat during the first of 45 min after injection of carbachol. A stage 1 seizure was observed during part of that time. Note the increase in uptake in the injected amygdala (carbachol 2.7 nmol)

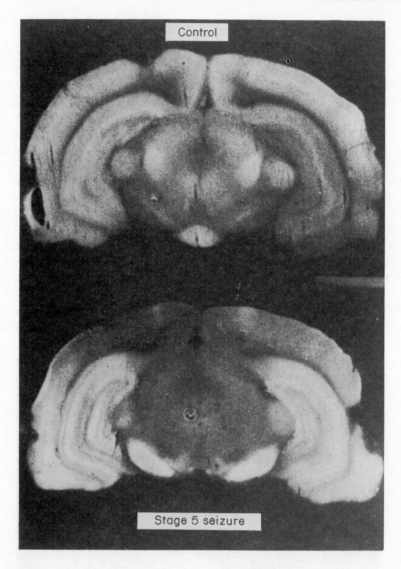

Figure 6. Autoradiogram of [^{14}C]2-deoxyglucose uptake in the brain of a control animal and of an animal which was fully kindled and undergoing kindled seizures during the uptake period. [^{14}C]2-deoxyglucose was injected immediately prior to carbachol. The accumulation of radioactivity reflects an average of ictal and post-ictal periods. This may explain why uptake in some brain regions seems to be decreased by seizures. The increased metabolic activity in substantia nigra, hippo-campus and entorhinal cortex is associated with seizure activity

or chemical. Some common agonists should facilitate all kinds of kindling, because they involve enhancement of synaptic excitability in this final common circuit; other drugs should inhibit all kinds of kindling because they inhibit synapses which are part of that final common circuit. Indeed potentiators of GABAergic inhibition, regardless of their precise site of action ((GABA receptor: GABA, muscimol; benzodiazepine allosteric site: diazepam, clonazepam, RO15–1788; or chloride channel: barbiturates), uniformly inhibit kindling of many types. Supporting the same generalization, positive transfer has been observed between many different types of kindling, both electrical and chemical (Table 3). At the same time, there exists a number of examples of extreme anatomical specificity. For example, we could obtain carbachol kindling in the amygdala but not in cortex (Table 4) and we reached some degree of bicuculline kindling in cortex but not in amygdala, in spite of the fact that both muscarinic and GABA receptors are abundant in both structures (Wasterlain, Farber and Fairchild, 1986). Since we injected pharmacological agents directly into the brain, bypassing any barriers, it is likely that simple adaptive changes in receptors (e.g. desensitization or denervation supersensitivity) would not have shown the anatomical specificity observed, and therefore cannot alone be responsible for the kindled trace. Specificity did not seem to be the simple expression of the presence of bicuculline-sensitive GABA receptors or of muscarinic receptors, which were abundant in both kindling-sensitive and kindling-resistant struc-

Table 3. Positive transfer

	Reference
El Am – El Am	Racine (1978)
Carbachol Am – Musc – ABM Am	Wasterlain and Jonec (1983)
Carbachol Am – El Septal	Wasterlain and Fairchild (1985)
Pilocarpine – El Am	Buterbaugh, Michelson and Keyser (1986)
Metrazol – El Am	Cain (1982)
Picrotoxin – El Am	Cain (1987)
Glu Asp – El Am	Mori and Wada (1987)

El, electrical stimulation; Am, amygdala; Musc, muscarine; ABM, acetyl-beta-methylcholine.

Table 4. Failures of transfer

	Reference
Metrazol – audiogenic	Vergnes et al. (1987)
Cocaine – El Am	Kilbey, Ellinwood and Easter (1970)
Bicuculline Am – carbachol Am	Wasterlain, Morin and Jonec (1982a)
Hip El – Hip El	Burchfield, Applegate and Konkol (1986)
Carbachol Am – El Am	Wasterlain, Morin and Jonec (1982b)

Hip, hippocampus; other abbreviations as in Table 3.

Table 5. Partial transfer

	Reference
Flurothyl – El Am	Okada *et al.* (1985)
CRF – El Am	Weiss *et al.* (1986)

Abbreviations as in Table 3.

tures. It probably reflects a considerable degree of anatomical specificity within a particular group of chemical synapses.

CHEMICAL SPECIFICITY OF KINDLING CIRCUITS

The many examples of transfer between kindling types support the commonality of chemical circuitry in the later stages of kindling seizures. However, many exceptions highlight a great deal of chemical specificity which differs from one kindling type to another. For example, carbachol kindling in the amygdala decreases seizure threshold and after-discharge thresholds for carbachol, muscarine and acetylbetamethylcholine, but not those for bicuculline. Injections of physiological GABA antagonists into cortex decreased seizure thresholds locally for picrotoxin, bicuculline and penicillin, without affecting carbachol seizure thresholds in the same location. The most parsimonious conclusion is that a considerable expanse of common circuitry exists which is shared in the final stages of the kindling seizure, but that access to that circuit depends on synaptic components which are specific for specific kindling types. Transfer of kindling persists even when the primary kindled site is destroyed (Goddard, 1981), supporting this hypothesis, and cross neuronal graft experiments (Messenheimet *et al.*, 1979; Barry *et al.*, 1987) showed that increased excitability can be transferred through appropriate sprouting.

CELLULAR CHANGES ASSOCIATED WITH KINDLING

In the brains of fully kindled animals, a widespread enhancement of evoked potentials is observed (Tuff, Racine and Adamec, 1983). This enhancement is specific for kindled pathways and it is not observed by nonspecific stimulation of adjacent areas. Several mechanisms seem to underlie this enhancement of evoked potentials (Table 6). The first component appears to be synaptic and resembles long-term potentiation (LTP) (Morimoto and Goddard, 1986). However, there are major differences between LTP and kindling (Goddard, 1981). Long-term potentiation seems to be part of some specific types of kindling in some specific locations, but it is certainly not the only mechanism of enhanced excitability in kindling, is less long-lasting and is often absent in synapses which participate in the kindled seizures. For example, LTP of the perforant path facilitates kindling (Sutula and Steward,

Table 6. Cellular changes in kindled brains

	References
Potentiation of EC–GC synpases	Maru and Goddard (1987)
Increased GC excitability	Sutula and Steward (1986)
	Maru and Goddard (1987)
Increased recurrent inhibition GC	Voskuyl and Albus (1987)
Rhythmic spiking AM	Morimoto and Goddard (1986)
Participation of GC NMDA receptors	Mody and Heinemann (1987)
Increased Ca^{2+} entry CA1	Wadman et al. (1985)
Enhanced NMDA-like responses CA1	Wadman et al. (1985)
Decreased recurrent inhibition CA1	Heinemann et al. (1986)
Increased low K^+ bursts CA2–3	King et al (1985)
	Piredda et al. (1986)
	Oliver et al. (1980)
Increased burst firing Am	Tsuru (1985)

1986); the first component of amygdaloid kindling resembles LTP (Morimoto and Goddard, 1986); but LTP is not seen following entorhinal cortex kindling in the first synapse that would be expected to participate in the seizures, namely the entorhinal–granule cell synapse (Giacchino et al., 1984). Similarly, in chemical kindling with metrazol, no LTP of dentate gyrus synapses was observed (Piredda et al., 1986).

A second synaptic component of the change in excitability seen in kindling involves the role of recurrent inhibition. As tested by paired pulse inhibition in dentate gyrus of kindled brains, recurrent GABAergic circuits are enhanced in both amygdala kindling and entorhinal cortex–angular bundle kindling (Voskuyl and Albus, 1987; Maru and Goddard, 1987b; DeJong and Racine, 1985). However, other studies using stimulation of the Schaeffer collaterals observed a reduction of recurrent inhibition in CA1 as kindling progressed (Heinemann et al., 1986). A similar collapse of inhibition has also been observed in late kindling in the amygdala (Morimoto and Goddard, 1986). Therefore, changes in opposite directions can be seen in different types of kindling, even in the same region. Similarly, our studies of calmodulin kinase activity in kindled hippocampus revealed an enhancement of calmodulin kinase-like immunoreactivity in some animals in CA2 and a decreased activity and immunoreactivity in most other hippocampal areas (Bronstein, 1987). Perhaps it is the relative balance of inhibition between various regions which is the key to epileptogenesis rather than the absolute changes in any one particular location. A third component of synaptic excitability that changes with kindling involves excitatory glutamate receptors of the NMDA type (Mody and Heinemann, 1987). In the dentate gyrus, these receptors in spite of their abundance do not normally participate in low frequency neurotransmission (Monaghan and Cotman, 1985; Morris et al., 1986; Crunelli, Forda and Kelly, 1983; Mody and Heinemann, 1986). After kindling of either the amygdala or the hippocampal commissure, the contribution of those receptors to synaptic potentials was studied in hippocampal slices (Mody and Heinemann, 1987).

In slices from kindled rats, the excitatory post-synaptic potentials of granule cells displayed a prominent NMDA receptor-mediated component, which could be blocked by 2-amino-5-phosphonovaleric acid (APV). Basic neuronal membrane properties were not altered. In low magnesium medium, this change resulted, in the kindled slices only, in APV-sensitive burst firing of dentate granule cells in response to single volleys in the perforant path. Since NMDA receptors are coupled to calcium-permeable cationic channels, these changes could underlie the marked changes in extracellular calcium seen upon stimulation in kindled brains (Heinemann et al., 1986) and the changes in calcium binding proteins associated with kindling (Wasterlain and Farber, 1984; Miller et al., 1986). Indeed, after kindling by stimulation of stratum radiatum–stratum moleculare of hippocampus, studies with calcium-sensitive electrodes in hippocampal slices revealed marked changes in extracellular calcium in response to stimulation. Passsage of electrical current through the stimulating electrode, or perfusion of excitatory amino acids, produced a measurable decline in extracellular calcium, presumably because of the opening of NMDA receptor-operated ionic channels through which calcium enters the neurons. In kindled slices, calcium responses were much larger than in normal slices, throughout the dendritic tree of CA1 neurons. This difference persisted in the presence of bicuculline, suggesting that loss of GABAergic control alone cannot explain it. While it is not yet clear whether these changes in calcium conductances are the direct result of the opening of ionic channels permeable to calcium or are secondary to other changes, they could be an important determinant of the paroxysmal firing too often seen in the kindled brain.

An increase in neuronal excitability has also been observed in kindled brains independently of the changes in synaptic function. The population excitatory post-synaptic potential and the amplitude of the population spike of dentate granule cells were measured throughout the course of entorhinal cortex kindling (Sutula and Steward, 1986). In response to the same excitatory post-synaptic potential, reflecting the same degree of synaptic excitation, kindled granule cells responded by larger population spikes than controls. This implies that the kindled dentate granule cells were more likely to fire in response to a given stimulus than their controls, and that even after subtraction of synaptic components cell excitability was increased by kindling.

In summary, at least four different components of synaptic and cellular excitability change during kindling, and different type of kindling result in different types of changes in at least some of those components. The net result, however, is a widespread increase in neuronal excitability expressed in different kindling paradigms by the rhythmic spiking of amygdala neurons

(Morimoto and Goddard, 1986), an increase in spontaneous burst firing in the amygdala (Tsuru, 1985) and in evoked bursts in pyriform cortex (McIntyre and Racine, 1986; McIntyre and Wong, 1986), increased spontaneous burst firing in CA1 (Heinemann et al., 1986) and CA2–3 (Oliver, Hoffer and Wyatt, 1980; Piredda et al., 1986) and an increase in bursts induced in CA2–3 by metrazol (Piredda et al., 1986) or by low potassium (King et al., 1985). These physiological changes, which we are just beginning to unravel, illustrate the extraordinary complexity of the kindling phenomenon. It is likely that both synaptic and cellular chemical changes underlie kindling, and that they vary biochemically and anatomically between varying kindling types. The diversity of the epilepsies is thus paralleled by the diversity of kindling phenomena.

ACKNOWLEDGEMENTS

Supported by the Research Service of the Veterans Administration and by Research Grant NS 13515 from NINDS.

REFERENCES

Barry, D. I., Kikvadze, I., Brundin, P., Bolwig, T. G., Björklund, A. and Lindvall, O. (1987). Grafted noradrenergic neurons suppress seizure development in kindling-induced epilepsy. *Proc. Natl Acad. Sci. USA*, **84**, 8412–8417.

Bronstein, J. (1987). Calmodulin kinase II: Studies of its role in physiology and pathology. Ph.D. thesis, University of California, Los Angeles.

Burchfield, J. L., Applegate, C. D. and Konkol, R. J. (1986). Kindling antagonism: a role for norepinephrine in seizure suppression. In: *Kindling 3* (ed. J. Wada), pp. 213–226. Raven Press, New York.

Buterbaugh, G. G., Michelson, H. B. and Keyser, D. O. (1986). Status epilepticus facilitated by pilocarpine in amygdala-kindled rats. *Exp. Neurol.*, **94**, 91–102.

Cain, D. P. (1980). Effects of kindling or brain stimulation on pentylenetetrazol-induced convulsions susceptibility. *Epilepsia*, **21**, 243–249.

Cain, D. P. (1981a). Kindling: Recent studies and new directions. In: *Kindling 2* (ed. J. Wada), pp. 49–62. Raven Press, New York.

Cain, D. P. (1981b). Transfer of pentylenetetrazol sensitization to amygdaloid kindling. *Pharmacol. Biochem. Behav.*, **15**, 533–536.

Cain, D. P. (1982). Bidirectional transfer of intracerebrally administered pentylenetetrazol and electrical kindling. *Pharmacol. Biochem. Behav.*, **17**, 1111–1113.

Cain, D. P. (1987). Kindling by repeated intraperitoneal or intracerebral injection of picrotoxin transfers to electrical kindling. *Exp. Neurol.*, **97**, 243–254.

Cain, D. P. and Corcoran, M. E. (1985). Epileptiform effects of met-enkephalin, beta-endorphin and morphine: kindling of generalized seizures and potentiation of epileptiform effects by handling. *Brain Res.*, **338**, 327–336.

Collins, R. C. (1978). Kindling of neuroanatomic pathways during recurrent focal penicillin seizures. *Brain Res.*, **150**, 503–517.

Corcoran, M. E., Urstad, H., McGaughran, J. A. J. and Wada, J. A. (1976). Frontal lobe and kindling in the rat. In: *Kindling* (ed. J. Wada), pp. 215–228. Raven Press, New York.

Corcoran, M. E., Cain, D. P., Finlay, J. M. and Gillis, B. J. (1984). Vasopressin and the kindling of seizures. Life Sci., 35, 947–952.

Crunelli, V., Forda, S. and Kelly, J. S. (1983). Blockade of amino acid-induced depolarizations and inhibition of excitatory post-synaptic poentials in rat dentate gyrus. J. Physiol. Lond., 341, 627–640.

DeJong, M. and Racine, R. (1985). The effects of repeated induction of longterm potentiation in the dentate gyrus. Brain Res., 328, 181–185.

Delgado, J. M. R. and Sevillano, M. (1961). Evolution of repeated hippocampal seizures in the cat. Electroencephalogr. Clin. Neurophysiol., 13, 722–733.

Diehl, R. G., Smialowski, A. and Totwo, T. (1984). Development and persistence of kindled seizures after repeated injections of pentylenetetrazol. Epilepsia, 24(4), 506–510.

Downs, A. W. and Eddy, N. B. (1932a). The effect of repeated doses of cocaine on the dog. J. Pharmacol. Exp. Ther., 46, 196–198.

Downs, A. W. and Eddy, N. B. (1932b). The effect of repeated doses of cocaine on the rat. J. Pharmacol. Exp. Ther., 36., 401–410.

Engel, J., Wofson, L. and Brown, L. (1978). Anatomical correlates of electrical and behavioral events related to amygdaloid kindling. Ann. Neurol., 3, 558–544.

Fabisiak, J. P. and Schwark, W. S. (1982). Aspects of the pentylenetetrazol kindling model of epileptogenesis in the rat. Exp. Neurol., 78, 7–14.

Frenk, H., Liban, A., Balamuth, R. and Urca, G. (1982). Opiate and non-opiate aspects of morphine induced seizures. Brain Res., 253, 253–261.

Giacchino, J. L., Somjen, G. G., Frush, D. P. and McNamara, J. O. (1984). Lateral entorhinal cortical kindling can be established without potentiation of the entorhinal-granule cell synapse. Exp. Neurol., 86, 483–492.

Gilbert, M. E. and Cain, D. P. (1985). A single neonatal pentylenetetrazol or hyperthermia convulsion increases kindling susceptibility in the adult rat. Dev. Brain Res., 22, 169–180.

Girgis, M. (1981). Electrical vs. cholinergic kindling. Electroencephalogr. Clin. Neurophysiol., 51, 403–416.

Goddard, G. V. (1969). Analysis of avoidance conditioning following cholinergic stimulation of the amygdala. J. Comp. Physiol. Psychol., 2, 1–18.

Goddard, G. V. (1981). The continuing search for mechanism. In: Kindling 2 (ed. J. Wada), pp. 1–14. Raven Press, New York.

Goddard, G. V., McIntyre, D. C. and Leech, C. K. (1969). A permanent change in brain function resulting from daily electrical stimulation. Exp. Neurol., 25, 295–330.

Heinemann, U., Konnerth, A., Pumain, R. and Wadman, W. T. (1986): Extracellular calcium and potassium concentration changes in chronic epileptic brain tissue. Adv. Neurol., 44, 641–661.

Ito, T., Hori, M., Yoshida, K. and Shimizu, M. (1977). Effect of anticonvulsants on seizure developing in the course of daily administration of pentetrazol to rats. Eur. J. Pharmacol., 45, 165–172.

Kilbey, M. M., Ellinwood, E. H. and Easler, M. E. (1970). The effect of chronic cocaine pretreatment on kindled seizures and behavioral stereotypes. Exp. Neurol., 64, 306–314.

King, G. L., Dingledine, R., Giacchhino, J. L. and McNamara, J. O. (1985). Abnormal neuronal excitability in hippocampal slices from kindled rats. J. Neurophysiol., 54(5), 1295–1304.

Little, H. I., Null, D. J. and Taylor, S. C. (1987). Selective changes in the in vivo effects of benzodiazepine receptor ligands after chemical kindling with FG 7142. Neuropharmacology, 26, 25–31.

Maru, E. and Goddard, G. V. (1987a). Alteration in dentate neuronal activities associated with perforant path kindling. I. Long-term potentiation of excitatory synaptic transmission. *Exp. Neurol.*, **96**, 19–32.

Maru, E. and Goddard, G. V. (1987b). Alteration in dentate neuronal activities associated with perforant path kindling. III. Enhancement of synaptic inhibition. *Exp. Neurol*, **96**, 46–60.

McIntyre, D. C. and Racine, R. J. (1986). Kindling mechanisms: current progress on an experimental epilepsy model. *Prog. Neurobiol.*, **27**, 1–12.

McIntyre, D. C. and Wong, R. C. (1986). Cellular and synaptic properties of amygdala-kindled pyriform cortex *in vitro*. *J. Neurophysiol.*, **55(6)**, 1295–1307.

Messenheimet, J. A., Harris, E. W. and Steward, O. (1979). Sprouting fibers gain access to circuitry transsynaptically altered by kindling. *Exp. Neurol.*, **64**, 469–481.

Miller, J. J., Baimbridge, K. G. and Mody, I. (1986). Calcium regulation in kindling-induced epilepsy. In: *Kindling 3* (ed. J. Wada), pp. 301–318. Raven Press, New York.

Mody, I. and Heinemann, U. (1986). Laminate profiles of the change in extracellular calcium concentration induced by repetitive stimulation and excitatory amino acids in the rat dentate gyrus. *Neurosci. Lett.*, **69**, 137–142.

Mody, I. and Heinemann, U. (1987). NMDA receptors of dentate gyrus granule cells participate in synaptic transmission following kindling. *Nature*, **326**, 701–704.

Monaghan, D. T. and Cotman, C. W. (1985). Distribution of N-methyl-d-aspartate-sensitive I ^{3}H-glutamate-binding sites in rat brain. *J. Neurosci.*, **5**, 2909–2919.

Mori, N. and Wada, J. A. (1987). Bidirectional transfer between kindling induced by excitatory amino acids and electrical stimulation. *Brain Res.*, **425**, 45–48.

Morin, A. M. (1984). Beta-carboline kindling of the benzodiazepine receptors. *Brain Res.*, **321**, 151–154.

Morin, A. M., Watson, A. L. and Wasterlain, C. G. (1983). Kindling of seizures with norhaman alpha-beta-carboline ligand of benzodiazepine receptors. *Eur. J. Pharmacol.*, **88**, 131–134.

Morimoto, K. and Goddard, G. V. (1986). Kindling induced changes in EEG recorded during stimulation from the site of stimulation: collapse of GABA-mediated inhibition and onset of rhythmic synchronous burst. *Exp. Neurol.*, **94**, 571–584.

Morrell, F. (1960). Secondar epileptogenic lesions. *Epilepsia*, **1**, 538–560.

Morrell, F. (1979). Human secondary epileptogenic lesions. *Neurology*, **29**, 558.

Morris, R. G. M., Anderson, E., Lynch, G. S. and Baudry, M. (1986). Selective impairment of learning and blockade of long-term potentiation by an N-methyl-D-aspartate receptor antagonist AP5. *Nature*, **319**, 774–776.

Nutt, E., Cowen, P., Batts, C., Smith, D. and Green, A. (1982). Rejected administration of subconvulsant doses of GABA antagonist drugs. I. Effect on seizures threshold (Kindling). *Psychopharmacology*, **76**, 84–89.

Okada, R., Solomon, L. M., Ono, K. and Albala, B. J. (1985). Unidirectional interaction between flurothyl seizures and amygdala kindling. *Brain Res.*, **344**, 103–108.

Oliver, A. P., Hoffer, B. J. and Wyatt, R. J. (1980). Kindling induces long-lasting alterations in response of hippocampal neurons to elevated potassium levels *in vitro*. *Science*, **208**, 1264–1265.

Peterson, D. W., Collins, J. F. and Bradford, H. F. (1984). Anticonvulsant action of amino acid antagonists against kindled hippocampal seizures. *Brain Res.*, **311**, 176–180.

Pinel, J. P. J. and Cheung, K. F. (1977). Brief communication: Controlled demonstration of metrazol kindling. *Pharmacol. Biochem. Behav.*, **6**, 599–600.

Pinel, J. P. J. and Van Oot, P. H. (1975). Generality of the kindling phenomenon: Some clinical implications. *Can. J. Neurol. Sci.*, **2**, 467–475.

Piredda, S., Yonekawa, W., Whittingham, T. S. and Kupferberg, H. J. (1986). Enhanced bursting activity in the CA3 region of the mouse hippocampal slice without long-term potentiation in the dentate gyrus after systemic pentylenetetrazole kindling. *Exp. Neurol.*, **94**, 659–669.

Post, R. M. (1981). Lidocaine-kindled limbic seizures: Behavioral implications. In: *Kindling 2* (ed. J. Wada), pp. 149–157. Raven Press, New York.

Post, R. M. and Kopanda, R. T. (1975). Cocaine, kindling and reverse tolerance. *Lancet*, **i**, 409–410.

Post, R. M. and Kopanda, R. T. (1976). Cocaine, kindling and psychosis. *Am. J. Psychiat.*, **133**, 627–634.

Post, R. M., Kopanda, R. T. and Black, K. E. (1976). Progressive effects of cocaine on behavior and central amine metabolism in rhesus monkeys: Relationship to kindling and psychosis. *Biol. Psychiat.*, **11**, 403–419.

Post, R. M., Kopanda, R. T. and Lee, A. (1975). Progressive behavioral changes during chronic lidocaine administration: relationship to kindling. *Life Sci.*, **17**, 943–950.

Racine, R. J. (1972a). Modification of seizure activity by electrical stimulation. I. After discharge threshold. *Electroencephalogr. Clin. Neurophysiol.*, **32**, 269–279.

Racine, R. J. (1972b). Modification of seizure activity by electrical stimulation. II. Motor seizures. *Electroencephalogr. Clin. Neurophysiol.*, **32**, 281–294.

Racine, R. J. (1978). Kindling: the first decade. *Neurosurgery*, **3**, 234–252.

Sato, M. and Okamoto, M. (1981). Dopaminergic and electrical kindling. In: *Kindling 2* (ed. J. Wada), pp. 105–119. Raven Press, New York.

Solviter, R. S., and Dempster, A. D. (1985). Epileptic brain damage is replicated qualitatively in rat hippocampus by central injection glutamate or aspartate but not GABA or acetylcholine. *Brain Res. Bull.*, **15**, 39–60.

Sutula, T. and Steward, O. (1986). Quantitative analysis of synaptic potentiation during kindling of the perforant path. *J. Neurophysiol.*, **56(3)**, 732–746.

Tsuru, N. (1985). Neuronal firing pattern following amygdaloid kindling in unrestrained rats. *Epilepsia*, **26(5)**, 488–492.

Tuff, L. P., Racine, R. J. and Adamec, R. (1983). The effects of kindling on GABA-mediated inhibition in the dentate gyrus of the rat. I. Paired-pulse depression. *Brain Res.*, **277**, 79–90.

Vergnes, M., Kiesmann, M., Marescaus, C., Depaulis, A., Micheletti, G. and Warter, J. (1987). Kindling of audiogenic seizures in the rat. *Int. J. Neurosci.*, **36**, 167–176.

Voskuyl, R. A. and Albus, H. (1987). Enhancement of recurrent inhibition by angular bundle kindling is retained in hippocampal slices. *Int. J. Neurosci.*, **36**, 153–166.

Vosu, H. and Wise, R. A. (1975). Cholinergic seizure kindling in the rat: comparison of caudate, amygdala, and hippocampus. *Behav. Biol.*, **13**, 491–495.

Wadman, W. T., Heinemann, U., Konnerth, A. and Neuhaus, S. (1985). Hippocampal slices of kindled rats reveal calcium involvement in epileptogenesis. *Exp. Brain Res.*, **57**, 404–407.

Wagman, I. H., deJong, R. H., Prince, D. A. (1967). Effects of lidocaine on the central nervous system. *Anesthesiology*, **28**, 155–172.

Wasterlain, C. G. and Fairchild, M. D. (1985). Transfer between chemical and electrical kindling in the septal-hippocampal system. *Brain Res.*, **331**, 261–266.

Wasterlain, C. G. and Farber, D. B. (1984). Kindling alters the calcium/calmodulin-dependent phosphorylation of synaptic plasma membrane proteins in rat hippocampus. *Proc. Natl Acad. Sci. USA*, **81**, 1253–1257.

Wasterlain, C. G. and Jonec, V. (1983). Chemical kindling by muscarinic amygdaloid stimulation in the rat. *Brain Res.*, **271**, 311–323.

Wasterlain, C. G., Farber, D. B. and Fairchild, M. D. (1986). Synaptic mechanisms in the kindled epileptic focus: a speculative synthesis. *Adv. Neurol.*, **44**, 411–433.

Wasterlain, C. G., Morin, A. M. and Jonec, V. (1982a). Kindling: a pharmacological approach. *Electroencephalogr. Clin. Neurophysiol, Suppl.*, **36**, 264–273.

Wasterlain, C. G., Morin, A. M. and Jonec, V. (1982b). Interactions between chemical and electrical kindling of the rat amygdala. *Brain Res.*, **247**, 341–346.

Wasterlain, C. G., Faichild, M. D., Bronstein, J. M. and Farber, D. B. (1986). Molecular changes in the synaptic apparatus associated with septal kindling. In: *Kindling 3* (ed. J. Wada), pp. 55–71. Raven Press, New York.

Weiss, S. R. B., Post, R. M., Gold, P. W., Chrousos, G., Sullivan, T. L., Walker, D. and Pert, A. (1986). CRF-Induced seizures and behavior: interaction with amygdala kindling. *Brain Res.*, **372**, 345–351.

The Clinical Relevance of Kindling
Edited by T. G. Bolwig and M. R. Trimble
© 1989 John Wiley & Sons Ltd

4

Kindling and antiepileptic drugs

M. Schmutz and K. Klebs
*Research and Development Department, Pharmaceuticals Division, Ciba-
Geigy Ltd, CH-4002 Basel, Switzerland*

PROLOGUE

This review deals with the effects of antiepileptic drugs on (1) kindling evolution following electrical stimulation and on (2) the kindled-seizure condition.

Phenobarbital and the benzodiazepines delayed kindling evolution most efficaciously, whereas the effects of valproate, ethosuximide and acetazolamide were somewhat less pronounced. Surprisingly, phenytoin, carbamazepine and oxcarbazepine did not affect rat kindling development or even enhanced it at higher doses, at least with regard to the EEG after-discharges. The evolution of cat and/or baboon kindling was delayed by phenobarbital and also by carbamazepine and valproate; phenytoin was not effective under the above experimental conditions.

Unlike their effect on kindling evolution, all antiepileptics studied suppressed rat amygdaloid and cortically kindled seizures to a certain degree. However, phenobarbital, trimethadione, valproate and diazepam were more efficacious than the other antiepileptics against rat amygdaloid kindled seizures. Only a limited number of animals and drugs have been included in cat and baboon studies. Phenobarbital, phenytoin and carbamazepine inhibited kindled seizures in these species, whereas ethosuximide exacerbated cat kindled seizures.

In addition to the above findings a hypothesis is proposed to explain why antiepileptics can inhibit or even enhance kindling evolution. Finally, the clinical significance of kindling is discussed with regard to antiepileptic drug activity, animal behaviour and electroencephalography.

INTRODUCTION

Since the publication of Goddard (1987), describing the development of seizures in animals through brain stimulation at low intensity, the kindling phenomenon has attracted the attention of many scientists from a variety of disciplines (see e.g. Schmutz, 1986 and 1987). One research direction deals with the influence of antiepileptic drugs on the evolution of kindling as well as on the kindled seizure condition. But contrary to many expectations, not all antiepileptics delay the evolution of kindling and, in addition, they differ in their efficacy to suppress kindled seizures. Divergent effects were, for instance, observed with carbamazepine and phenytoin. Depending on the animal species and experimental conditions, these compounds delayed, did not affect or enhanced the evolution of kindling. Carbamazepine delayed the development of seizures during amygdala kindling in cats and baboons. In these species without medication tonic–clonic convulsions occur following kindling (Wada, 1977, 1980; Wada *et al.*, 1976b). In rats, on the other hand, this substance did not influence or accelerate kindling (Albertson, Jay and Stark, 1984; Baltzer, Klebs and Schmutz, 1981; Schmutz, Klebs and Baltzer, 1988; Wada, 1977). Phenytoin was reported to be ineffective or to accelerate amygdaloid kindling (Baltzer, Klebs and Schmutz, 1981; Ehle, 1980; Racine, Livingston and Joaquin, 1975; Schmutz, Klebs and Baltzer, 1988; Wada, 1980; Wada *et al.*, 1976b; Wise and Chinerman, 1974) but to delay neocortical kindling (Racine, Livingston and Joaquin, 1975) in the rat.

This review is the first one since that of Wada in 1977 on this topic; it offers a comprehensive summary on the published literature and hitherto unpublished results from our own laboratory concerning the influence of antiepileptic drugs on the *evolution of electrically induced kindling* and on the *kindled seizure condition*. In addition we try to explain why, under certain circumstances, antiepileptics can inhibit or even enhance kindling evolution and discuss the clinical significance of this animal model with regard to antiepileptic drug activity, animal behaviour and electroencephalography.

RESULTS

Phenytoin

In a number of studies phenytoin (see Table 1) proved to be ineffective or even enhanced the evolution of amygdaloid kindling in rats, cats and baboons. In experiments on rats for instance, the high dose of 60 mg kg^{-1} day^{-1} p.o. resulted in a marked increase in duration of after-discharges, the maximal discharge duration being about 70 s compared to roughly 40 s of a placebo group. The dose of 20 mg kg^{-1} day^{-1} p.o. only led to a non-significant trend to increase the duration of afterdischarges, whereas lower doses of

Table 1. Effects of phenytoin, carbamazepine and oxcarbazepine on amygdaloid-kindling evolution

Drug/reference	Animal	Effects
Phenytoin		
Baltzer, Klebs and Schmutz (1981)	rat	enhancement (p.o.; ADs)
Ehle (1980)	rat	equivocal (p.o.; ADs ↓ ; R0)
Racine, Livingston and Joaquin (1975)	rat	enhancement (p.o.; ADs + R)
Schmutz, Klebs, Baltzer (1988)	rat	enhancement (p.o.; ADs ↑ ; R(↑))
Wise and Chinerman (1974)	rat	ineffective (s.c.)
Wada *et al.* (1976b)	cat	equivocal (i.m.; ADs(↓); R0)
Wada (1980)	baboon	ineffective (p.o.; few data)
Carbamazepine		
Albertson, Joy and Stark (1984)	rat	ineffective (i.p.; ADs0; R(↓))
Baltzer, Klebs and Schmutz (1981)	rat	enhancement (p.o.; ADs)
Schmutz, Klebs and Baltzer (1988)	rat	enhancement (p.o; ADs)
Wada (1977)	rat	ineffective
Wada *et al.* (1976b)	cat	inhibition (p.o.; ADs + R)
Wada (1977, 1980)	baboon	inhibition (p.o.; ADs + R)
Oxcarbazepine		
Schmutz, Klebs and Baltzer (1988)	rat	slight enhancement (p.o.; ADs)

ADs, after discharges; R, Racine scale; 0, no effect; ↓ , inhibition; ↑ , enhancement; (↑), (↓), slight effect.

phenytoin were without effect on kindling development (Schmutz, Klebs and Baltzer, 1988).

On the other hand, phenytoin suppressed amygdaloid-kindled seizures in cats and baboons, but was ineffective in rabbits. In rats this antiepileptic generally attenuated amygdaloid-kindled seizures, although ineffectiveness or even an exacerbation of seizures was observed in some studies (see Table 4). Effects of phenytoin on neocortically kindled seizures were reported also (see Table 10). All data indicate that neocortically kindled seizures were more potently or efficaciously attenuated by this antiepileptic than seizures kindled by electrical stimulation of the amygdala.

Carbamazepine, oxcarbazepine

With regard to the evolution of rat amygdaloid kindling, carbamazepine showed the same results as phenytoin, i.e. it was ineffective or enhanced

Table 2. Effects of phenobarbital, valproate and ethosuximide on
amygdaloid-kindling evolution

Drug/reference	Animal	Effect
Phenobarbital		
Schmutz, Klebs and Baltzer (1988)	rat	inhibition
Wise and Chinerman (1974)	rat	inhibition
Wada (1977)	cat	inhibition
Wada (1977, 1980)	baboon	inhibition
Valproate		
Leviel and Naquet (1977)	rat	inhibition
Salt, Tulloch and Walter (1980)	rat	inhibition
Schmutz and Klebs (1982)	rat	inhibition
Schmutz, Klebs and Baltzer (1988)	rat	inhibition
Tanaka and Lange (1975)	rat	inhibition
Wada (1977)	cat	inhibition
Ethosuximide		
Schmutz, Klebs and Baltzer (1988)	rat	inhibition

Table 3. Effects of diazepam, clonazepam, clobazam and
acetazolamide on amygdaloid-kindling evolution

Drug/reference	Animal	Effect
Diazepam		
Racine, Livingston and Joaquin (1975)	rat	inhibition
Schmutz, Klebs and Baltzer (1988)	rat	inhibition
Schmutz et al. (1985)	rat	inhibition
Schwark and Haluska (1987)	rat	inhibition
Wise and Chinerman (1974)	rat	inhibition
Clonazepam		
Schmutz, Klebs and Baltzer (1988)	rat	inhibition
Clobazam		
Schmutz, Klebs and Baltzer (1988)	rat	inhibition
Acetazolamide		
Schmutz, Klebs and Baltzer (1988)	rat	inhibition

kindling development (see Table 1). A slight enhancement was also observed
for oxcarbazepine, a structurally related antiepileptic, at the high dose of
100 mg kg^{-1} day^{-1} p.o. (Schmutz, Klebs and Baltzer, 1988). Unlike phenytoin,
however, carbamazepine seemed to delay kindling development in cats and
baboons (see Table 1), although less potently than did phenobarbital.

Carbamazepine generally suppressed amygdaloid-kindled seizures in rats,
cats and baboons (Table 5); neocortically kindled seizures in rats were attenu-

Table 4. Effects of phenytoin on amygdaloid-kindled seizures

Reference	Animal	Effects
Albertson, Peterson and Stark (1980)	rat	weak suppression (ADs only)
Albright and Burnham (1980)	rat	suppression (ADs + R)
Ashton and Wauquier (1979)	rat	suppression (forepaw clonus)
Babington and Wedeking (1973)	rat	suppression (high dose; ADs)
Callaghan and Schwark (1980)	rat	exacerbation (ADs + R)
Howe et al. (1981)	rat	ineffective (p.o.; ADs + R)
Howe et al. (1981)	rat	weak suppression (i.p.; R)
Kamei et al. (1981)	rat	ineffective (p.o.; ADs)
Kamei et al. (1981)	rat	weak suppression (i.v.; ADs)
Klebs and Schmutz (unpublished data)	rat	suppression (high dose; R)
Löscher, Jaeckel and Czuczwar (1986)	rat	suppression (ADs < R)
Pinel (1983)	rat	weak suppression (i.p.; R)
Racine, Livingston and Joaquin (1975)	rat	weak suppression (i.p.; ADs)
Wise and Chinerman (1974)	rat	ineffective (s.c.; ADs + R)
Tanaka (1972)	rabbit	ineffective
Wada et al. (1976a)	cat	suppression (i.m.; ADs)
Wada et al. (1976a)	baboon	suppression (p.o.; ADs + R)

ADs, after-discharges; R, Racine scale.

Table 5. Effects of carbamazepine on amygdaloid-kindled seizures

Reference	Animal	Effects
Albertson, Peterson and Stark (1980)	rat	moderate suppression (R)
Albertson, Joy and Stark (1984)	rat	suppression (ADs + R)
Albright and Burnham (1980)	rat	suppression (ADs + R)
Ashton and Wauquier (1979)	rat	suppression (forepaw clonus)
Howe et al. (1981)	rat	weak suppression (p.o.; R)
Howe et al. (1981)	rat	suppression (i.p.; ADs + R)
Kamei et al. (1981)	rat	moderate suppression (high dose)
Klebs and Schmutz (unpubl. data)	rat	suppression (high dose; R)
Löscher, Jaeckel and Czuczwar (1986)	rat	suppression (ADs < R)
Wada (1977)	rat	equivocal results
Wada et al. (1976a)	cat	suppression (ADs > R)
Wada et al. (1976a)	baboon	suppression (ADs + R)

ADs, after discharges; R, Racine scale.

ated also by this drug, in some cases more potently than amygdaloid-kindled seizures (see Table 10).

Phenobarbital

Phenobarbital efficaciously inhibited the evolution of rat amygdaloid kindling in all species tested, i.e. in rats, cats and baboons (see Table 2). In the study of Schmutz, Klebs and Baltzer (1988), for example, at the dose of 20 mg kg^{-1} day^{-1} p.o. the after-discharge duration did not increase during the treatment period of 25 days and the behavioural symptoms were restricted to the Racine stages 1 and 2.

Phenobarbital also significantly suppressed amygdala- and neocortically kindled seizures in rats and in addition amygdala-kindled seizures in rabbits, cats and baboons (see Tables 6, 10).

Table 6. Effects of phenobarbital on amygdaloid-kindled seizures

Reference	Animal	Effects
Albertson, Peterson and Stark (1980)	rat	suppression (ADs + R)
Albright and Burnham (1980)	rat	suppression (ADs + R)
Babington and Wedeking (1973)	rat	suppression (ADs)
Callaghan and Schwark (1980)	rat	suppression (ADs + R)
Howe et al. (1981)	rat	suppression (ADs + R)
Kamei et al. (1981)	rat	moderate suppression (ADs)
Klebs and Schmutz (unpublished data)	rat	suppression (ADs + R)
Löscher, Jaeckel and Czuczwar (1986)	rat	suppression (ADs + R)
Wise and Chinerman (1974)	rat	suppression (ADs + R)
Tanaka (1972)	rabbit	suppression
Wada (1976a)	cat	suppression (ADs + R)
Wada (1976a)	baboon	suppression (ADs + R)

ADs, after-discharges; R, Racine scale.

Valproate

Valproate delayed the evolution of rat and cat amygdala kindling (see Table 2) and suppressed amygdaloid- as well as neocortically kindled seizures in rats (see Tables 7, 10). Qualitatively, these effects were comparable to those of phenobarbital; quantitatively, however, i.e. with regard to potency and efficacy, the anticonvulsant effects of phenobarbital proved to be superior to those of valproate (see also Schmutz, Klebs and Baltzer, 1988).

Ethosuximide

The few studies dealing with ethosuximide and kindling indicate that this antiepileptic inhibits rat amygdaloid kindling development (see Table 2) and moderately attenuates amygdaloid- as well as neocortically kindled seizures in rats (see Tables 8, 10). It is interesting to note, however, that the compound exacerbates convulsions of amygdala-kindled cats. Such a profile is opposite to that of carbamazepine which has been shown to suppress convulsions of amygdala-kindled cats and to enhance rat amygdaloid kindling evolution (see Tables 1, 5).

Table 7. Effects or valproate on amygdaloid-kindled seizures

Reference	Animal	Effects
Albertson, Peterson and Stark (1980)	rat	suppression (ADs + R)
Albright and Burnham (1980)	rat	suppression (ADs + R)
Ashton and Wauquier (1979)	rat	suppression (forepaw clonus)
Kamei *et al.* (1981)	rat	moderate suppression (high dose)
Löscher, Jaeckel and Czuczwar (1986)	rat	suppression (ADs + R)
Schmutz and Klebs (1982)	rat	suppression (ADs + R)
Tanaka and Lange (1975)	rat	suppression (ADs + R)
Wada (1977)	rat	suppression
Wada (1977, 1980)	cat	suppression (ADs + R)
Wada (1977)	baboon	suppression
Wada (1977)	rhesus	suppression

ADs, after-discharges; R, Racine scale.

Table 8. Effects of ethosuximide, trimethadione and acetazolamide on amygdaloid-kindled seizures

Drug/reference	Animal	Effects
Ethosuximide		
Albertson, Peterson and Stark (1980)	rat	weak suppression (ADs + R)
Albright and Burnham (1980)	rat	moderate suppression (ADs + R)
Klebs and Schmutz (unpublished data)	rat	suppression (high dose; ADs + R)
Wada (1980)	cat	exacerbation (ADs + R)
Trimethadione		
Albertson, Peterson and Stark (1980)	rat	suppression (high dose; ADs + R)
Ashton and Wauquier (1979)	rat	suppression (forepaw clonus)
Callaghan and Schwark (1980)	rat	suppression (ADs + R)
Klebs and Schmutz (unpublished data)	rat	suppression (high dose; ADs + R)
Acetazolamide		
Albertson, Peterson and Stark (1980)	rat	moderate suppression (ADs only)
Ashton and Wauquier (1979)	rat	suppression (forepaw clonus)

ADs, after-discharges; R, Racine scale.

Trimethadione, acetazolamide

Both drugs, which are only rarely used as antiepileptics today, have been reported to suppress rat amygdaloid-kindled convulsions (see Table 8). Acetazolamide also inhibited the evolution of rat amygdaloid kindling (see Table 3).

Benzodiazepines

Diazepam, clonazepam and clobazam potently and efficaciously inhibited the development of rat amygdaloid kindling (see Table 3) and suppressed amygdaloid kindled seizures in rats and, diazepam only, in rabbits (see Table 9). For diazepam and clonazepam it could be shown that they also attenuated rat neocortically kindled seizures (see Table 10).

Table 9. Effects of diazepam, clonazepam and clobazam on amygdaloid-kindled seizures

Drug/reference	Animal	Effects
Diazepam		
Albertson, Peterson and Stark (1980)	rat	suppression (ADs + R)
Albright and Burnham (1980)	rat	suppression (ADs + R)
Ashton and Wauquier (1979)	rat	suppression (forepaw clonus)
Babington and Wedeking (1973)	rat	suppression (ADs)
Callaghan and Schwark (1980)	rat	suppression (ADs + R)
Ichimaru, Gomita and Moriyama (1987)	rat	suppression (ADs + R)
Kamei et al. (1981)	rat	suppression (ADs)
Klebs and Schmutz (unpublished data)	rat	suppression (ADs + R)
Löscher, Jaeckel and Czuczwar (1986)	rat	suppression (ADs + R)
Pinel (1983)	rat	suppression (R)
Racine, Livingston and Joaquin (1975)	rat	suppression (ADs)
Wise and Chinerman (1974)	rat	suppression (ADs + R)
Tanaka (1972)	rabbit	suppression
Clonazepam		
Albertson, Peterson and Stark (1980)	rat	suppression (ADs + R)
Albright and Burnham (1980)	rat	suppression (ADs + R)
Ashton and Wauquier (1979)	rat	suppression (forepaw clonus)
Klebs and Schmutz unpublished data)	rat	suppression (ADs + R)
Löscher, Jaeckel and Czuczwar (1986)	rat	suppression (ADs + R)
Clobazam		
Ichimaru, Gomita and Moriyama (1987)	rat	suppression (ADs + R)

ADs, after discharges; R, Racine scale.

DISCUSSION

Effects of antiepileptics on kindling evolution

The diversity of the above results, especially with regard to drug effects on kindling development, is surprising: phenobarbital (rat, cat, baboon) and

Table 10. Comparative suppression of generalized amygdaloid- and neocortically kindled seizures by antiepileptic drugs

Drug/reference	Comparative suppression
Phenytoin	
Albright and Burnham (1980)	amygdala<neocortex
Babington and Wedeking (1973)	amygdala≤neocortex
Kamei et al. (1981)	amygdala<neocortex
Klebs and Schmutz (unpublished data)	amygdala<neocortex
Carbamazepine	
Albright and Burnham (1980)	amygdala≥neocortex
Kamei et al. (1981)	amygdala<neocortex
Klebs and Schmutz (unpublished data)	amygdala<neocortex
Phenobarbital	
Albright and Burnham (1980)	amygdala=neocortex
Babington and Wedeking (1973)	amygdala=neocortex
Kamei et al. (1981)	amygdala<neocortex
Valproate	
Albright and Burnham (1980)	amygdala=neocortex
Kamei et al. (1981)	amygdala<neocortex
Ethosuximide	
Albright and Burnham (1980)	amygdala≤neocortex
Diazepam	
Albright and Burnham (1980)	amygdala>neocortex
Babington and Wedeking (1973)	amygdala<neocortex
Kamei et al. (1981)	amygdala≤neocortex
Clonazepam	
Albright and Burnham (1980)	amygdala>neocortex

the benzodiazepines (rat) delay kindling evolution most efficaciously; the respective effects of valproate, ethosuximide and acetazolamide are somewhat less pronounced. On the other hand, phenytoin, carbamazepine and oxcarbazepine did not affect or even enhanced rat kindling development, at least with regard to the EEG after-discharges; the evolution of cat and baboon kindling was delayed by carbamazepine, however.

The publication of Schmutz, Klebs and Baltzer (1988) is the most comprehensive systematic study, describing the effects of a variety of antiepileptics on rat kindling evolution under identical experimental conditions. For this reason and in order to discuss the finding that, under certain circumstances, antiepileptics can inhibit or enhance kindling evolution, it is worthwhile to review some of their results. They are in line with those of other authors in that carbamazepine, oxcarbazepine and phenytoin, in contrast to all other antiepileptics studied, did not inhibit the development of rat kindling. In fact, at rather high doses these drugs accelerated the evolution of after-discharges, leaving the behavioural epileptiform symptoms uninfluenced or even increasing their expression in some cases. By contrast, diazepam, clonazepam, clobazam, phenobarbital, acetazolamide, valproate and ethosuximide delayed the evolution of after-discharges and behavioural epileptiform symptoms. Similarly, Racine, Livingston and Joaquin (1975) have shown that phenytoin increased the rate of seizure development whereas diazepam delayed amygdaloid kindling.

These findings thus discriminate between drugs such as carbamazepine and phenytoin, which are mainly active against generalized tonic–clonic and partial seizures and those drugs which have in common an anti-absence and/or anti-myoclonic component. Engel et al. (1981) proposed a hypothesis which may offer at least a partial explanation for this differential activity of antiepileptics in the kindling situation described. They postulated that absence seizures are the result of an excessive activity of inhibitory processes and termed them 'inhibitory seizures'. Factors supporting their inhibitory nature are the observation that in absence seizures an arrest of ongoing mental activity occurs (e.g. Penry, Porter and Dreifuss, 1975), and that during the wave component of spike-wave-activity cortical neurons are subject to inhibitory post-synaptic potentials (Pollen, 1964). In addition, synaptic inhibition seems to require a greater energy expenditure than excitation and it is during absence seizures that the most striking increase in glucose metabolism is observed (Ackermann et al., 1984; Engel et al., 1985).

Schmutz, Klebs and Baltzer (1988) now propose that under physiological conditions hitherto unknown 'endogenous' inhibitory processes can be activated to counteract emerging seizure activity, but that under pathological conditions these inhibitory processes overshoot and build up self-sustained trains of 3 Hz spike-wave complexes, resulting in myoclonic/absence-type-seizures. Daily rat amygdaloid threshold stimulation, which produces clonic-seizures as well as generalized spike-wave complexes of, on the average, 2–4 Hz in the EEG (see above publication), seems to represent such a pathological condition. According to the above line of thinking, antiepileptics which have an anti-absence and/or anti-myoclonic component should therefore suppress the overshooting inhibitory activity which leads to the observed trains of spike-wave complexes and thus inhibit rat kindling development. Antiepileptics without an anti-absence/anti-myoclonic component such as phenytoin or carbamazepine should leave these inhibitory processes uninfluenced or even sustain them (in case these processes are initiated to counteract partial and tonic–clonic seizures), thus consequently accelerating their development to self-sustained spike-wave discharges and enhancing the evolution of kindling.

Compatible with the above hypothesis and findings are the results of experiments by Fromm and Terrence (1985) and Micheletti *et al.* (1985). The former authors reported that the anti-absence drugs ethosuximide and valproate suppress segmental neuronal inhibition evoked by conditioned maxillary nerve stimulation in the trigeminal nucleus of the cat. On the other hand, carbamazepine and phenytoin intensified segmental neuronal inhibition under identical experimental conditions. The latter authors used rats with spike and wave-like EEG discharges. Drugs with an anti-absence component suppressed these EEG-discharges, whereas carbamazepine and phenytoin were ineffective or aggravated them at higher doses.

The concepts of Engel *et al.* (1981) and Schmutz, Klebs and Baltzer (1988) would also explain the clinical observation that phenytoin and carbamazepine may sometimes precipitate absence-type seizures (e.g. Paine, 1965; Snead and Hosey, 1985), whereas anti-absence drugs such as ethosuximide or trime-thadione can facilitate generalized tonic–clonic seizures (e.g. Lennox, 1947; Lorentz de Haas and Kuilman, 1964). They are also in accordance with the fact that carbamazepine delays amygdaloid kindling evolution in cats and baboons which — contrary to rats — culminates in generalized tonic–clonic seizures. However, only few animals were investigated and replication of these data would be helpful, especially since the ineffectiveness of phenytoin under such conditions cannot be explained for the moment (phenytoin, however, suppresses amygdaloid-kindled seizures in cats and baboons; see below).

The data available on antiepileptics and kindling evolution suggest that rat amygdaloid kindling represents a model for the development of generalized absence/myoclonic-type seizures whereas kindling in cats and baboons represents a model for the development of generalized tonic–clonic seizures. The assumption that kindling evolution in Rhesus monkeys is an animal model for complex partial seizures (Wada, 1980) remains to be further explored.

Effects of antiepileptic drugs on kindled seizures

In general, all antiepileptics investigated suppressed the components of rat amygdaloid-kindled seizures, i.e. after-discharge duration and behavioural symptoms, to a certain degree. The observed differences in efficacy become most evident when the papers by Albertson, Peterson and Stark (1980), Albright and Burnham (1980), Ashton and Wauquier (1979), Kamei *et al.* (1981) and Löscher, Jaeckel and Czuczwar (1986) are examined, since each of these groups reported on the effects of at least five antiepileptics on after-discharge duration and/or behavioural symptoms (Racine scale). Taken together, phenobarbital, trimethadione, valproate and diazepam seem to suppress rat amygdaloid-kindled seizures more efficaciously than clon-azepam, carbamazepine, acetazolamide, phenytoin and ethosuximide. It is of interest to note that those drugs which have the most marked impact on after-discharge duration were also those which suppressed the behavioural symptoms most efficaciously. Differences in 'drug ranking' between the before-mentioned publications exist; they may be due to different routes of administration and/or to differences in the experimental protocols.

Concerning drug effects, electroencephalography and clinical significance, it seems questionable whether or not a specific human seizure type is mimicked by rat amygdaloid kindled seizures. Some authors tend to define the Racine stages 1 to 3 as 'partial seizure' stages and their suppression by anticonvulsants as indicative of activity against partial seizures with complex symptomatology. However, (secondary) generalization of seizure activity can be observed already at stage 1 of Racine; furthermore, the spike-wave EEG pattern and the above-described drug ranking do not convincingly argue in favour of this assumption. Even less is known about the clinical significance of kindled seizure suppression in cats and baboons because only a limited number of drugs and animals have been included in the respective studies. Phenobarbital and, to a lesser degree, phenytoin and carbamazepine inhibited kindled seizures in these species, whereas ethosuximide exacerbated cat kindled seizures. These data and the fact that amygdaloid kindling in cats and baboons culminates in tonic–clonic convulsions indicate that, in these two species, kindled seizures may be a model of human (secondary) generalized tonic–clonic convulsions. Nevertheless, as with rabbits and Rhesus monkeys, where even less data are available, additional experiments would be needed to confirm such an assumption. With regard to the seizure-types elicited and the species under investigation, the necessity to perform additional experiments should be carefully weighed against ethical considerations.

ACKNOWLEDGEMENT

The authors wish to thank Mrs Chantal Portet for her efficient secretarial assistance in preparing this manuscript.

REFERENCES

Ackermann, R. F., Finch, D. M., Babb, T. L. and Engel Jr, J. (1984). Increased glucose metabolism during long-duration recurrent inhibition of hippocampal pyramidal cells. *J. Neurosci.*, **4**, 251–264.

Albertson, T. E., Joy, R. M. and Stark, L. G. (1984). Carbamazepine: a pharmacological study in the kindling model of epilepsy. *Neuropharmacology*, **23**, 1117–1123.

Albertson, T. E., Peterson, S. L. and Stark, L. G. (1980). Anticonvulsant drugs and their antagonism of kindled amygdaloid seizures in rats. *Neuropharmacology*, **19**, 643–652.

Albright, P. S. and Burnham, W. M. (1980). Development of a new pharmacological seizure model: effects of anticonvulsants on cortical- and amygdala-kindled seizures in the rat. *Epilepsia*, **21**, 681–689.

Ashton, D. and Wauquier, A. (1979). Behavioral analysis of the effects of 15 anticonvulsants in the amygdaloid kindled rat. *Psychopharmacology*, **65**, 7–13.

Babington, R. G. and Wedeking, P. W. (1973). The pharmacology of seizures induced by sensitization with low intensity brain stimulation. *Pharmacol. Biochem. Behav.*, **1**, 461–467.

Baltzer, V., Klebs, K. and Schmutz, M. (1981). Effects of oxcarbazepine, a compound related to carbamazepine, and of GP 47 779, its main metabolite in man, on the evolution of amygdaloid-kindled seizures in the rat. In: *13th Epilepsy International Congress*. Kyoto, 1981, Abstracts, p. 151.

Callaghan, D. A. and Schwark, W. S. (1980). Pharmacological modification of amygdaloid-kindled seizures. *Neuropharmacology*, **19**, 1131–1136.

Ehle, A. L. (1980). Effects of phenytoin on amygdaloid kindled seizures in the rat. *Electroencephalogr. Clin. Neurophysiol.*, **48**, 102–105.

Engel Jr, J., Ackerman, R. F., Caldecott-Hazard, S, and Kuhl, D. E. (1981). Epileptic activation of antagonistic systems may explain paradoxical features of experimental and human epilepsy: a review and hypothesis. In: *Kindling 2* (ed. J. A. Wada), pp. 193–217, Raven Press, New York.

Engel Jr, J., Lubens, P., Kuhl, D. E. and Phelps, M. E. (1985). Local cerebral metabolic rate for glucose during petit mal absences. *Ann. Neurol.*, **17**, 121–128.

Fromm, G. H. and Terrence, C. F. (1985). Trigeminal nucleus as a model for testing antiepileptic drugs. In: *Epilepsy and GABA Receptor Agonists: Basic and Therapeutic Research* (eds G. Bartholini, L. Bossi, K. G. Lloyd and P. L. Morselli), pp. 149–157. Raven Press, New York.

Goddard, G. V. (1967). Development of epileptic seizures through brain stimulation at low intensity. *Nature* (London.), **214**, 1020–1021.

Howe, S. J., Salt, T. E., Tulloch, I. and Walter, D. S. (1981). Effect of anti-grand mal drugs on kindled epilepsy in the rat. *Br. J. Pharmacol.*, **72**, 501–502P.

Ichimaru, Y., Gomita, Y. and Moriyama, M. (1987). Effects of clobazam on amygdaloid and hippocampal kindled seizures in rats. *J. Pharmacobiodyn.*, **10**, 189–194.

Kamei, C., Oka, M., Masuda, Y., Yoshida, K. and Shimizu, M. (1981). Effects of 3-sulfamoylmethyl-1, 2-benzisoxazole (AD–810) and some antiepileptics on the kindled seizures in the neocortex, hippocampus and amygdala in rats. *Arch. Int. Pharmacodyn. Ther.*, **249**, 164–176.

Lennox, W. G. (1947). Tridione in the treatment epilepsy. *J. Am. Med. Assoc.*, **134**, 138–143.

Leviel, V. and Naquet, R. (1977). A study of the action of valproic acid on the kindling effect. *Epilepsia*, **18**, 229–234.

Löscher, W., Jaeckel, R. and Czuczwar, S. J. (1986). Is amygdala kindling in rats a model for drug-resistant partial epilepsy? *Exp. Neurol.*, **93**, 211–226.

Lorentz de Haas, A. M. and Kuilman, M. (1964). Ethosuximide (alpha-ethyl-alpha-methyl-succin-imide) and grand mal. *Epilepsia*, **5**, 90–96.

Micheletti, G., Vergnes, M., Marescaux, C., Reis, J., Depaulis, A., Rumbach, L. and Warter, J. M. (1985). Antiepileptic drug evaluation in a new animal model: spontaneous petit mal epilepsy in the rat. *Drug. Res.*, **35**: 483–485.

Paine, R. S. (1965). Neurology grand rounds: petit mal, myoclonic and akinetic seizures, infantile spasms. *Clin. Proc. Child. Hosp. (Washington)*, **21**, 61–77.

Penry, J. K., Porter, R. J. and Dreifuss, F. E. (1975). Simultaneous recording of absence seizures with video tape and electroencephalography. *Brain*, **98**, 427–440.

Pinel, J. P. J. (1983). Effects of diazepam and diphenylhydantoin on elicited and spontaneous seizures in kindled rats: a double dissociation. *Pharmacol. Biochem. Behav.*, **18**, 61–63.

Pollen, D. A. (1964). Intracellular studies of cortical neurons during thalamic induced wave and spike. *Electroencephalogr. Clin. Neurophysiol.*, **17**, 398–404.

Racine, R. J., Livingston, K. and Joaquin, A. (1975). Effects of procaine hydrochloride, diazepam, and diphenylhydantoin on seizure development in cortical and subcortical structures in rats. *Electroencephalogr. Clin. Neurophysiol.*, **38**, 355–365.

Salt, T., Tulloch, I. and Walter, D. (1980). Anti-epileptic properties of sodium valproate in rat amygdaloid kindling. *Br. J. Pharmacol.*, **68**, 134P.

Schmutz, M. (1986). The significance of kindling. In: *What is Epilepsy?* (eds M. R. Trimble and E. H. Reynolds), pp. 251–264. Churchill Livingstone, Edinburgh.

Schmutz, M. (1987). Relevance of kindling and related processes to human epileptogensis. *Prog. Neuropsychopharmacol. Biol. Psychiat.*, **11**, 505–525.

Schmutz, M. and Klebs, K. (1982). Effects of valproate sodium on amygdaloid kindling and amygdaloid kindled seizures in the rat. In: *Physiology and Pharmacology of Epileptogenic Phenomena* (eds M. R. Klee, H. D. Lux and E. J. Speckmann), p. 391. Raven Press, New York.

Schmutz, M., Klebs, K. and Baltzer, V. (1988). Inhibition or enhancement of kindling evolution by antiepileptics. *J. Neural Transm.*, **72**, 245–257.

Schmutz, M., Klein, M., Klebs, K., Bernasconi, R., Bittiger, H. and Baltzer, V. (1985). Pharmacological and neurochemical aspects of kindling. *J. Neural Transm.*, **63**, 143–156.

Schwark, W. S. and Haluska, M. (1987). Prophylaxis of amygdala kindling-induced epileptogenesis: Comparison of a GABA uptake inhibitor and diazepam. *Epilepsy Res.*, **1**, 63–69.

Snead III, O. C. and Hosey, L. C. (1985). Exacerbation of seizures in children by carbamazepine. *N. Engl. J. Med.*, **313**, 916–921.

Tanaka, A. (1972). Progressive changes of behavioral and electroencephalographic responses to daily amygdaloid stimulation in rabbits. *Fukuoka Med. J.*, **63**, 152–164.

Tanaka, T. and Lange, H. (1975). L'effet d'embrasement (kindling effect) par stimulation amygdalienne chez le chat et le rat. *Rev. Electroencephalogr. Neurophysiol. Clin.*, **5**, 41–44.

Wada, J. A. (1977). Pharmacological prophylaxis in the kindling model for epilepsy. *Arch. Neurol.*, **34**, 389–395.

Wada, J. A. (1980). Kindling, antiepileptic drugs, seizure susceptibility and a warning. In: *Epilepsy Updated: Causes and Treatment* (ed. P. Robb), pp. 51–69. Year Book Medical Publishers, Chicago.

Wada, J. A., Osawa, T., Sato, M., Wake, A., Corcoran, M. E. and Troupin, A. S. (1976a). Acute anticonvulsant effects of diphenylhydantoin, phenobarbital, and carbamazepine: a combined electroclinical and serum level study in amygdaloid kindled cats and baboons. *Epilepsia*, **17**, 77–88.

Wada, J. A., Sato, M., Wake, A., Green, J. R. and Troupin, A. S. (1976b). Prophylactic effects of phenytoin, phenobarbital, and carbamazepine examined in kindling cat preparations. *Arch. Neurol.*, **33**, 426–434.

Wise, R. A. and Chinerman, J. (1974). Effects of diazepam and phenobarbital on electrically-induced amygdaloid seizures and seizure development. *Exp. Neurol.*, **45**, 355–363.

The Clinical Relevance of Kindling
Edited by T. G. Bolwig and M. R. Trimble
© 1989 John Wiley & Sons Ltd

Discussion — Session 1

THE KINDLING PHENOMENON

R. Adamec One thing that has always been intriguing about kindling stems from the initial report that kindling was really not associated with damage. Some people suggested that it might really be a good model for spread or development of epilepsy and also as a model for perhaps idiopathic epilepsy, as idiopathic epilepsy is not dependent upon damage. How do you interpret the astrocyte data? It might suggest that when you kindle an animal you are really producing some very extensive damage.

R. Racine There was a lot of work initially, in kindling, on the anatomy using Nissl-stains, Golgi-stains, electron microscopy and so on, and there were no reports of cell damage from those studies. Although some of that work was done by our laboratory, I am still not convinced that there is no cell damage, that there are no degenerative effects with kindling. I think more work needs to be done. It is possible, for example, that there might be a subset of cells that show some damage that might not have been detected in earlier experiments. It is also possible there may be some damage to synaptic contact that has been missed in previous experiments.

On the other hand, although the astrocyte activation definitely accompanies cell damage, it does not mean that there is necessarily cell damage. One of the functions of the astrocyte is presumably to remove excess potassium from the astrocytal fluid. So it is quite possible that astrocyte hypertrophy might occur simply as a result of repeated exposure to excess potasssium.

J. Majkowski Is there any correlation between the localization of the gliosis and the spread of the discharges?

R. Racine We have just begun work on the astrocytes, so I cannot be certain of the ultimate pattern we will find.

Question Could you comment on the time course of the appearance of the reactive astrocytosis in relation to the development of kindling.

R. Racine We have looked so far at 24 h and one week. We have animals that are now being prepared with delays of one month and two months. The astrocyte activation begins to appear very rapidly, it increases rapidly, and it continues to develop over a long period of time. You can see increases in astrocyte hypertrophy, certainly up to one month, and perhaps even longer than that.

Question Is your piriform cortex the area that Karen Gale has looked at and calls the area tempesta. Will animals kindle just as fast if you remove that area?

R. Racine The whole piriform region seems to be equivalent in terms of reactivity — with one possible exception which may relate to this so-called area tempesta, and that is the endopiriform nucleus. The area tempesta is a deep piriform region that is not, as far as I can recall, associated with any obvious structure, but it is at least close to the endopiriform nucleus.

I. Rosén Is the increase of the mass electrical discharge in the tissue you have shown by activating pathways to an area due to an increased synaptic current, or is it due to activation or spread of the activity to more cellular elements in the area?

R. Racine The increase of *duration* of the discharge is due in part to activation of other sites. An interesting thing is that kindling-induced potentiation looks very similar to the phenomenon of long-term potentiation (LTP), but there are some definite differences. One of the most striking is that kindling-induced potentiation is very long lasting — it lasts for months — whereas LTP tends to decay over a period measured in weeks.

Question Is LTP related to post-synaptic change?

R. Racine By potentiation I mean a change in the strength of efficacy at the synapse, the change in the conductivity between cells. It has been shown by several people to be a synaptic mechanism. Kindling-induced potentiation, I believe, is also a synaptic mechanism, although the proof is not so compelling.

Question Is LTP necessary for kindling to occur?

R. Racine We and several other laboratories have monitored evoked responses and a number of different pathways during kindling, and it is often the case that animals kindle with no potentiation. In fact, in some cases, the amplitude of the response actually is lower than it was before kindling began. There may be an initial increase of the amplitude of the response, followed by a decline, and the response may end up *below* baseline — so potentiation does not always accompany kindling.

R. Adamec Can you be certain that when you kindle an animal there is no potentiation elsewhere in the brain?

R. Racine There is a possibility, because we cannot cover all the parts of the brain; but we have placed multiple electrodes in the brain to monitor the amplitude of responses before and after kindling, and generally, if you see potentiation, you see potentiation at all the target sites. If you don't see potentiation, you don't see it at any of the target sites. It is either there, or it's not there.

R. Adamec Have you looked at astrocyte staining, when you partially kindle the animals?

R. Racine No.

J. Majkowski We know that in the most severe cases of head trauma, post-traumatic epilepsy develops in 50%. Would it be possible to suggest that the development of epilepsy is related to a competition between the epileptic force which is spreading or discharging, and the development of a wall of glioses, which helps prevent it?

C. G. Wasterlain Racine and several others have shown that there is a build-up of inhibition at the same time as excitation in the kindled brain. The relationship to glioses, I do not know.

R. Adamec With respect to post-traumatic epilepsy: I know that Graham Goddard wrote a review on this, suggesting that the fact that there is a delay in the onset of seizures might suggest that a kindling process is involved.

C. G. Wasterlain I would not want to make too much of the analogy between post-traumatic epilepsy and kindling. We really have no evidence that the two are in any way related. It is tempting to build an analogy because of the delay in many cases of post-traumatic epilepsy, but that is just a superficial resemblance. *If* it is true that it is a kindling-like phenomenon, it should be possible to block it with anticonvulsants. In Czechoslovakia a very large, uncontrolled study was carried out in which they gave phenobarbitol and diphenylhydantoin, both in small amounts, to patients after surgery. They had a very significant reduction of the incidence of post-traumatic epilepsy. That study was uncontrolled; but it would support the notion that it is possible to prevent post-traumatic epilepsy with anticonvulsants. The other major piece of evidence is the experience from the Vietnam and Korean wars. In war injuries, the incidence of epilepsy after penetrating head injuries is over 50%. In Korea, the head-injured American soldiers were *not* treated with anticonvulsants. In Vietnam, they were routinely given them. There was no check on whether or not they took it, but in a large population, such as was surveyed, some of them must have taken it, and there should be a statistically significant difference, if an effect existed. The fact is that the incidence of post-traumatic epilepsy in the two groups was precisely the same.

There are, however, three ways to interpret that data. One is that there was no effect: or the wrong anticonvulsant was used. Of all anticonvulsants, there is one which is very poor at preventing kindling, and that is phenytoin, which was used! The third possibility is that the head injuries were not the same. In Korea, the vast majority of the head injuries were bullet wounds. In Vietnam, surprisingly for this was a guerilla conflict, most of them were shrapnel from shells. Only 7% of head injuries to American soldiers in Vietnam were bullet wounds. 93% were shrapnel wounds. The wounds due to shrapnel were more severe and they should lead to a higher incidence of post-traumatic epilepsy, which was prevented by the phenytoin. There have been several attempts to run controlled studies, which failed for lack of patients.

KINDLING AND ANTICONVULSANTS

G. Wasterlain Dr Schmutz, surely seizures are excitatory and anticonvulsants are inhibitory?

M. Schmutz I talked about petit-mal seizures and spike-wave complexes as inhibitory events. There are indications that during spike-wave complexes inhibition takes place. You have inhibitory post-synaptic potentials on cortical neurons during the wave of the spike-wave complex. You also have some arrest of mental activity in petit-mal seizures. Finally, energy expenditure, which is greatest in petit-mal, is greater during synaptic inhibition than during synaptic excitation. I think it is worthwhile to consider petit-mal seizures as events which share inhibitory mechanisms.

C. Wasterlain That is an interesting answer. I cannot agree with the fact that inhibition produces higher metabolic rates than excitation. Ackermann and Engel showed that while the inhibitory state in the hippocampus seemed to consume more energy than the unstimulated state, it was not nearly as much as seizure excitation.

Question　I was interested by your new classification of seizures based on the use of the antiepileptic drugs. You told us that phenobarbital was a drug which is effective against absences. That is not the case, in the patients at least. On the contrary, it can *provoke* absences. But here it was classified together with valproate and ethosuximide, being able to hinder the development of kindling. How much similarity is there between these models and patients?

M. Schmutz　In fact, Engel *et al.* (1985) found that the local cerebral metabolic rate for glucose was higher in patients during absence seizures than in patients during partial or generalized tonic–clonic seizures. It may, however, be the case that this difference reflects the fact that absence seizures are not associated with a postictal depression. Concerning the word 'petit mal' I use this and not absences because I wanted to include myoclonic seizure in this group, and phenobarbital is active at least to some degree, against myoclonic seizures.

5

Kindling and neurotransmitter systems: seizure suppression by intracerebral grafting of fetal neurons

DAVID I. BARRY, JØRN KRAGH and BENEDIKTE WANSCHER
Neurobiology Research Group, Department of Psychiatry, Rigshospitalet, University of Copenhagen, DK-2100 Copenhagen, Denmark

INTRODUCTION

Elucidation of the underlying defect in epilepsy necessitates a better understanding of the neurotransmitter systems, both inhibitory and excitatory, that influence the firing of neurones in normal and epileptic brain tissue. Evidence is accumulating that the basic defect in the epileptic focus might involve the loss of inhibitory synapses (Ribak, Bradburne and Harris, 1982) and/or the loss of basket cell activating systems that activate inhibitory neurones (Sloviter, 1987). It is thus clear that pharmacological and surgical approaches to the treatment of epilepsy can at best be palliative, but never curative. As a supplement to these two approaches, a possible third approach could be to replace the lost inhibitory synapses, or their activating systems, either by promoting spontaneous regeneration or by effective reinnervation through the intracerebral grafting of the missing or damaged neurones (Ward, 1985).

The present article examines the use of intracerebral grafting of fetal neural tissue as a means of seizure suppression in the kindling model of epilepsy. As kindling is discussed in detail elsewhere in this volume, suffice it to say that kindling is the process whereby repeated administration of an initially subconvulsive electrical stimulus results in progressive intensification of stimulus-induced electrical activity, culminating in generalized seizures (Goddard, McIntyre and Leech, 1969; Racine, 1972). The mechanisms responsible for the kindling, which have a permanent effect on brain tissue (Wada and Sato, 1974) have not been clarified, although valid hypotheses exist (Racine, 1978; McIntyre and Racine, 1986; Cain, 1989). The role of neurotransmitter systems in kindling has been extensively studied. The influence of the catecholaminergic system will be outlined here as the background to studies of transplantation of fetal noradrenergic neurones. The serotoninergic system will be briefly mentioned in relation to a study involving transplantation of serontoninergic neurones. The gamma-aminobutyric acid (GABA) system, although perhaps of the greatest importance in kindling, is not discussed because no studies on transplantation of GABA-ergic neurones appear to have been published.

KINDLING AND CATECHOLAMINES

Some of the earliest studies of the kindling phenomenon concerned the role of central catecholamines. Kindling rate was found to increase markedly after intracerebroventricular administration of 6-hydroxydopamine (6-OHDA) (Arnold, Racine and Wise, 1973; Corcoran et al., 1974). 6-Hydroxy-dopamine is taken up into cells by the transport mechanisms for catecholamines and is oxidized to a cytotoxic indol (Breese, 1975; Cohen, 1986), with resultant degeneration of catecholmainergic nerve terminals and central depletion of dopamine and noradrenaline. 6-Hydroxydopamine does not influence the GABA or serotonin content (Björklund, Segal and Stenevi, 1979; Björklund, Nornes and Gage, 1986; Uretsky and Iversen, 1970). The effect of 6-OHDA is seen with both hippocampal (McIntyre and Edson, 1982) and amygdala kindling (McIntyre, Saari and Pappas, 1979; McIntyre, 1980; McIntyre and Racine, 1986; Corcoran and Mason, 1980). A similar effect on kindling rate was also seen after central depletion of dopamine and noradrenaline by reserpine pretreatment (Arnold, Racine and Wise, 1973) or by the catecholamine synthesis inhibitor alpha-methyl-para-tyrosine (Callaghan and Schwark, 1979).

The effects of catecholamine depletion on kindling rate result from destruction of noradrenergic neurons, there being ample evidence that dopaminergic systems are not involved. For example, pretreatment with desmethylimipramine, which selectively protects noradrenergic neurones from the effects of 6-OHDA, prevents the expected facilitation of the kindling rate even though dopaminergic neurones are destroyed (McIntyre, Saari and Pappas, 1979; McIntyre and Edson, 1981). Selective noradrenergic depletion with N-[2-chloroethyl]-N-ethyl-2-bromidbenzylamine has the same effect on the kindling rate (Bortolotto and Cavalheiro, 1986) as 6-OHDA. Local injection of 6-OHDA into the amygdala, which reduces the level of noradrenaline, but not dopamine, facilitates amygdala kindling to the same extent as forebrain catecholamine depletion with intracerebroventricular 6-OHDA. Selective lesions of the ascending noradrenergic pathways from the locus coeruleus by intracerebral injection of 6-OHDA facilitate kindling whereas selective depletion of forebrain dopamine or lesions of the serotoninergic pathways do not (Corcoran and Mason, 1980; Araki et al., 1983).

The 6-OHDA-induced facilitation of kindling seems primarily to result from damage to ascending noradrenergic innervation originating in the locus coeruleus. This system dampens epileptic activity in the central nervous system in a wide range of experimental seizure models. Electrical stimulation of the locus coeruleus suppresses epileptiform EEG activity caused by penicillin (Neuman, 1986), cobalt, and pentylenetetrazol (Libet et al., 1977). In contrast to the effects of stimulation, selective 6-OHDA-induced lesions of the forebrain projections from the locus coeruleus potentiate electroshock-induced and pentylenetetrazol-induced seizures (Mason and Corcoran, 1979), cobalt-induced seizures (Trottier et al., 1987) and facilitate electrical kindling (Corcoran and Mason, 1980).

Although the locus coeruleus system suppresses the development of kindling, it does not influence the severity of duration of established kindled seizures (Westerberg, Lewis and Corcoran, 1984). Furthermore, although kindling is associated with reduced noradrenergic inhibition of the limbic system (McIntyre and Racine, 1986), this does not result from inhibition of noradrenergic activity in the locus coeruleus as the latter is normal during kindling (Bonhaus and McNamara, 1987).

The exact role that the locus coeruleus noradrenergic innervation of the forebrain plays in kindling remains to be elucidated. However, as described below, the facilitation of kindling after 6-OHDA-induced noradrenergic depletion has proven a useful model with which to attempt to answer the question — could intracerebral grafting of inhibitory neurones be used as a new tool to modify the excitability of a brain region sufficiently to dampen the development or spread of seizure activity?

KINDLING AND INTRACEREBRAL GRAFTING OF FETAL NEURONES

The idea of using intracerebral grafting of fetal neural tissue as a means of seizure suppression is relatively new (Ward, 1985). The few studies that have so far been published will be summarized. The first to demonstrate that grafts of fetal neural tisue could suppress the development of kindling (Barry et al., 1987a, b) will be discussed in detail.

Olfactory bulb kindling and grafting of serotoninergic neurones

The inhibitory effect of serotonin on epileptic activity has been demonstrated in a variety of epilepsy models, including kindling. Destruction of the serotoninergic innervation of the olfactory bulb by intracerebral injection of 5,7-dihydroxytryptamine enhances kindling rate and increases the duration of stimulus-induced electrical activity (after-discharge) (Lerner-Natoli, 1987). Two studies have examined transplantation of serotoninergic neurones to olfactory bulb, one in intact rats and one in lesioned rats. Although the data are not published, these studies are included here because of their interest.

A study of the effect on olfactory bulb kindling of transplatation of raphe cells has been mentioned in a meeting report (Lerner-Natoli, 1987). The cells were taken from 14-day-old rat fetuses and grafted into the olfactory bulb of intact adult rats. Kindling was started 3 weeks later, and took 1 week. There was no difference in kindling rate or after-discharge duration between transplanted and control rats. However, stimulation threshold was higher in the transplanted rats (although this does not necessarily reflect a physiological inhibitory effect as was suggested — it could as well be a reflection of damage etc.). The short time between grafting and kindling might account for the lack of effect, although it was claimed that, 5 weeks after grafting, 'the morphology of serotonin neurons in the olfactory bulb was like that of adult neurons in the raphe, with branched dendrites and axons ending far from the injection site. . .'.

The same model was used in the second study, so far only published in abstract form (Camu and Privat, 1988). Camu and Privat reported that grafted serotoninergic neurones were able to restore normal excitability to olfactory neurones previously deprived of their intrinsic serotoninergic supply. They transplanted either raphe cells or neopallial cells from 14-day-old fetuses into the olfactory bulb of 5,7-dihydroxytryptamine-lesioned rats. After a 2 week recovery period, control, lesioned and grafted rats were kindled in the olfactory bulb. As expected, lesioned rats kindled more quickly than control rats. Rats with grafts of cortical cells were reported to kindle as quickly as lesioned rats, whereas rats with grafts of raphe cells exhibited a kindling course and duration of after-discharge similar to control rats. Despite the short time between transplantation and kindling, extensive reinnervation of the olfactory bulb, especially the glomerular area, was reported. Although no data were given in the abstract (Camu and Privat, 1988), this study lends support to the concept of using the grafting of fetal neurones as a means of seizure suppression.

Amygdala kindling and grafting of neocortical tissue

As was mentioned in the introduction, eventual transplantation therapy for epilepsy needs to take into consideration not just grafting of new neurones, but also reinnervation, through the promotion of spontaneous regeneration. This is because the effects of neural transplantation may result not only from the correction of anatomical connections or the production of missing hormones and neurotransmitters, but also from the effects of trophic factors produced by both graft and host tissue (Björklund and Stenevi, 1984). These aspects were considered in an interesting, albeit negative, study of amygdala kindling and transplantation of neocortical tissue to hippocampus (Holmes *et al.*, 1987). Neocortical tissue was chosen for the grafts because it is rich in nerve growth factor; hippocampus was chosen as the implantation site because it has a high content of neurotrophic factor and because of the numerous connections between hippocampus and amygdala. No attempt was made to interfere with any of the inhibitory neurotransmitter systems; transplantation was undertaken to intact brain. Two aspects of kindling were examined — initial kindling rate and transfer kindling. The latter refers to the phenomenon whereby, following kindling of a particular structure in one hemisphere, the contralateral same structure, or even another structure (ipsi- or contralateral), will kindle more rapidly than normal i.e. following kindling of the left amygdala, the right amygdala will kindle more rapidly. The transplantation was undertaken in very young (19-day-old) rats, a group of which had been subjected to so-called rapid kindling of the right amygdala. At 12 weeks the rats were kindled in the left amygdala. The study thus examined the influence of transplants of neocortical tissue on both transfer kindling of the amygdala, and on initial kindling of the amygdala. The transplanted rats did not kindle differently from sham kindled controls. However, because of the many unconventional aspects of the methodology (i.e. the kindling methods used, the young age of graft recipients, lack of suitable recovery period after electrode implantation, large areas of necrosis, long time interval between initial and transfer kindling etc.) and the fact that no transfer kindling was demonstrated in the sham group, little can be concluded from the study about grafting and kindling. Despite this the study remains interesting for the ideas behind it, and as one of the first published studies of transplantation and kindling.

Hippocampal kindling and grafting of noradrenergic neurons

The question behind the present article is whether intracerebral grafting of neurones could be used as a new tool to modify the excitability of a brain region sufficiently to dampen the development or spread of seizure activity. Although the clinical perspectives are in the epilepsy, the field is very new and so far only animal studies have been undertaken. The study which established the principle that grafting of fetal neurones could be used to modulate the excitability of epileptic brain regions (Barry *et al.*, 1987a, b), was instigated by the Swedish neurosurgeon Olle Lindvall, who has since undertaken some of the first transplants of human fetal tissue to Parkinson's disease patients (Lindvall *et al.*, 1988). The study used as a test model the well-described facilitation of kindling following 6-OHDA-induced dener- vation of the rat forebrain noradrenergic innervation from the locus coeruleus (*vide supra*). Since it had been established that grafts of fetal noradrenergic neurones are able to re-establish fairly normal terminal innervation patterns in the hippocampus and reinstate noradrenaline turnover and metabolism (Björklund, Nornes and Gage, 1986), it was postulated that restoration of noradrenergic innervation to previously noradrenaline-depleted hippocampus would prevent the expected facilitation of kindling. In other words, whereas kindling is much quicker in noradrenaline-depleted rats than in normal rats, kindling would be slower in grafted rats, perhaps even as slow as control rats (Barry et al., 1987b).

To test the hypothesis, hippocampal kindling was chosen because it takes much longer than amygdala kindling (25–30 days as compared with 10–15 days) and the difference in kindling rate between control rats, and 6-OHDA-lesioned rats, is greater. Thus there was a greater chance of detecting any effect of the grafts. Hippocampal kindling was undertaken in three groups of aged matched adult rats; a control group, a 6-OHDA-lesioned group, and a 6-OHDA-lesioned group that received grafts of fetal pontine locus coeruleus bilaterally into the hippocampus. Sufficient time was allowed for the grafts to effectively reinnervate the hippocampus (6–11 months) before kindling electrodes were implanted. Kindling was undertaken using the standard method of daily stimulation until a generalized motor seizure had occurred. This took only 8 days in 6-OHDA-lesioned rats, compared with 31 days in controls. The transplanted lesioned rats, in which the hippocampus had been reinnervated by fetal noradrenergic neurones, kindled almost as slowly as controls, taking 22 days. The restorative effect of the reinnervation is even more clearly demonstrated by correlating the kindling rate in the transplanted rats with the degree of graft-derived reinnervation of the stimulated hippocampus — there was a significant linear relationship between the two. Thus rats with poor reinnervation kindled more quickly than the group mean and rats with good reinnervation kindled more slowly than the group mean. It should be remembered that the 6-OHDA lesion used here depletes the whole forebrain of noradrenergic innervation, yet only the hippocampus was reinnervated by the fetal noradrenergic neurones. Thus there was clear evidence that graft derived reinstatement of noradrenergic transmission in the area surrounding the kindling electrode is sufficient to suppress kindling in norepinephrine-depleted rats (Barry et al., 1987b).

The amygdala–pyriform cortex area is considered to be of central importance in kindling and hippocampal kindling is thought to involve the amygdala (McIntyre and Racine, 1986). Specific noradrenergic denervation of the amygdala (by local 6-OHDA injection) also facilitates kindling (McIntyre, Saari and Pappas, 1979). In our study, the whole of the rest of the forebrain, including the amygdala, was devoid of noradrenergic innervation: only the hippocampus was reinnervated. We thus wondered why, if the amygdala was so important in hippocampal kindling, was reinnervation around the hippocampal electrode sufficient to suppress kindling. Was the reinnervation effectively preventing involvement of the amygdala in the facilitation of kindling in the lesioned brain? Would reinnervation of just the amygdala/pyriform cortex in rats depleted of forebrain noradrenergic innervation have any effect on kindling by hippocampal stimulation, given that the hippocampus remained denervated? These two questions have been answered affirmatively by a recent study in which the facilitation of hippocampal kindling seen in 6-OHDA-lesioned rats was almost completely suppressed by simple reinnervation of the amygdala/pyriform cortex, without any reinnervation around the stimulating electrode (Wanscher *et al.*, 1989). This finding suggests that grafting of inhibitory neurones to a site distant from the stimulation focus, but important for the generalization and spread of seizure, can modulate the effects of epileptic activity in the focus. It also confirms that the amygdala/pyriform area is of central importance in kindling-epilepsy.

The above-mentioned studies relate to a single model, i.e. the facilitation of kindling by noradrenergic denervation, and aimed only to establish the principle that grafted neurones can modulate the excitability of epileptic brain regions. For these initial studies it was useful to have a clear lesion/repair model with which to work. It is not proposed that transplantation of noradrenergic neurones would be useful in epilepsy. Other inhibitory neurones, especially GABA-ergic, are much more likely candidates. However, studies of the effects of transplantation of GABA-ergic neurones on kindling have not yet been published, and much useful basic work remains to be done with noradrenergic neurones. Normal noradrenergic innervation appears to have little or no effect on established kindling. Despite that, it would clearly be of interest to investigate kindling following graft-derived hyperinnervation of relevant structures. One problem with the kindling model of epilepsy is that it is only possible to kindle once (transfer kindling excepted) and so it is not possible to compare kindling before and after grafting in individual animals. Another is that the testing of graft effects on seizures in kindled animals is difficult because of the technical problems associated with grafting to animals with implanted electrodes. Thus many important questions concerning the ability of grafted neurones to modulate the excitability of epileptic brain regions must be answered using other models. One such study has recently shown that intrahippocampal grafts of fetal noradrenergic neurones protect subcortically denervated seizure-prone rats from picrotoxin-induced seizures and reduce the frequency of interictal spiking (Buzsàki *et al.*, 1988).

FUTURE POSSIBILITIES

The use of transplantation therapy in epilepsy is clearly a scenario for the future. Basic science has only recently approached the concept and much background work remains to be done before clinical experimental studies can begin. However, it is quite clear that this concept will become reality, and given the explosive growth in the field of central nervous tissue transplantation, the first clinical studies could be expected in a decade. Clearly, not even the type of neurone to be transplanted has yet been identified. In spite of whatever results are achieved in animal models, until the first clinical studies have been undertaken, it will be impossible to predict whether transplantation therapy will be effective in epilepsy, and indeed, what types of epilepsy will be amenable to transplantation therapy. That the concept of transplanting human fetal dopaminergic neurones in Parkinson's disease patients progressed from animal to clinical studies in 10 years (Lindvall et al., 1988) lends support to the notion that transplantation will be attempted in epilepsy within the next decade. The fact that the defect in Parkinson's disease was clearly defined, whereas that in epilepsy is as yet undefined, does not undermine the validity of the prediction given the rapid pace of research in this area and that some neurosurgeons are already thinking along these lines (Ward, 1985).

The ethical aspects of transplanting human fetal nervous tissue to man are presently being debated in relation to transplantation in Parkinson's disease patients. In epilepsy, especially, ethical consideration must be given not only to the use of human fetal tissue, but to the possible side-effects on the recipients personality, etc. By the time that clinical trials of transplantation in epilepsy will be attempted, many of these ethical problems will have been overcome. Donor tissue of direct fetal origin will be replaced by cultured lines of a single neurone type which will have been genetically modified so that the cells produce only the required substance (i.e. neurotransmitter, growth factor etc.), with the production of unwanted substances having been switched off. This will overcome the ethical problems associated with the use of aborted fetal tissue, and, because the donor material will be of a very specific cell type, minimize the problems associated with transplantation of very heterogeneous fetal nervous tissue.

Establishment of neural cell lines for transplantation requires, firstly, that the cells be immortalized and secondly, that immortalization can be reversed prior to transplantation (in order to prevent tumour formation). Neural cell lines have now been established following immortalization by oncogene transduction (Cepko, 1988) and the first study of grafting of neural cells that have been genetically modified by gene transfer has been undertaken (Gage et al., 1987). Although not yet applied to neural cell lines, immortalization oncogenes are available that are either photo- or temperature-sensitive, and can thus be switched off (as would be necessary prior to transplantation). As a further safeguard against tumour formation, so-called suicide-oncogenes could be inserted which would destroy any cell which started to divide, for instance if the immortalization oncogene failed to switch off. The application of molecular genetics to clinical neuroscience is a rapidly expanding field, with the molecular mechanisms underlying phenotypic expression of a number of neurological diseases having been identified (Martin, 1987). Grafting of genetically modified cells might thus become a therapeutic approach not just in epilepsy, but in a wide range of conditions.

CONCLUSION

Intracerebral grafting of fetal neurones as a means of seizure suppression is a relatively new concept and as yet only few experimental studies have been undertaken. However, it has already been clearly demonstrated that transplanted neurones are able to establish functional synaptic neurotransmission with host brain cells and that, at least for noradrenergic innervation, functional reinnervation can be achieved which can modulate the excitability of an epileptic brain region (Barry et al., 1987b; Buzsàki et al., 1988). Apart from the promise of a new therapeutic approach to the treatment of epilepsy, studies of kindling and intracerebral grafting of fetal neurones may prove a useful tool with which investigate the 'missing pieces in the epilepsy puzzle' (Ward, 1985).

REFERENCES

Araki, H., Aihara, H., Watanabe, S., Yamamoto, T. and Ueki, S. (1983). Effects of reserpine, alpha-methyl-p-tyrosine, p-chlorophenylalanine and 5,7-dihydroxytryptamine on the hippocampal kindling effect in rats. Jpn J. Pharmacol., 33, 1177–1182.

Arnold, P. S., Racine, R. J. and Wise, R. A. (1973). Effects of atropine, reserpine, 6-hydroxydopamine, and handling on seizure development in the rat. Exp. Neurol., 40, 457–470.

Barry, D. I., Kikvadze, I., Lindvall, O., Björklund, A., Brundin, P., Kragh, J. and Bolwig, T. G. (1987a). Functional reinnervation of denervated rat hippocampus by grafts of foetal locus coeruleus. Eur. J. Clin. Invest., 17, 2(II), A3.

Barry, D. I., Kikvadze, I., Brundin, P., Bolwig, T. G., Björklund, A. and Lindvall, O. (1987b). Grafted noradrenergic neurons suppress seizure development in kindling-induced epilepsy. Proc. Natl Acad. Sci. USA, 84, 8712–8715.

Björklund, A. and Stenevi, U. (1984). Intracerebral neural implants: neuronal replacement and reconstruction of damaged circuitries. Annu. Rev. Neurosci., 7, 279–308.

Björklund, A., Nornes, H. and Gage, F. H. (1986). Cell suspension grafts of noradrenergic locus coeruleus neurons in rat hippocampus and spinal cord: reinnervation and transmitter turnover. Neuroscience, 18, 685–698.

Björklund, A., Segal, M. and Stenevi, U. (1979). Functional reinnervation of rat hippocampus by locus coeruleus implants. Brain Res., 170, 409–426.

Bonhaus, D. W. and McNamara, J. O. (1987). Activity of locus coeruleus neurons in amygdala kindled rats: role in the suppression of afterdischarge. Brain Res., 407, 102–109.

Bortolotto, Z. A. and Cavalheiro, E. A. (1986). Effect of DSP4 on hippocampal kindling in rats. Pharmacol. Biochem. Behav., 24, 777–779.

Breese, G. R. (1975). Chemical and immunochemical lesions by specific neurotoxic substances and antisera. In: *Handbook of Psychopharmacology*, Vol. 1, *Basic Neuropharmacology* (eds L. L. Iversen, S. D. Iversen and S. H. Snyder), pp. 137–139. Plenum Press, New York.

Buszàki, G., Ponomareff, G., Bayardo, F., Shaw, T. and Gage, F. H. (1988). Suppression and induction of epileptic activity by neuronal grafts. *Proc. Natl. Acad. Sci.*, **85**, 9327–9330.

Cain, D. P. (1989). Long-term potentiation and kindling: how similar are the mechanisms? *TINS*, **12**, 6–10.

Callaghan, D. A. and Schwark, W. S. (1979). Involvement of catecholamines in kindled amygdaloid convulsions in the rat. *Neuropharmacology*, **18**, 541–545.

Camu, W. and Privat, A. (1988). Transplantation of serotoninergic neurons into the 5-7 DHT lesioned rat olfactory bulb restore the parameters of kindling. *Eur. J. Neurosci., Suppl.*, 307.

Cepko, C. (1988). Immortalization of neural cells via oncogene transduction. *TINS*, **11**, 6–8.

Cohen, G. (1986). Monoamine oxidase, hydrogen peroxide and Parkinson's disease. *Adv. Neurol.*, **45**, 119–215.

Corcoran, M. E. and Mason, S. T. (1980). Role of forebrain catecholamines in amygdaloid kindling. *Brain Res.*, **190**, 473–484.

Corcoran, M. E., Fibiger, H. C., McCaughran, J. A. J. and Wada, J. A. (1974). Potentiation of amygdaloid kindling and metrazol-induced seizures by 6-hydroxydopamine in rats. *Exp. Neurol.*, **45**, 118–133.

Gage, F. H., Wolff, J. A., Rosenberg, M. B., Xu, L., Yee, J. K., Shults, C. and Friedman, T. (1987). Grafting genetically modified cells to the brain: possibilities for the future. Neuroscience, **23**, 795–807.

Goddard, G. V., McIntyre, D. C. and Leech, C. K. (1969). A permanent change in brain function resulting from daily electrical stimulation. *Exp. Neurol.*, **25**, 295–330.

Holmes, G. L., Thompson, J. L., Smeyne, R. J. and Wallace, R. B. (1987). Failure of neocortical transplants to alter seizure susceptibility in previously kindled rats. *Epilepsia*, **28**, 242–250.

Lerner-Natoli, M. (1987). Serotonin and kindling development. *Int. J. Neurosci.*, **36**, 139–151.

Libet, B., Gleason, C. A., Wright, E. W. and Feinstein, B. (1979). Suppression of epileptiform type of electrocortical activity in the rat by stimulation in the vicinity of locus coeruleus. *Epilepsia*, **18**, 451–462.

Lindvall, O. *et al.* (1988). Fetal dopamine-rich mesencephalic grafts in Parkinson's disease. *Lancet*, **ii**, 1483–1484.

Martin, J. B. (1987). Molecular genetics: application to the clinical neuroscience. *Science*, **238**, 765–772.

Mason, S. T. and Corcoran, M. E. (1979). Catecholamines and convulsions. *Brain Res.*, **170**, 497–507.

McIntyre, D. C. (1980). Amygdala kindling in rats: facilitation after local amygdala norepinephrine depletion with 6-hydroxydopamine. *Exp. Neurol.*, **69**, 395–407.

McIntyre, D. C. and Edson, N. (1982). Effect of norepinephrine depletion on dorsal hippocampus kindling in rats. *Exp. Neurol.*, **77**, 700–704.

McIntyre, D. C. and Racine, R. J. (1986). Kindling mechanisms: current progress on an experimental epilepsy model. *Prog. Neurobiol.*, **27**, 1–12.

McIntyre, D. C., Saari, M. and Pappas, B. A. (1979). Potentiation of amygdala kindling in adult or infant rats by injections of 6-hydroxydopamine. *Exp. Neurol.*, **63**, 527–544.

Neuman, R. S. (1986). Suppression of penicillin-induced focal epileptiform activity by locus coeruleus stimulations: Mediation by an alpha-adrenoreceptor. *Epilepsia*, **27**, 359–366.

Racine, R. J. (1972). Modification of seizure activity by electrical stimulation: II. motor seizure. *Electroencephalogr. Clin. Neurophysiol.*, **32**, 281–294.

Racine, R. J. (1978). Kindling: the first decade. *Neurosurgery*, **3**, 234–252.

Ribak, C. E., Bradburne, R. M. and Harris, A. B. (1982). A preferential loss of gabaergic symmetric synapses in epileptic foci: a quantitative ultrastructural analysis of monkey neocortex. *J. Neurosci.*, **2**, 1725–1735.

Sloviter, R. S. (1987). Decreased hippocampal inhibition and a selective loss of interneurons in experimental epilepsy. *Science*, **235**, 73–76.

Trottier, S., Lindvall, O., Chauvel, P. and Björklund, A. (1987). Facilitation of focal cobalt-induced epilepsy after lesions of the noradrenergic locus coeruleus system. *Brain Res.*, **454**, 308–314.

Uretsky, N. J. and Iversen, L. L. (1970). Effects of 6-hydroxydopamine oncatecholamine containing neurones in the rat brain. *J. Neurochem.*, **17**, 269–278.

Wada, J. A. and Sato, M. (1974). Generalized convulsive seizure induced by daily electrical stimulation of the amygdala in cats: correlative electrographic and behavioral features. *Neurology*, **24**, 565–574.

Wanscher, B., Barry, D. I., Kragh, J., Bolwig, T. G., Kokaia, K., Brundin, P., Björklund, A. and Lindvall, O. (1989). Reinnervation of the amygdala-pyriform cortex by fetal locus coeruleus neurones suppresses hippocampal kindling-epilepsy in catecholamine depleted rats. *Eur. J. Clin. Invest.*, **19**, 2(II), 50.

Ward, A. A. J. (1985). Missing pieces in the epilepsy puzzle. *Appl. Neurophysiol.*, **48**, 384–394.

Westerberg, V., Lewis, J. and Corcoran, M. E. (1984). Depletion of noradrenaline fails to affect kindled seizures. *Exp. Neurol.*, **84**, 237–240.

The Clinical Relevance of Kindling
Edited by T. G. Bolwig and M. R. Trimble
© 1989 John Wiley & Sons Ltd

6

Kindling and memory

JERZY MAJKOWSKI
*Laboratory of Experimental Neurology, Department of Neurology and
Epileptology, Medical Center for Postgraduate Education, Czerniakowska
231, 00-416 Warszawa, Poland*

INTRODUCTION

In current epileptology the relation between learning and memory on one
side and epilepsy on the other has become an important clinical research
problem. We realize today that the relation presents a complex interaction
of a number of factors, which has been shown during last decade (1979–1985)
in four Gothenburg workshops on Memory Functions and Epilepsy. The
associations between epilepsy and memory deal with two most complex
groups of variables. Epilepsies in humans or in animal models are extremely
heterogenous in their pathomechanisms and in the diversity of their
behavioral manifestations. The same can be said about memory. Clinical
neurological studies have shown independent and selective impairment of
different memory systems in brain-damaged patients. Each system has its
own functional and structural properties and localization. The idea of multiple memory systems has been supported by clinical and electrophysiological
findings (Rolls *et al.*, 1981; Warrington, 1981; Weiskrantz, 1981).

The complex relation between memory and epilepsy received promising
new insights from the phenomenon of kindling, giving it research and concepts. Whether this or any experimental model truly simulates human related
problems in physiology and pathology, remains an open question. However,
the validity of a model grows with the number of verifiable features the
model shares with human disorders. The main problem, however, is the
appropriate choice of a model for the clinical question we ask. Kindling is a
rather well defined phenomenon. However, it is surprisingly difficult to define
memory, despite the fact that everybody is familiar with it. For the purpose

of this discussion the term memory will be used as the relatively long-lasting neuronal alterations, often called neuronal plasticity, induced by interaction between the brain and environmental stimulation. These alterations can be indirectly measured by a change in the behavior of the subject or a change in some physiological responses. Learning processes underly memory traces and from an electrophysiological point of view it is difficult to establish the borderline between these processes; they overlap.

THE RELATION BETWEEN KINDLING AND MEMORY

It is a rather general agreement that kindling produces simultaneously two types of phenomena: (1) local, of an epileptogenic nature, and (2) widespread neuronal plastic changes. The spatial distribution of the network of brain structures containing the alterations responsible for these two kindling phenomena are not known.

Major hypotheses based on neurophysiological and autoradiographic studies have been proposed to address the issue: one locally oriented hypothesis suggests that the neural reorganization responsible for kindling involves neurons restricted to the area of the kindling electrode. Another hypothesis claims that alterations in neurons remote from the kindled area contribute to the kindling effect (Post and Kopanda, 1976; Collins, 1978; Messenheimer, Harris and Steward, 1979). However, both hypotheses are questionable (McNamara, 1986). Moreover, it is not clear whether these remote alterations are essential to the primary local changes, and whether they are of an epileptic or a nonepileptic nature. In many aspects they are similar to learning or memory consolidation processes. This brings us to the problem of the relationship between epileptogenesis and epilepsy on one hand, and learning and memory on the other. This relation can be viewed in three ways:

(1) similarities between epileptogenesis and memory consolidation;
(2) interference between epileptogenesis and memory consolidation;
(3) relationship between epileptic discharges or seizures and memory retrieval.

Similarities between kindled epileptogenesis and memory consolidation

Most publications deal with kindling as a model for epilepsy. However, for a long time some authors emphasized that kindling can be a model for learning and memory, and similarities between learning and kindling were suggested at the very early stages of research on the kindling phenomenon (Goddard, McIntyre and Leech, 1969).

Each of the processes involves relatively permanent and widespread neuronal activity changes resulting from repeated stimulations; both involve trans-synaptic changes in function; both demonstrate positive transfer effects; in both cases the acquisition of a new response results in retroactive interference with old responses; and in both the limbic system plays an important role. Also, both procedures, kindling and conditioning require similar principles in order to obtain optimal results. Gaito (1974) provides some evidence suggesting that kindling is a better model of learning than other techniques for several reasons.

Kindling is associated with a long-term enhancement of synaptic responses quite similar to long-term potentiation (LTP) of synaptic efficacy obtained following brief bursts of high-frequency stimulation. It is suggested that both kindling and LTP share similar cellular and biochemical mechanisms and changes (Rutledge, Wright and Duncan, 1974; Van Harreveld and Fitkova, 1975; Racine and Zaide, 1978; Baundry, 1986). There are suggestions that learning and memory also require LTP.

Widespread and long-lasting neuronal plastic changes produced by kindling can be seen in modification of behavior (Adamec, 1975; Goddard, 1980) and in studies of direct or sensory-specific evoked potentials (EP) (Racine, Gartner and Burnham, 1972; Kwast and Majkowski, 1979; Majkowski and Kwast, 1981; Tsuru et al., 1981; Tsuru and Shimada, 1984). It has been shown that EP modification occurring during kindling is of a similar type to that observed during conditioning (Majkowski and Sobieszek, 1975; John et al., 1973). In both situations the changes occur gradually as both procedures progress. These EP modifications to visual or somato-sensory stimulation occur in cats (Majkowski and Kwast, 1981), or guinea pigs (Lidsky, Majkowski and Budek, 1984, 1985; Majkowski, Lidsky and Budek, 1985) during hippocampal or cortical kindling. These strikingly similar changes consist mainly of the occurrence of new components of the EP with a latency of 80–105 ms, and a shorter duration of the late component of latency of about 300 ms, indicating involvement of polysynaptic pathways (Figure 1). In differently designed studies, Tsuru and Shimada (1984) observed changes in visual and auditory EP in subcortical nuclei (lateral and medial geniculate bodies) within 20–50 ms, in amygdala kindling.

It is an interesting question whether EP modification, expressing long-lasting synaptic changes, represents an epileptogenic phenomenon as does interictal spiking, afterdischarges or seizures produced by kindling. The Japanese authors related these EP changes to secondary epileptogenesis in the subcortical modality specific structures following amygdala kindling. An alternative hypothesis may assume that the widespread and long-lasting changes in EP represent a process of a nonepileptic nature, and is rather more general, like LTP, which underlies learning and memory consolidation.

A number of facts seems to support the latter hypothesis. The EP modifications are not correlated with (1) type of kindling (neocortical, hippocampal, amygdala), (2) afterdischarge (AD) duration and their EEG patterns, or (3)

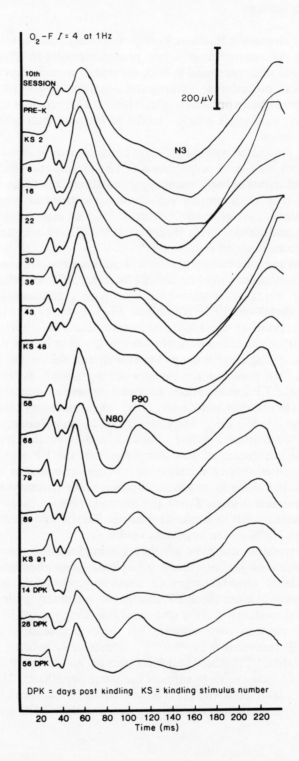

O_2-F $I = 4$ at 1Hz

200 μV

10th
SESSION

PRE-K

KS 2   N3

8

16

22

30

36

43

KS 48

58   P90

N80

68

79

89

KS 91

14 DPK

28 DPK

56 DPK

DPK = days post kindling   KS = kindling stimulus number

20 40 60 80 100 120 140 160 180 200 220
Time (ms)

type of seizure occurrence. Also, studies with hippocampal self-stimulation in rats support this point of view (Campbell, Milgram and Christoff, 1978). In such studies there was no relationship between seizure development and acquisition of hippocampal self-stimulation. On the contrary, seizures interfered with bar pressing for brain stimulation (Milgram, Smith and Chong, 1978).

Interference between epileptogenesis and learning or memory consolidation

The interference seems to operate both ways. It has been found that kindling may affect learning, e.g. passive avoidance learning (McIntyre and Molino, 1972); predatory behavior in cats (Adamec, 1975); reactivity to tail pinch in rats (Pinel, Treit and Rovner, 1977); bar pressing for hippocampal stimulation (Campbell, Milgram and Christoff, 1978); and the acquisition of taste and odor aversions (Mikulka and Freeman, 1984). We found that formation of the avoidance conditioned reflex was severely retarded (Sobieszek and Majkowski, 1988). The learning deficit was related to the duration of AD and partial complex seizures in hippocampally kindled cats.

Only a few studies have investigated the potential effects of environmental stimulation on kindling. Kindling was affected by maze bright and maze dull traits (Zaide, 1974) and by strain differences in learning ability under massed vs spaced practice in mice (Leech and McIntyre, 1976). Pinel, Phillips and MacNeill (1973) found that when intense footshocks were administered to previously kindled rats, seizures were blocked. In the study of Freeman and Mikulka (1986) it appeared that the white condition (box) had a facilitatory effect on kindling. Intermittent photic stimulation has also been shown to facilitate the development of cortical (visual) kindling (Baba, 1982). In our study, interictal spiking in hippocampally kindled cats was blocked by a conditioning stimulus (CS), while a differential stimulus had no such effect. Thus, the experiments suggest that environmental cues can affect the development of kindled seizures and AD duration. This effect may be inhibitory or facilitatory.

In relation to this discussion it is interesting to discuss experiments dealing with conditioning of kindling, that is to pair a CS with kindling electrical stimulation. Wyler and Heavner (1979) found that the CS significantly retarded the rate of kindling and there was no evidence for the conditioning

Figure 1. Changes in cortical evoked potentials to light flashes at frequency 1/s, before, during and after kindling termination. Note occurrence of N80–P90 complex during kindling which lasts for 56 days after last kindled stimulation. Recording from right occipital cortex. Averaging of 64 evoked potentials. Hippocampal kindling in guinea pig (From Lidsky and Majkowski, unpublished data)

of behavioral seizures, AD, or interictal spiking actvity. This is in agreement within another study (Myslobodsky *et al.*, 1983). The only positive findings were reported by Janowsky *et al.* (1980). However, there are a number of methodological problems in their study and positive results were obtained in only two cats. Thus, there is no evidence that a CS paired with a kindling stimulation can elicit a seizure.

Relationship between epileptic subclinical EEG discharges and/or seizures, and memory retrieval

It is generally assumed that in all experimental models of epilepsy, epileptiform activity is a valid equivalent of clinical or subclinical seizures. It seems to be justified that in both animals and humans, local epileptic discharges produced experimentally or occurring spontaneously, can be treated as a sign of temporary functional blocking of this structure. However, from a neurophysiological point of view there seems to be a basic difference between a single seizure produced acutely experimentally, and seizures spontaneously reoccurring or in a chronic model of kindling.

The effect of brain electrical stimulation can be of a twofold nature: depending on the brain site stimulation, it can impair acquisition and/or retention of a conditioned reflex or it can improve learning or memory storage and retention. This problem has been discussed elsewhere (Majkowski, 1981).

All these studies show that memory-storage processes may remain susceptible to modulating influences over long posttraining intervals if an appropriate stimulation is used. However, in the majority of brain electrical stimulations the effect of the stimulation is poorly documented in terms of the intensity and the duration of the AD, as is the relation between the EEG patterns of AD and their effects on cognitive functions.

INTERICTAL HIPPOCAMPAL SPIKING AND MEMORY RETRIEVAL

We found that bilateral interictal hippocampal spiking, produced by hippocampal kindling in cats, does not interfere with memory retrieval of the conditional avoidance reflex (CAR) established prior to the hippocampal kindling. Moveover, presentation of the CS, before the kindling stimulation when the number of spikes was relatively low (17 per 10 min) and after hippocampal stimulation when the number of spikes was several times higher (112 per 10 min), resulted in the same (above 90) percentage of correct responses. In other words, there is no influence of interictal hippocampal spiking on retrieval and performance of the established CAR.

EFFECT OF THE AFTERDISCHARGE (AD) ON MEMORY RETRIEVAL

The effect of the AD on the CAR performance is more complex and depends on the duration of the AD. Presentation of the CS during an AD shorter than 10 s resulted in about 75% of correct responses. However, presentation of the CS during an AD longer than 10 s, but without associated seizures, resulted in 25% of correct responses (Figure 2). The CS was presented within first 6 s after termination of hippocampal stimulation.

Usually, in later stages of kindling, longer ADs are associated with partial simple or complex seizures. Presentation of the CS within the range of 20–100 s of the AD, which is associated with a complex partial seizure, results in no response. However, when the CS was presented just after seizure termination, it resulted, in the majority, in correct responses, thus indicating no after-effect and full recovery of the animal.

In the final stages of kindling, when complex partial seizures have secondarily generalized to tonic–clonic seizures, presentation of the CS during 20 min after termination of the seizures resulted in a dramatic decrease of percentage of the CAR. If the seizures were occurring on successive days the performance of the CAR dropped to zero. Occasionally, the CS produced an orienting response and forepaw extension instead of flexion.

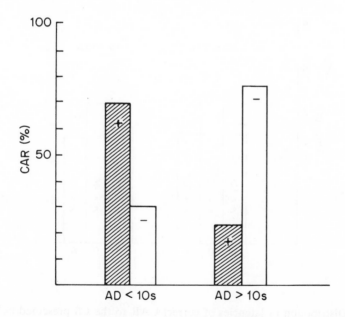

Figure 2. Distribution of correct (+) and no (−) responses to the CS presentation within 2–6 s after hippocampal stimulation. [Reproduced with permission from Majkowski and Sobieszek (1988)]

EFFECTS OF AD ON CAR LATENCY

In addition to yes and no response to the CS, we analyzed latency of the CAR, during shorter and longer AD, in comparison to response latency obtained before and after hippocampal stimulation. An analysis of variance showed significant differences between the distribution in the group of ADs, both shorter and longer than 10 s. The application of the Duncan test indicated that regardless of the AD duration, latencies of responses during AD were significantly longer than before and after hippocampal stimulation (Figure 3).

EEG PATTERNS OF AD AND THEIR EFFECT ON CAR PERFORMANCE

The studies of the effects of AD duration on the memory retrieval and on latency suggested that AD duration was not the only factor critical for impairment of memory retrieval. We asked whether the EEG pattern of AD was not also contributing to the AD effect. Five types of EEG pattern of AD were identified (Figures 4 and 5). The distribution of percent values of

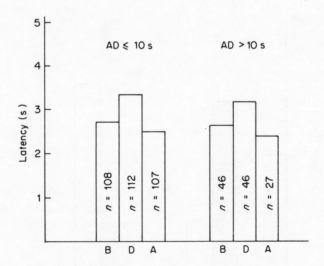

Figure 3. Distribution of latencies of correct CAR to the CS presented before (B), during (D) and after (A) hippocampal afterdischarges shorter and longer than 10 s. Differences are significant at the P < 0.01 level for D vs B and at the P < 0.001 level for D vs A latency groups. [Reproduced with permission from Majkowski et al., 1989]

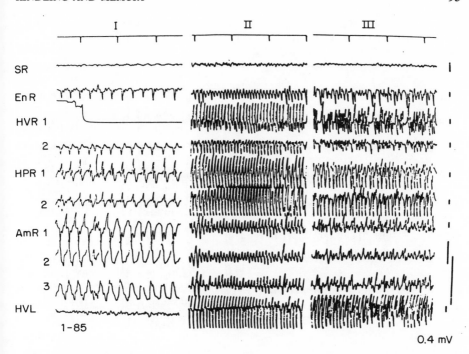

Figure 4. Examples of types I, II and III of the EEG patterns of afterdischarges (SR, right somatomotor cortex; EnR, right entorhinal cortex; HVR, HVL, right and left ventral hippocampus; HPR, right posterior hippocampus; AmR, right amygdala). [Reproduced with permission from Majkowski *et al.* (1989)]

each type of the EEG patterns of AD in the two groups of AD, shorter and longer than 10 s, was significantly different.

The distribution of the correct CAR and failures to the CS presentation in relation to the type of the EEG patterns is shown on Table 1. It can be

Table 1. Relation between AMCR performance and EEG afterdischarge types (I–III)*

AD type	conditioned response present	no response	ratio of response failures to correct responses
	(*n*)	(*n*)	
I	16	22	1.4
II	58	165	2.8
III	42	186	4.4

* Significance level $P < 0.01$; $\chi^2 = 11.3$; df 2.
AMCR, advanced motor conditioned reflex.
Reproduced with permission from Majkowski, Sobieszek and Dlawichowska (1988).

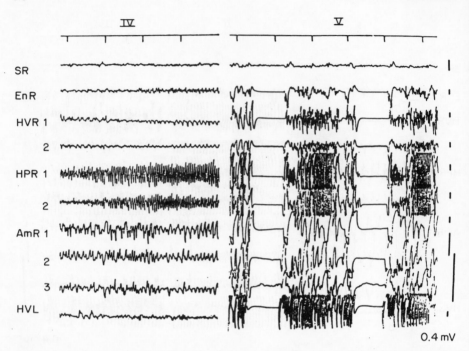

Figure 5. Examples of types IV and V of the EEG patterns of afterdischarges (SR, right somatomotor cortex; EnR, right entorhinal cortex; HVR, HVL, right and left ventral hippocampus; HPR, right posterior hippocampus; AmR, right amygdala). [Reproduced with permission from Majkowski *et al.* (1989)]

seen that the number of failures evidently increases from type I to III EEG pattern of AD.

Since the sequence of the identified types of EEG pattern of AD and their duration varies during each AD, we analyzed the effect of different EEG patterns on memory retrieval in three situations: (A) types of EEG patterns at the CS onset, only; (B) types of EEG patterns at the CS termination, only. In these two situations termination of the CS in (A) and onset of the CS in B were associated with different types of EEG patterns. In the third (C) situation, the EEG pattern was not changed from onset to termination of the CS. Figure 6 shows percentages of the CAR performance to the CS onset presented during types I–IV EEG patterns of AD. Significant failure of memory retrieval was observed during type II and III. Figure 7 shows the effect of EEG patterns of AD on memory retrieval at the moment of the CS termination. A significant negative effect was observed during the type III EEG pattern.

If the onset and termination of the CS was within the same type of EEG

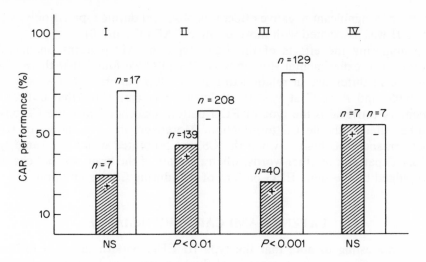

Figure 6. Effect of types of the EEG pattern of afterdischarges (I, II, III, IV), associated with the CS onset, on memory retrieval of the CAR. + = correct response; − = no response. [Reproduced with permission from Majkowski, Sobieszek and Dławichowska (1988)]

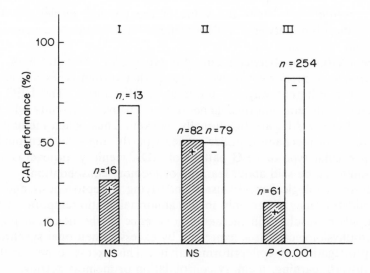

Figure 7. Effect of types of the EEG pattern of afterdischarges, associated with the CS termination, on memory retrieval. [Reproduced with permission from Majkowski, Sobieszek and Dławichowska (1988)]

pattern, a significant negative effect was observed during type III only, while type II was associated with more positive CARs (Figure 8).

Comparing the effects of the EEG types of AD patterns on memory retrieval in experimental situations A, B and C we found that there was a significant difference in relation to type II EEG pattern only (A vs B at P < 0.05, and A vs C at P < 0.001 level). The data show that critical for memory retrieval is the type of EEG pattern associated with the CS onset, rather than with the CS termination. Moreover, the percentage of CAR performance was highest when the CS was presented within the same type II EEG pattern; in other words, when the state of the brain was not changed as judged by the same EEG pattern of AD during CS presentation.

LATENCY AND CAR PERFORMANCE

It is interesting to note that the type III EEG pattern that had the most negative effect on memory retrieval, had no effect on latency of the CAR performance. This was in contrast to the type II EEG pattern which significantly increased the CAR latency in comparison to a control group and type III EEG pattern of AD (Figure 9).

CONCLUSION

The presented data show the value of the kindling model for studies of the relationship between epileptogenesis and memory consolidation or retrieval.

The relationship between different types of EEG pattern of AD and impairment of memory retrieval suggests that certain types of memory are affected in different ways by different EEG patterns. The EEG patterns represent different neuronal generators or neuronal circuits which, being involved in the AD, are functionally blocked. Thus, when memory storage or a read-out mechanism utilize, at least partly, the same neuronal circuits as a particular type of EEG pattern of ADs, memory retrieval is impaired. The same can be said about learning or memory consolidation.

Neurophysiological mechanisms underlying epileptogenesis and memory consolidation may differ only in the abnormal spatio-temporal distribution of impulses, resulting in increased coherence of the neuronal population. Electrophysiologically it is expressed by excessive neuronal synchronization and propagation of epileptiform activity. This excessive neuronal activity may disturb learning, memory consolidation or memory retrieval. The final product of this interfering interaction may depend on the dynamic localization of cognitive processes and overlapping epileptic discharges in the same neuronal circuits.

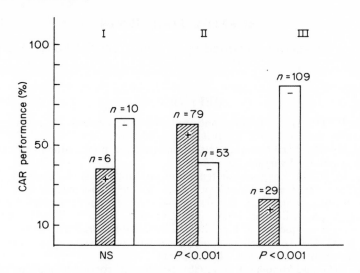

Figure 8. Effect of types of the EEG pattern associated with the CS presentation. Type I, II and III was not changed during the whole period of the CS presentation. [Reproduced with permission from Majkowski, Sobieszek and Dławichowska (1988)]

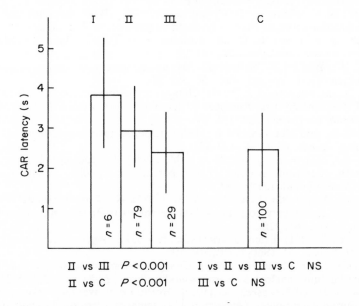

Figure 9. Effect of types I, II and III of the EEG pattern of afterdischarges on latency of CAR in comparison to control (C) group (the CS was presented before hippocampal stimulation). [Reproduced with permission from Majkowski, Sobieszek and Dławichowska (1988)]

ACKNOWLEDGEMENTS

This paper was partly supported by a grant from the Polish Academy of Sciences.

REFERENCES

Adamec, R. (1975). Behavioral and epileptic determinants of predatory attack behavior in the cat. *Can. J. Neurol. Sci.*, **2**, 457–466.

Baba, H. (1982). Facilitatory effects of intermittent photic stimulation on visual cortical kindling. *Epilepsia*, **23**, 663–670.

Baundry, M. (1986). Long-term potentiation and kindling: smilar biochemical mechanisms? In: *Advances in Neurology* (eds A. V. Delgado-Escueta, A. A. Ward Jr, D. M. Woodbury and R. J. Porter), pp. 401–410. Raven Press, New York.

Campbell, K. A., Milgram, N. W. and Christoff, J. K. (1978). Plasticity in the reinforcing consequences of hippocampal stimulation. *Brain Res.*, **159**, 458–462.

Collins, R. C. (1978). Kindling of neuroanatomic pathways during recurrent focal penicillin seizures. *Brain Res.*, **150**, 503–517.

Freeman, F. G. and Mikulka, P. J. (1986). Differential conditioning of environmental cues with amygdala kindling. *Epilepsia*, **27**, 189–193.

Gaito, J. (1974). The kindling effect. *Physiol. Psychol.*, **2**, 45–50.

Goddard, G. V. (1980). The kindling model of limbic epilepsy. In: *Limbic Epilepsy and the Dyscontrol Syndrome* (eds M. Girgis and L. G. Kiloh), pp. 107–116. Elsevier/North Holland Biomedical Press.

Goddard, G. V., McIntyre, D. C. and Leech, C. K. (1969). A permanent change in brain function resulting from daily electrical stimulation. *Exp. Neurol.*, **25**, 295–330.

Janowsky, J. S., Laxer, K. D. and Rushmer, D. S. (1980). Classical conditioning of kindled seizures. *Epilepsia*, **21**, 393–398.

John, E. R., Bartlett, F., Shimokochi, M. and Kleinman, D. (1973). Neural readout from memory. *J. Neurophysiol.*, **36**, 893–924.

Kwast, O. and Majkowski, J. (1979). Changes in the somatosensory evoked potentials (SSEP) in kindled cats. Analogon of learning? *Wiss. Zeitsch Ernst-Moritz-Arndt-Universität Greifswald.*, **28**, 133–136.

Leech, C. K. and McIntyre, D. C. (1976). Kindling rates inbred mice: an analog of learning? *Behav. Biol.*, **16**, 439–452.

Lidsky, A., Majkowski, J. and Budek, M. (1984). Hippocampal kindling produces longterm alterations in visual evoked potential morphology. *Electroencephalogr. Clin. Neurophysiol. (abstr)*, **57**, 1.

Lidsky, A., Majkowski, J. and Budek, M. (1985). Kindling as a model for neuronal plasticity. II. Sensory cortical evoked potentials (EP). *Electroencephalogr. Clin. Neurophysiol.*, **61**, 518.

Majkowski, J. (1981). Brain electrical stimulation: kindling and memory aspects. *Acta Neurol. Scand.*, **64**, (Suppl. 89), 101–108.

Majkowski, J. and Kwast, O. (1981). Changes in somatonsensory evoked potentials during kindling: analogy to learning modifications. *Epilepsia*, **22**, 276–274.

Majkowski, J. and Sobieszek, A. (1975). Evolution of average evoked potentials in cats during conditioning before and after tegmental lesions. *Physiol. Behav.*, **14**, 123–131.

Majkowski, J. and Sobieszek, A. (1988). Effects of hippocampal kindled afterdischarges and complex partial seizures on previously established avoidance response in cats. *Acta Neurobiol. Exp.*, **48**, 295–309.

Majkowski, J., Lidsky, A. and Budek, M. (1985). Kindling as a model for neuronal plasticity. I. Epileptic afterdischarges (AD). *Electroencephalogr. Clin. Neurophysiol.*, **61**, 555.

Majkowski, J., Sobieszek, A. and Dławichowska, E. (1988). EEG afterdischarge patterns and performance of the avoidance response in hippocampally kindled cats. *Acta Neurobiol. Exp.* (accepted for publication).

McIntyre, D. C. and Molino, A. (1972). Amygdala lesions and CER learning: long term effect of kindling. *Physiol. Behav.*, **8**, 1055–1058.

McNamara, J. O. (1986). Kindling model of epilepsy. In: *Advances in Neurology* (eds A. V. Delgado-Escueta, A. A. Ward Jr, D. M. Woodbury, and R. J. Porter), pp. 303–318. Raven Press, New York.

Messenheimer, J. A., Harris, E. W. and Steward, O. (1979). Sprouting fibers gain access to circuitry transsynaptically altered by kindling. *Exp. Neurol.*, **64**, 469–481.

Mikulka, P. J. and Freeman, F. G. (1984). The effect of amygdala kindled seizures on the acquisition of taste and odor aversions. *Physiol. Behav.*, **32** 967–972.

Milgram, N. W., Smith, H. L. and Chong, S. M. (1978). Rapid development of motor seizures in rats bar pressing for electrical stimulation of the preoptic area. *Physiol. Psychol.*, **6**, 57–60.

Myslobodsky, M. S., Mintz, M., Lerner, T. and Mostofsky, D. I. (1983). Amygdala kindling in the classical paradigm. *Epilepsia*, **24**, 275–283.

Pinel, J. P., Phillips, A. G. and MacNeill, B. (1973). Blockage of highly-stable 'kindled' seizures in rats by antecedent footshock. *Epilepsia*, **14**, 29–37.

Pinel, J. P., Treit, D. and Rovner, L. I. (1977). Temporal lobe aggression in rats. *Science*, **197**, 1088–1089.

Post, R. M. and Kopanda, R. T. (1976). Cocaine, kindling and psychosis. *Am. J. Psychiat.*, **133**, 627–634.

Racine, R. and Zaide, J. (1978). A further investigation into the mechanisms underlying the kindling phenomena. In: *Limbic Mechanisms* (eds K. E. Livingston and O. Horynkiewicz), pp. 457–493. Plenum Press, New York.

Racine, R. J., Gartner, J. G. and Burnham, W. M. (1972). Epileptiform activity and neural plasticity in limbic structures. *Brain Res.*, **47**, 262–268.

Rolls, E. T., Woody, C. A., Perrett, D. I. and Wilson, F. A. (1981). Neural activity related to long-term memory. *Acta Neurol. Scand.*, **64** (Suppl. 89), 121–124.

Rutledge, L. T., Wright, C. and Duncan, J. (1974). Morphological changes in pyramidal cells of mammalian neocortex associated with increased use. *Exp. Neurol.*, **44**, 209–228.

Sobieszek, A. and Majkowski, J. (1988). Influence of hippocampal kindling on avoidance learning in cats. *Acta Neurobiol. Exp.*, **48**, 311–322.

Tsuru, N. and Shimada, Y. (1984). Changes in subcortical visual and auditory evoked potentials following amygdaloid kindling in cats. *Epilepsia*, **25**, 288–291.

Tsuru, N., Ninomiya, H., Fukuoka, H. and Nakahara, D. (1981). The effect of excitability curve of the auditory cortex and auditory evoked responses of the medial geniculate nuclei amygdaloid kindling in cats. *Jap. J. EEG EMG.*, **9**, 270–277.

Van Harreveld, A. and Fifkova, E. (1975). Swelling of dendritic spines in the fascia dentata after stimulation of the perforant fibers as a mechanism of post-tetanic potentiation. *Exp. Neurol.*, **49**, 736–749.

Warrington, E. K. (1981). Neuropsychological evidence for multiple memory systems. *Acta Neurol. Scand.*, **64** (Suppl. 89), 13–19.

Weiskrantz, L. (1981). Introduction to neurophysiology and neuropharmacology of memory functions. *Acta Neurol. Scand.*, **64** (Suppl. 89), 85.

Wyler, A. and Heavner, J. E. (1979). Kindling phenomenon: impairment by auditory stimuli. *Epilepsia*, **20**, 333–338.
Zaide, J. (1974). Differences between Tyron Bright and Dull rats in seizure activity evoked by amygdala stimulation. *Physiol. Behav.*, **12**, 527–534.

The Clinical Relevance of Kindling
Edited by T. G. Bolwig and M. R. Trimble
© 1989 John Wiley & Sons Ltd

7

Kindling, behaviour and memory

J. Mellanby and L. Sundstrom
Department of Experimental Psychology, University of Oxford, South Parks Road, Oxford OX1 3UD, UK

In epilepsy there is a tendency to have spontaneous seizures. Does this mean that the brain of a person suffering from epilepsy has been kindled? (Goddard, 1967; Goddard, McIntyre and Leech, 1969). There are three particularly relevant points about experimentally kindled animals: they have a lowered seizure threshold to electrical or chemical convulsants; this change is apparently irreversible; they may, though need not, exhibit spontaneous seizures. When a brain produces a seizure, there is abnormally synchronous firing of neurons, and the neurons which normally would generate single action potentials fire in bursts. Such activity may result from an imbalance between excitation and inhibition in the CNS. The primary epileptogenic change could lie in facilitation of excitatory mechanisms — the N-methyl-D-aspartate (NMDA) receptor (Herron *et al.*, 1986) has been a recent prime candidate (Mody and Heinemann, 1987) — or in a reduction in inhibitory mechanisms such as those employing gamma-aminobutyric acid (GABA) as a transmitter (but see Higashima, 1988). Recent work has suggested that these may actually be interrelated, since activation of NMDA receptors via repetitive stimulation leading to entry of large amounts of calcium may result in a desensitization of GABA receptors (Stelzer, Slater and ten-Bruggencate, 1987) — thus reducing the normal recurrent inhibitory check on excess excitation. We do not at present know whether in clinical epilepsies changes in GABA or glutamate transmission do occur, although post-mortem data have suggested that GABA neurones may sometimes be deficient. Such changes could cause the epilepsy or be caused by it. It is often said that 'fits beget fits' but it also must be remembered that the most likely prognosis for someone who has a seizure is that he will not have any more. There are, however, many patients in whom the severity and frequency of seizures increase over time — does this mean that we are observing a kindling phenomenon in which the kindling stimulus is the abnormal electrical activity of the brain itself? It is well known that in epilepsy permanent physical damage in terms of Ammon's horn sclerosis for example, is likely to result from prolonged status epilepticus, and indeed Sloviter (1987) has shown that in rats after 24 h of low frequency stimulation of the perforant path there is loss of CA3 pyramidal cells and of one class of inter-neurone, somatostatin-containing cells (but not of GABA-containing cells). Such damage has not actually been found in kindled rats, which seem to sustain their abnormally convulsive brains without any gross anatomical damage. This contrasts with kainic acid treated animals, which show a chronic epileptiform syndrome which is associated with widespread cell loss (Ben-Ari, Tremblay and Ottersen, 1980; Ben-Ari et al., 1981; Kessler and Markowitsch, 1983). Many other chronic experimental epilepsies in which spontaneous seizures occur do also involve gross neuropathology, but in contrast the tetanus toxin induced model of hippocampal epilepsy (which we have been exploiting for some years) does not (Mellanby et al., 1977, 1981, 1982, 1985a, b; Hawkins, Mellanby and Brown, 1985; George and Mellanby, 1982). It thus seems that spontaneous seizures can occur without gross structural damage (Kessler and Markowitsch, 1983). The permanence of the kindled change (after electrical or chemical kindling) is therefore the result of some more subtle neurophysiological change than merely a result of cell damage.

Many workers have noted that the permanence of kindling is reminiscent of the time-scale of long-term memory and conceivably the mechanisms by which they are established might be similar. Such a proposition fits also with the idea that formation of at least some sorts of memory may first involve the process of long-term potentiation (LTP; Bliss and Lomo, 1973; Teyler and Discenna, 1984) in the hippocampus, and that the engram may then pass to other parts of the brain. Block of long-term potentiation with drugs which block the NMDA receptor has been shown to parallel a block in the ability of animals to learn a spatial task (Morris et al., 1986). NMDA receptors are also involved in the hippocampus in the induction of kindling (Mody and Heinemann, 1987) and indeed the type of repetitive stimulation which produces LTP will eventually (if repeated at intervals over a period of several weeks) produce kindling. One might indeed ask 'How do we learn without having a fit?' It is of interest that many of the drugs which apparently facilitate memory (e.g. strychnine, picrotoxin, pentylenetetrazol, bemegride, physostigmine, see McGaugh, 1973) can cause convulsions. This was interpreted percipiently by George (1976) as suggesting that 'a close proximity to the seizure threshold' is optimal for remembering. Kindling might be LTP 'gone over the top'. It would be expected that seizure activity might interfere with the ability of an animal to learn (George and Mellanby, 1982; Hesse and Teyler, 1976; Majkowski, this volume), and might also affect the stability of long-term memories if the kindled changes spread to areas of the brain that are involved in storing memory (Flexner *et al.*, 1985).

Curiously, memory and learning in kindled animals have not yet been systematically investigated. Some work on general behaviour has however been done and long-term changes in emotional responses have been reported both in kindled animals (Adamec and Stark-Adamec, 1983 and this volume) and in kainate-injected animals (Griffith, Engel and Bandler, 1987). In our laboratory we have carried out a systematic study of the chronic epilepsy that is produced by injecting minute amounts of tetanus toxin into the hippocampus of rats. Although Griffith, Engel and Bandler (1987) have stated that this is not a good model of temporal lobe epilepsy, the seizures appear very comparable to human complex partial seizures, and the changes in behaviour, including hyper-reactivity, social passivity and problems in learning and memory have many parallels in the human illness (Glaser, 1975; Mellanby *et al.*, 1985b). The toxin is injected stereotaxically into the hippocampus under anaesthesia. Continuous EEG and simultaneous video (Hawkins and Mellanby, 1988) recordings of the rats over periods of up to 7 weeks after the injections have shown that during the first 24–48 h after operation the hippocampus starts to generate small bursts of epileptiform activity; over the next 1–2 days, these become more frequent and lengthen to produce after-discharges lasting up to 2 min. By 2–3 days after operation, some of these seizure discharges do not seem to produce abnormal behaviour, others are associated with cessation of movement, flattening of the ears and twitching of jaws and vibrissae and some are associated with a motor fit, involving clonic jerks of the forepaws, rearing and falling. Whether or not a fit occurs does not seem to be related to the nature of the focal discharge but is determined by the effectiveness of damping in other parts of the brain. Focal seizure activity, as recorded with an implanted electrode, often appears remarkably similar during many consecutive seizures, regardless of whether a motor fit occurs, and the similarity gives the superficial impression that the same neuronal circuitry might be activated each time (Figure 1). A striking feature of this syndrome is that the epilepsy then usually wanes for a few days and then returns again and there may be three or more such cycles of waxing and waning. Then, by about 3 weeks after operation most rats stop having overt fits, but seizure discharges continue to occur for two or three more weeks. Thus at this stage, while there is still an active focus in the hippocampus, the brain has effectively stopped the spread of seizure activity to motor areas. After this the brain successfully recovers from the epilepsy and the EEG apparently returns to normal. During the period of 4–6 weeks when the EEG is epileptiform the animals' general behaviour is abnormal — in particular, they are extremely hyper-reactive. After the EEG normalizes, they become much easier to handle (though they are more difficult to tame

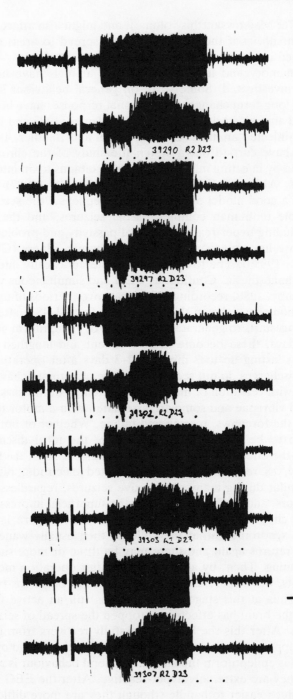

39290 R2 D23

39297 R2 D23

39292 R2 D23

39303 R2 D23

39307 R2 D23

than their controls and occasionally bite). During the period of active epilepsy the limbic system of the rats appears to be in some sense kindled (Mellanby *et al.*, 1981): 75 mg/kg intraperitoneal pentylenetetrazol produces characteristic limbic fits at times when controls respond with a tonic convulsion. (The rest of the CNS is, however, more resistant to seizure, since there is a marked delay in the epileptic animals in the onset of tonic convulsions.) Once the rats have recovered from epilepsy, however, the differences are no longer present — thus we must argue that the limbic system is not actually kindled since the lowered seizure threshold is not permanent.

However, although the recovered rats are not kindled, they do exhibit some apparently permanent changes in general behaviour and in learning and memory. Thus they remain abnormally passive in social interaction (Mellanby *et al.*, 1985a), they are impaired in performing a discrimination task (in a Y-maze) which they had learned before operation and they are impaired in learning a number of tasks believed to require hippocampal function [e.g. delayed alternation (Mellanby *et al.*, 1982), the radial arm maze (Brace, Jefferys and Mellanby, 1985), DRL-20 (H. Brace and J. Tanner, unpublished)]. Interestingly the impairment in memory and on the DRL-20 task correlate with the number of overt fits which the rats have experienced whereas the radial arm maze impairment does not (Brace, Jefferys and Mellanby, 1985). (DRL-20 is a task carried out in a Skinner box in which a rat presses a lever to obtain a pellet. When the rat presses the lever, it resets a timing device so that it will not receive another reward pellet for 20 s. Hence, if the animal presses in less than 20 s, it does not receive a reward and resets the meter again. Animals can learn to wait the requisite 20 s before pressing the bar if they are trained daily in 10-min sessions for about 30 consecutive days.) This could be interpreted as meaning that spread of seizure activity outside the hippocampus is relevant to the subsequent deficits in memory and DRL but that the learning deficit on the radial arm maze is related to a hippocampal abnormality.

These behavioural changes are accompanied by neurophysiological changes in the hippocampus. These changes are still present more than a year after the original toxin injection and are thus also essentially permanent. In particular there is a reduction in the excitability of hippocampal CA3 cells and granule cells of the dentate gyrus (Brace, Jefferys and Mellanby, 1985; Mellanby and Sundstrom, 1985; Jefferys and Williams, 1987) (see Table 1)

Figure 1. Electroencephalogram recorded with electrodes implanted in the left and right ventral hippocampus (top and each alternate record from left) 23 days after injection of tetanus toxin (= 12 mouse LD_{50}), into the left ventral hippocampus of rat. This illustrates the remarkable superficial similarity beween successive hippocampal seizure discharges from the uninjected hippocampus (right). [Calibrations: vertical bar just before seizure record = 1000 μV; horizontal bar = 50 s]

Table 1. Long-term effect of tetanus toxin-induced epilepsy on excitation in the rat dentate gyrus

	n	Population spike at 12 volts	Maximum spike	Population EPSP at 12 volts	Maximum EPSP	Slope of linear portion of spike/EPSP
Controls	12	5.92 (±1.49)	11.08 (±1.73)	5.54 (±0.73)	7.37 (±0.82)	2.83 (±0.37)
Toxin	9	2.66 (±0.71)	6.47 (±1.13)	5.07 (±1.06)	6.78 (±1.12)	1.63 (±0.31)

Acute electrophysiology under urethane anaesthesia was carried out 11–14 months after the original bilateral toxin (or control) injection into the ventral hippocampus. Field potentials of granule cells of the dentate gyrus in the dorsal hippocampus were recorded in response to stimuli from 0–30 V applied to the perforant path.
Values are given ±SEM.

and at the same time a reduction in recurrent inhibition (as induced by paired pulse stimulation of the perforant path) of dentate granule cells (Table 2) (Mellanby and Sundstrom, 1986) and hippocampal pyramidal cells (Williams and Jefferys, 1985). The decreased excitability could be considered part of the successful damping process; on the other hand, a reduction in inhibition might be expected to lead to lowered seizure threshold. It seems that the balance between excitation and inhibition may have been restored at the cost of a reduction in both. Interestingly, similar electrophysiological changes have been reported by King et al. (1985) in the dentate gyrus of amygdala-kindled rats. Perhaps in this case though both are reduced, the balance is somehow left favouring excitation.

Table 2. Long-term effect of tetanus toxin-induced epilepsy on inhibition in the rat dentate gyrus

	n	C spike for 50% inhibition	C stimulus for 50% inhibition	Maximum inhibition
Buffer	7	2.32 (±0.63)	11.21 (±1.12)	89.71 (±3.46)
Toxin	7	4.81 (±1.83)	13.29 (±1.42)	72.57 (±6.81)

Acute electrophysiology under stereotaxic urethane anaesthesia was carried out 11–14 months after the original bilateral stereotaxic toxin (or control) injection into the ventral hippocampus. Field potentials of granule cells of the dentate gyrus in the dorsal hippocampus were recorded in response to stimulation of the perforant path. Paired pulse inhibition was produced by delivering pairs to stimuli at 15 ms separation. The first stimulus (C, conditioning) was varied from 0–20 V; the second (T test) stimulus was fixed at 20 V. The percentage inhibition of the population spike was calculated with respect to the mean of six responses to single 20 V stimuli.
Values are given ±SEM.

In the toxin rats the neurophysiological changes in the dentate granule cells do not correlate with the impairments in learning either DRL or the radial arm maze; however the reduction in excitability of CA3 neurons has been shown to correlate with the impairment in the radial arm maze (Brace, Jefferys and Mellanby, 1985). It is tempting to speculate that the dentate gyrus is acting as a 'gate', permitting or preventing the flow of seizure activity around the hippocampal circuit (Collins, Tearse and Lothman, 1983), while it is the CA3 region whose responses are actually important in learning of 'hippocampal' tasks. Both regions of the hippocampal formation respond to seizure activity by reducing both excitation and inhibition — in this model, damping wins, but at a cost to the organism in terms of subsequent plasticity. If this is also the case in human epilepsy, then we have a rational basis for our belief that we should treat seizures with medication — not just to reduce the inconvenience of having fits but also to prevent the brain from activating its own damping mechanisms which are themselves damaging. Future work on kindled animals of the sort already carried out in the toxin 'model' should show whether being 'kindled' is more or less damaging in behavioural terms than having been successful in damping fits.

ACKNOWLEDGEMENTS

We would like to thank the British Epilepsy Research Foundation, CIBA-GEIGY pharmaceuticals and St Hilda's College, Oxford, for financial support.

REFERENCES

Adamec, R. E. and Stark-Adamec, C. (1983). Limbic kindling and animal behaviour — implications for human psychopathology associated with complex partial seizures. *Biol. Psychiat.*, **18**, 269–293.

Ben-Ari, Y., Tremblay, E. and Ottersen, O. P. (1980). Injections of Kainic acid into the amygdaloid complex of the rat: an electrographic clinical and histological study in relation to the pathology of epilepsy. *Neuroscience*, **5**, 515–528.

Ben-Ari, Y., Tremblay, E., Riche, D., Ghilini, G. and Naquier, R. (1981). Electrographic, clinical and pathological alterations following systemic administration of Kainic acid, bicuculline or pentetrazol: metabolic, mapping using the deoxyglucose method with special reference to the pathology of epilepsy. *Neuroscience*, **6**, 1361–1392.

Bliss, T. V. P. and Lomo, T. (1973). Long-lasting potentiation of synaptic transmission in the dentate area of the anaesthetized rabbit following stimulation of the perforant path. *J. Physiol. (Lond.)*, **232**, 331–356.

Brace, H., Jefferys, J. and Mellanby, J. (1985). Long-term changes in hippocampal physiology and learning ability of rats after intrahippocampal tetanus toxin. *J. Physiol. (Lond.)*, **368**, 343–357.

Collins, R. C., Tearse, R. G. and Lothman, E. W. (1983). Functional anatomy of limbic seizures; Focal discharges from medial entorhinal cortex in rats. *Brain Res.*, **280**, 25–40.

Flexner, J. F., Flexner, L. B., Church, A. C., Rainbow, T. C. and Brunswick, D. J. (1985). Blockade of beta 1 but not beta 2 adrenergic receptors replicates propranolol's suppression of the cerebral spread of the engram in mice. *Proc. Natl. Acad. Sci. USA*, **82**, 7458–7461.

George, G. (1976). Some pharmacological studies on learning and memory in rats. D. Phil. thesis, p. 1.18, University of Oxford.

George, G. and Mellanby, J. (1982). Memory deficits in an experimental hippocampal syndrome in rats. *Exp. Neurol.*, **75**, 678–689.

Glaser, G. H. (1975). Epilepsy: neuropsychological aspects. In: *American Handbook of Psychiatry* (ed. S. Arieti), pp. 314–355. Basic Books, New York.

Goddard, G. V. (1967). Development of epileptic seizures through brain stimulation at low intensity. *Nature (Lond.)*, **214**, 1020–1021.

Goddard, G. V., McIntyre, D. C. and Leech, C. K. (1969). A permanent change in brain function resulting from daily electrical stimulation. *Exp. Neurol.*, **25**, 295–330.

Griffith, N., Engel, J. and Bandler, R. (1987). Ictal and enduring inter-ictal disturbances in emotional behaviour in an animal model of temporal lobe epilepsy. *Brain Res.*, **400**, 360–364.

Hawkins, C. A. and Mellanby, J. H. (1988). Limbic epilepsy induced by tetanus toxin: a longitudinal electroencephalographic study. *Epilepsia*, **28**, 431–444.

Hawkins, C. A., Mellanby, J. and Brown, J. (1985). Antiepileptic effect of carbamazepine in an experimental epilepsy. *J. Neurol. Neurosurg. Psychiat.*, **48**, 459–468.

Herron, C. E., Lester, R. A. H., Coan, E. J. and Collingridge, G. L. (1986). Frequency-dependent involvement of NMDA receptors in the hippocampus: a novel synaptic mechanism. *Nature (Lond.)*, **322**, 265–267.

Hesse, G. M. and Teyler, T. J. (1976). Reversible loss of hippocampal long-term potentiation following electroconvulsive seizures. *Nature (Lond.)*, **264**, 562–564.

Higashima, M. (1988). Inhibitory processes in development of seizure activity in hippocampal slices. *Exp. Brain Res.*, **72**, 37–44.

Jefferys, J. G. R. and Williams, S. F. (1987). Physiological and behavioural consequences of seizures induced in rat by intrahippocampal tetanus toxin. *Brain*, **110**, 517–582.

Kessler, J. and Markowitsch, H. J. (1983). Different neuropathological effects of intrahippocampal injections of kainic acid and tetanus toxin. *Experimentia*, **39**, 922–924.

King, G. L., Dingledine, R., Giacchino, J. and McNamara, J. O. (1985). Abnormal neuronal excitability in hippocampal slices from kindled rats. *J. Neurophysiol.*, **54**, 1295–1304.

McGaugh, J. L. (1973). Drug facilitation of learning and memory. *Annu. Rev.Pharmacol.*, **13**, 229–241.

Mellanby, J. and Sundstrom, L. (1985). Long-term reduction in excitability of rat dentate granule cells after tetanus toxin. *J. Physiol.*, **371**, 49P.

Mellanby, J. and Sundstrom, L. (1986). Long-term reduction in inhibition in rat dentate gyrus after intra-hippocampal tetanus toxin. *J. Physiol.*, **382**, 89P.

Mellanby, J., George, G., Robinson, A. and Thompson, P. A. (1977). Epileptiform syndrome in rats produced by injecting tetanus toxin into the hippocampus. *J. Neurol. Neurosurg. Psychiat.*, **40**, 404–414.

Mellanby, J., Strawbridge, P., Collingridge, G. I., George, G., Rands, G., Stroud, C. and Thompson, P. (1981). Behavioural correlates of an experimental hippocampal epileptiform syndrome in rats. *J. Neurol. Neurosurg. Psychiat.*, **44**, 1084–1093.

Mellanby, J., Renshaw, M., Cracknell, H., Rands, G. and Thompson, P. (1982). Long-term impairment of learning ability in rats after an experimental hippocampal epileptiform syndrome. *Exp. Neurol.*, **75**, 690–699.

Mellanby, J., Hawkins, C., Baillie-Hamilton, S., Bourne, M., Shepherd, L. and

Stroud, C. (1985a). Kindling, behaviour and anticonvulsant drugs. In: *Psychopharmacology of Epilepsy* (ed. M. Trimble), pp. 17–31. John Wiley, London.

Mellanby, J., Mellanby, H., Hawkins, C. A., Rawlins, J. N. P. and Impey, M. E. (1985b). Tetanus toxin as a tool for studying epilepsy. *J. Physiol. (Paris)*, **79**, 207–215.

Mody, I. and Heinemann, U. (1987). NMDA receptors of the dentate gyrus granule cells participate in synpatic transmission following kindling. *Nature (Lond.)*, **326**, 701–704.

Morris, R. G. M., Anderson, E., Lynch, G. S. and Baudry, M. (1986). Selective impairment of learning and blockade of long-term potentiation by an *N*-metyl-D-aspartate receptor antagonist, AP5. *Nature (Lond.)*, **319**, 774–776.

Sloviter, R. S. (1987). Decreased hippocampal inhibition and a selective loss of interneurons in experimental epilepsy. *Science*, **235**, 73–76.

Stelzer, A., Slater, N. T. and ten-Bruggencate, G. (1987). Activation of NMDA receptors blocks GABAergic inhibition in an in vitro model of epilepsy. *Nature (Lond.)*, **326**, 698–701.

Teyler, T. J. and Discenna, P. (1984). Long-term potentiation as a candidate mnemonic device. *Brain Res. Rev.*, **7**, 15–28.

Williams, S. F. and Jefferys, J. G. R. (1985). Inhibition and long-term neuronal depression after intrahippocampal tetanus toxin. *Neurosci. Lett.* (Suppl. 22), S510.

The Clinical Relevance of Kindling
Edited by T. G. Bolwig and M. R. Trimble
© 1989 John Wiley & Sons Ltd

Discussion — Session 2

KINDLING AND NEUROTRANSMITTER SYSTEMS

R. Adamec Dr Barry are you proposing the possibility of a nor-adrenergic transplant for epilepsy?

D. I. Barry No. What we were doing was trying to establish the principle that you can modify the epileptic activity of the brain, using transplanted neurons. In a first step we use fetal striatal cells, because they are able to reinstate the original nor-adrenergic innervation. We know that nor-adrenergic innervation affects kindling, and therefore we can show, in the transplanted animals, we can restore the situation to normal. I am not saying that in a clinical situation you can use nor-adrenergic transplants.

Question Does the transplant grow endlessly?

A. Björklund When grafting is done under these conditions, with this kind of tissue, there is no evidence that tissue can overgrow. It follows its normal embryogenetic growth and stops at approximately the same time as it would stop. Under other conditions, there have been reported excess overgrowth of tissue. That is, if you take very early fetal material, or contaminated fetal material which contains mesenchyme, then you can get tissue that grows to compress and destroy the tissue round the graft. In such instances there have been reported incidences of epileptic seizures. But that is under conditions that would not be representative for what is reported here.

A. Dam Was there a difference in the ability to kindle dependent on if you put the transplant in different parts of the hippocampus; in the anterior or the posterior, or in relation to H1, 2 or 3 regions?

D. I. Barry That I cannot answer.

113

R. Adamec Did you try to determine whether there were alpha or beta receptors involved in the transplantation restoration of normal kindling rate?

D. I. Barry No. We have not done that.

M. Trimble Dr Majkowski, in your animal model, you have suggested overlaps between epilepsy or seizure phenomena and learning. As clinicians, we are very familiar with something similar, namely that patients with certain types of seizure are prone to memory disorders. However, the reverse is less clear. In other words: you have suggested that learning may influence epileptogenesis. Does this have any relevance to the issue of control of seizures by behavioural techniques?

J. Majkowski Yes, and there are some groups trying to utilize behavioural techniques, like bio-feedback, for example. However, this bio-feedback is actually de-sensitization for reflex epilepsy, due to light flashes for example. I think that conditioning is something different, because this implies long-term changes in the brain, so that intensive learning might interfere with epileptogenesis. This is not epilepsy. When we are dealing with epileptic discharges, it is too late to influence that. I am talking about early stages when it is still possible to effect spiking which at that point in time is a relatively mild impairment of the brain function.

S. Thelander You have studied conditioned responses. I would think that it would be of interest to study a simpler model, that is: habituation of the orienting response.

J. Majkowski I studied habituation of evoked potentials, not *behaviour*.

S. Thelander Do we kindle some patients whom we give ECT?

J. Majkowski It is surprising that there is not much epilepsy due to that. I have personally two patients, who, not with electroshock, but with *stimulation* for spasticity with electrodes in the spinal cord developed seizures after a year of stimulation, very frequent stimulation.

I. Rosén Dr Mellanby, have you been looking at the morphological changes?

J. Mellanby Only rather crudely. There are no gross morphological changes. Cell counting we are doing, but we have not done any immunocyto-chemisty.

M. Trimble Dr Mellanby, there is a very important distinction between seizures and epilepsy touched on in your work. What are the consequences of temporal lobe lesions? Clearly, one of them is seizures, and if there are several clinical seizures, we say: well, that's epilepsy. But you reach the stage in your animals of no seizures, but they continue to have the effects of the temporal lobe pathological changes, namely behaviour and learning disturbances. They still have the pathology or the process, which caused the seizures. They still have pathological brain changes which lead to the behaviour problems. That is analogous to the clinical situation, where just because a patient is not having seizures does not mean to say that we have cleared up the whole problem of the temporal lobe pathology and indeed the whole problem of the epilepsy.

J. Mellanby We believe your interpretation is correct.

The Clinical Relevance of Kindling
Edited by T. G. Bolwig and M. R. Trimble
© 1989 John Wiley & Sons Ltd

8

Kindling, anxiety and personality

ROBERT E. ADAMEC
*Departments of Psychology and Basic Medical Science, Memorial
University, St John's, Newfoundland, Canada, A1B 3X9*

INTRODUCTION

Part of the clinical issue of the nature of psychopathology associated with
epilepsy is the question of the existence of the epileptic personality. This
question has had a controversial history (Hermann and Whitman, 1984 for
review). In this paper, recent attempts to define the epileptic personality
will be discussed. Then more recent clinical data indicating that the critical
psychopathology associated with limbic epilepsy is anxiety and depression
will be reviewed. It will then be contended that kindling-like processes in
human limbic epilepsy increase interictal vulnerability to response to the
stress of being an epileptic with anxiety and depression.

Animal parallels to the effects of human limbic epilepsy on anxiety will
then be considered. The relevance of the animal data to human personality
will be defined in terms of studies in primates and humans which suggest
that an anxious personality type exists in at least three species — cats,
monkeys and humans. It will also be shown how studies of the effects of
limbic kindling on both fearful behavior and the 'anxious personality' in the
cat may model the effects of limbic seizures on human anxiety.

THE EPILEPTIC PERSONALITY AND SEIZURE
PSYCHOPATHOLOGY

The most recent, and widely quoted, study of the 'epileptic personality' is
by Bear and Fedio (1977). These authors claimed to have statistically isolated
18 'traits' which define a behavioral syndrome associated with personality
alteration due specifically to temporal lobe epilepsy (TLE). Bear (1979) went

117

on to propose that persons suffering from TLE also suffer from sensory–limbic hyperconnection. He proposed that the behavioral traits enhanced by TLE reflect an increased responsiveness of limbic structures to complex sensory-ideational input from temporal cortical analyzers.

The idea of limbic hyperfunction has also appeared in studies of the physiological basis of the 'anxious personality' in both cats (Adamec, 1975, 1978; Adamec and Stark-Adamec, 1983a, b, c, d, 1984) and humans (Kagan, Reznick and Snidman, 1988). It has also been proposed to underlie the fear enhancing effects of limbic kindling in animals (Adamec and Stark-Adamec, 1983d). This correspondence of ideas from different lines of investigation is suggestive. Unfortunately, there are a number of empirical problems with Bear's hypothesis.

The original study by Bear and Fedio has been faulted on numerous methodological grounds (Hermann and Whitman, 1984; Stark-Adamec and Adamec, 1986). In addition, the consensus from subsequent studies using the Bear and Fedio personality behavior inventory (PBI) is that the PBI measures significant psychopathology among epileptics, but what it measures is not specific to seizure diagnosis (Hermann and Whitman, 1984). Such findings call into question the view that these traits are unique to a temporal lobe, and therefore, limbic, seizure disorder.

Another issue not addressed in this literature is the question of whether or not what is being measured are behavioral or personality traits at all. Of the 18 traits described by Bear and Fedio, only three correspond in name, at least, with two of the six 'robust' personality traits described by personality investigators (Digman and Inouye, 1986). These are emotional stability (or neuroticism with the dimensions calm–anxious, composed–excitable, poised–nervous, compared with Bear's emotionality) and agreeableness (or affection with the dimensions trusting–suspicious, affectionate–hostile, compared with Bear's aggression and paranoia). Of these two robust traits mentioned above, only one, neuroticism, is universally recognized (Brand, 1984). Moreover, Bear and Fedio did not demonstrate the nomothetic quality of the traits measured. That is they did not investigate the cross situational or temporal stability of the putative traits.

At this point, it cannot be said that there are any convincing data which define epileptic personality traits (see Strauss, 1988 for a more general review). Perhaps an alteration in personality is the wrong place to look for how epilepsy disturbs patients' behavior.

LIMBIC EPILEPSY, LIMBIC AURAS AND ANXIETY

A number of investigators have reported that between 25% and 35% of epileptics experience serious psychological problems (Betts, 1974; Graham and Rutter, 1968; Pond and Bidwell, 1960; Reynolds, 1981). Past attempts to ascribe these problems to TLE, however, have not consistently demonstrated a particular vulnerability to psychopathology of persons suffering from this subtype of epilepsy (Hermann and Whitman, 1984; Strauss, 1988).

Recently, psychological disturbance has been associated more directly with limbic epileptic disturbance. For example, Wieser (1983) reported that patients with temporal-limbic foci, verified by depth electrode recording, scored higher on a number of the PBI scales (circumstantiality and hypermoralism) than did patients with either temporal neocortical involvement only, or with foci located elsewhere. Dana-Haeri and Trimble (1984) found an association between levels of hypothalamo-pituitary hormones (prolactin and luteinizing hormone) secreted following a complex partial seizure and psychopathology (schizophrenia, depression and personality disorder). These data suggest that seizures which involve limbic structures with strong excitation of midline hypothalamic areas may predispose patients to interictal psychopathology. Somewhat less direct evidence of limbic involvement in seizure related psychopathology was demonstrated by Hermann et al. (1982). They found that TLE patients with fear auras scored higher than the other epileptic groups on, among others, the schizophrenia, paranoia and psychasthenia scales of the Minnesota Multiphasic Personality Inventory. Fear auras are considered to be markers of involvement of limbic structures, particularly the amygdala, in a seizure episode (Gloor et al., 1982).

These studies suggest that limbic involvement in seizure activity, rather than diagnosis, is more important in identifying epileptic patients at risk for interictal psychological disturbance. Unfortunately, all of these studies used small numbers of subjects, and did not have other criticial contrast groups, including normal, chronic illness and non-neurological psychiatric groups. Thus they cannot be said to have clearly delimited the nature of psychological disturbance particularly ascribable to a limbic epileptic disturbance.

A recently completed study (Stark-Adamec and Adamec, 1986; Adamec, Perry and Stark-Adamec, 1989), however, addresses the question of limbic involvement in epileptic psychopathology with larger group sizes and more contrast groups. This study permits a more detailed specification of the nature of limbic epileptic psychological disturbance.

A modified Bear and Fedio 101 item personal behavior inventory (PBI-2) was used. Unlike other studies with the PBI, the format was changed from true–false to the more reliable 7 point scale. The PBI-2 was completed by 114 epileptics of mixed diagnosis. The majority (82.5%) of the sample had complex partial seizures (CPS), CPS + secondary generalized or primary generalized seizures. The responses of 91 psychiatry patients of mixed diagnosis were also obtained. 'Sick person' controls were two chronic illness groups (kidney failure and diabetics: $n = 28$ and $n = 15$ respectively). There were 100 normal controls. With the exception of the epileptics, none of the participants had a history of neurological disturbance. All groups were matched with respect to age and education. Medical history data were taken and analyzed.

The nature of aura experiences of the epileptics was also examined. An aura questionnaire assessed frequency and intensity of 33 auras (on a 5 point scale) which have been associated in the literature with onset of epileptic attacks. As described above, certain types of auras may be classified as 'limbic auras' whose presence suggests an involvement of limbic circuits in the onset of seizure activity. Thus, aura data may provide a hidden variable, independent of seizure diagnosis, which predicts psychopathology in seizure disorders. We were also interested in the further question of whether presence or frequency and intensity of limbic auras best predicted psychopathology.

The study first investigated the nature of psychopathology uniquely associated with seizure disorder. This was done as follows. Item cluster analysis and subsequent jackknifed discriminant function analysis reduced the PBI-2 to 10 clusters of items which were statistically useful. These items were those which best predicted inclusion of participants in the study in seizure, psychiatry and non-patient groups. Psychiatry patients were grouped together, there being no differences in cluster scores among the different diagnostic categories.

The percentages of participants *correctly* classified by the discriminant function were then tabulated (Table 1). The percentage of correct classification of epileptics was not very good. However, it is of interest that three types of seizure patients emerged from the analysis: those correctly classified as seizure patients (S-seizure), those classified as psychiatry patients (S-psych); and those classified as non-patients (S-non-pat). Moreover, 24.6% were classified as psychiatry patients. This corresponds well with several reports that between 25 and 35% of seizure patients experience psychological problems (Betts, 1974; Graham and Rutter, 1968; Pond and Bidwell, 1960, Reynolds, 1981).

Table 1. Table of discriminant function classifications

Diagnostic group	Percent classified as:		
	Seizure	Psychiatry	Non-Patient
Seizure	47.4	24.6	28.1
Psychiatry	31.9	58.2	9.9
Non-Patient	24.0	3.0	73.0

The new groupings of seizure patients, as well as the different diagnostic groups, were investigated further. S-psych patients scored higher than other seizure patients, normal participants, and chronic illness controls, who did not differ, on Depression, Moody and Metaphysical (religious) clusters *only*.

S-psych patients were also equal to psychiatry patients on these clusters, and psychiatry patients scored higher than controls.

When seizure patients were grouped into the different seizure diagnostic categories, no differences in cluster scores were found between them or the other contrast groups. This is because equal numbers of CPS and primary generalized epileptics were classified as seizure, psychiatry or non-patients.

The problems experienced by S-psych patients may reflect an underlying anxious-depression. Depression, Moody and Metaphysical clusters are highly correlated with trait anxiety as measured by the Spielberger Trait Anxiety Scale (multiple $R = 0.861$, $P < 0.001$, $n = 15$; and with depression as measured by the Beck Depression Inventory (BDI, multiple $R = 0.728$, $P < 0.003$, $n = 15$; the correlations were calculated from a subset of seizure patients of all types).

If one uses the prediction equations from the subset to predict BDI and anxiety scores in the total sample, the different groupings appear as in Figure 1. S-psych and psychiatry patients are equal and higher than the remaining groups, who do not differ. These findings are consistent with other investigators who have reported elevated anxiety and depression in epileptic populations (see Hermann and Whitman, 1984 for review). For example, the BDI and Spielberger Trait Anxiety scores observed by Robertson, Trimble and Townsend (1987) among unipolar depressed epileptics ($n = 80$) of mixed seizure diagnoses (similar to those studied by Adamec, Perry and Stark-Adamec, 1989), correspond remarkably well with the predicted scores in the S-psychiatry subpopulation of Adamec, Perry and Stark-Adamec (1989; Figure 1). Moreover, Trimble and Perez (1980) found epileptics to be more anxious and depressed than controls and equal to or greater than a psychiatric contrast group. This study involved a large sample of epileptics ($n = 281$) of the same diagnoses examined by Adamec, Perry and Stark-Adamec (1989).

It is of interest that both Adamec, Perry and Stark-Adamec (1989) and Robertson, Trimble and Townsend (1987) found no association between diagnosis, seizure frequency or EEG abnormalities and psychopathology. Furthermore, Adamec, Perry and Stark-Adamec (1989) found no association between current anticonvulsant medication and psychopathology.

Taken together these findings indicate that:

(1) problems with depression, anxiety, moodiness and metaphysical concerns are unique to a particular subset of epileptics who are not identifiable by seizure diagnosis;
(2) these problems are not an outcome of being chronically ill;
(3) these problems are psychiatrically relevant since they are shared with psychiatric patients.

This last point is supported further by the fact that more S-psych patients

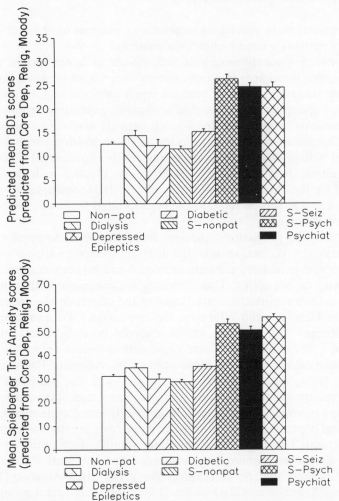

Figure 1. Mean (± standard error) predicted scores on the Beck Depression Inventory (BDI) and the Speilberger Trait Anxiety Scale are plotted for six patient groups described in the text and in Adamec, Perry and Stark-Adamec (1989). The six groups are non-patients (non-pat), dialysis, and diabetic controls, psychiatry patients (psychiat) and the seizure patients classified by the discriminant function analysis as: non-patients (S-nonpat), seizure patients (S-Seiz), and psychiatry patients (S-Psych) (see Table 1). Scores for each subject were calculated from multiple regression equations derived from a subset of seizure patients. These equations predict BDI and Speilberger scores from the Depression (Core Dep), Metaphysical Interpretation (Relig) and Moody clusters from the personal behavior inventory. These scores are contrasted with the observed mean BDI and Speilberger Anxiety Scale scores reported by Robertson, Trimble and Townsend (1987) in depressed epileptics (Depressed Epileptics). S-Psych, Psychiat and Depressed Epileptic patients do not differ from each other, but each differs from the remaining groups, which are equal to each other (Group Effect Anova plus Duncan Multiple Range Tests, all $P < 0.01$)

were hospitalized for psychiatric problems, were treated for psychiatric problems, and more often attempted suicide than other seizure patients (Adamec, Perry and Stark-Adamec, 1989).

One seizure-related variable did differentiate the groups in the Adamec and coworkers (1989) study, however. S-psych patients reported having 5 of the 33 aura experiences more intensely and frequently than other seizure patients, who did not differ. These appear to be limbic auras (Figure 2). Formed Images, Humming or Buzzing, and Irritability have been associated with epileptic, pharmacological or electrical stimulation of areas of the human limbic system (Halgren *et al.*, 1978; Kling *et al.*, 1987; Mark, Erwin and Sweet, 1972; Stark-Adamec *et al.*, 1982). The remaining two auras cluster with experiences associated with human limbic stimulation (Jamais Vu clusters with Formed Images and Time Changes clusters with Derealization).

These findings, together with the studies of Dana-Haeri and Trimble (1984) and Hermann *et al.* (1982), suggest that limbic activation during seizure attack is associated with intercital psychopathology. Moreover, the psychopathology resembles in many respects that seen in non-epileptic anxious and depressed people. Anxious patients report time changes, derealization and Jamais Vu (Harper and Roth, 1962), whereas depressed patients report formed images and derealization (Silberman *et al.*, 1985). These data suggest a shared non-ictal limbic disturbance between epileptic and non-epileptic patients experiencing anxiety and depression.

VULNERABILITY AND LIMBIC DISTURBANCE IN EPILEPTIC PSYCHOPATHOLOGY

It is likely that seizure-induced alteration of limbic function increases vulnerability to respond to the stresses of being an epileptic with anxiety and depression. For example, fears associated with their disorder, including fear of the consequences of the illness, fear of losing employment, as well as social withdrawal as a coping strategy, are prominent among epileptics (Mittan and Locke, 1982a, b). Illness, employment and family relation problems (which could be created by social withdrawal among epileptics) are social stressors which are among the most frequent predecessors of anxiety neuroses and depression in non-epileptics (Paykel, 1979; Takeuchi *et al.*, 1986).

Genetic predispositions likely play a role in addition to social stressors. Robertson, Trimble and Townsend (1987) report that 52% of depressed epileptics have family histories of predominately depression, and 42.4% are endogeneously depressed.

Medication is also a factor. Patients on phenobarbitone are more depressed (as measured by the Beck Depression Inventory) whereas patients on carbamazepine are less depressed and anxious (Robertson, Trimble and Townsend, 1987). Similar effects of anticonvulsants have been reported by others.

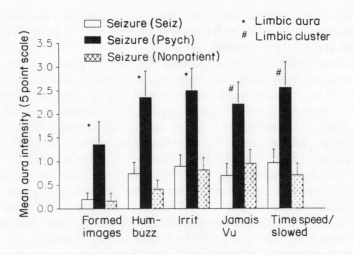

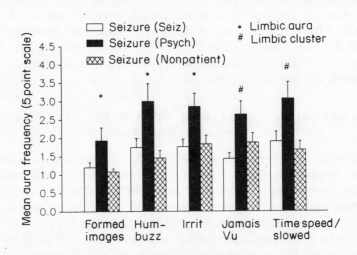

Figure 2. Means (± standard error) of self reported aura intensity and frequency scores are plotted for the three seizure patient groups classified by the discriminant function analysis as: non-patients [Seizure Nonpatient]; seizure patients [Seizure Seiz]; and psychiatry patients [Seizure Psych] (see Table 1). Scores are plotted for the five aura types on which Seizure Psych patients scored higher than the remaining seizure patients (who did not differ) (Manova, $P < 0.01$; Duncan Multiple Range Tests, all $P < 0.01$). IRRIT refers to the irritability aura. The remaining auras are self explanatory. Auras designated as 'Limbic aura' are those aura experiences which resemble subjective experiences produced by direct activation of the limbic system (see text). Auras labelled 'Limbic cluster' are aura experiences which cluster closely with limbic auras

These data could mean that social, genetic and medication factors alone contribute to anxious depression in epileptics independently of the pathophysiology of the seizure disorder. Alternately, one could conclude that these factors, together, interact with alterations in limbic function produced by limbic seizures to precipitate anxiety and depression. This latter concept makes more sense in view of the fact that only 25–30% of epileptics are troubled, whereas 49–65% of epileptic populations experience psychiatrically relevant social stresses (Mittan and Locke, 1982a, b), and 11% of troubled epileptics may be genetically prone to anxious depression (Robertson, Trimble and Townsend, 1987). These percentages suggest that not all epileptics will respond pathologically to social stress, nor are all troubled epileptics genetically predisposed to do so. Data which implicate limbic involvement in the seizure disorder as a predictor of psychopathology suggest that those patients who do respond pathologically to such stressors have, in addition, a seizure-induced alteration of limbic function.

These and other data are consistent with a kindling process, which alters limbic function. Repeated seizure invasion of limbic tissue in epileptics, signalled by limbic aura, could produce kindling-like changes which alter limbic function interictally and lastingly. This may be happening in the S-psych patients of Adamec, Perry and Stark-Adamec (1989). In these patients intensity and frequency of limbic auras are both highly intercorrelated (r range: 0.941–0.957, all $P < 0.0001$), and predict interictal psychopathology (Adamec, Perry and Stark-Adamec, 1989). There are two animal parallels to these findings in humans. The first is that the more limbic activation is repeated during kindling, the more the seizure discharge is intensified. [Intensification appears as increases in duration, amplitude of seizure and frequency of firing of limbic cells (Racine, 1978).] If intensity of subjective experience is related to intensity of limbic activation, then the kindling analogy is a viable one. The second animal parallel is that lasting interictal changes in limbic function, and in animal 'anxiety', are produced by, and require, *repeated* limbic seizures (Adamec, 1989a, b, c). In this formulation, the presence or absence of limbic participation in seizure onset is not the critical variable, rather it is *degree* of limbic activation that is important.

It is probable that a temporally stable anxiety is experienced by anxious and depressed epileptics who score high on the Spielberger trait scale. This scale has been shown to be stable on retest (Spielberger, Gorsuch and Lushere, 1971). Whether this represents a personality trait remains to be determined. Nevertheless, newly emerging data from humans and animals concerning an anxiety-like personality trait with possible genetic origins, suggest that another genetic predisposing factor to consider in human epileptics is the nature of premorbid anxiety trait characteristics.

The animal data concerning anxious traits in animals, and how limbic kindling affects this will now be considered. It will be contended that studies of the effects of limbic seizures on defensive behavior in the cat represent one of the better models of interictal human affective disturbance.

LASTING INTERICTAL BEHAVIORAL CHANGES — SEIZURE-INDUCED LIMBIC HYPERFUNCTION AND INTERICTAL ANXIETY

Feline defensive response to threat satisfies most of the criteria of Skolnick and Paul (1983) (Table 2) for an animal model of anxiety (Adamec, 1989a, b; Maeda, 1976; Stoddard et al., 1986a, b; Stoddard et al., 1987; Stoddard-Apter, Siegel and Levin, 1983; Wolgin and Servidio, 1979). If one adopts these criteria, then defensive behavior in the cat may be seen as a model of human anxiety.

Table 2. Critiera for animal models of anxiety

Animal behaviors which model human anxiety should:
1. Be species characteristic responses to threat
2. Be associated with somatic (e.g. tachycardia) and pituitary adrenal axis manifestations of human anxiety
3. Be suppressible by clinically effective anxiolytics
4. Be exacerbated by benzodiazepine inverse agonists which precipitate anxiety in humans

Three lines of investigation will be reviewed which indicate that repeated limbic seizures in the cat produce an interictal enhancement of defensive response to environmental threat. It will be contended that experimental limbic seizures lastingly potentiate the function of neural circuits participating in 'anxiety'.

Effects of seizures on cat anxiety — in a model of CPS

Interictal enhancement of feline defensiveness has been demonstrated in a model of recurrent, spontaneous complex partial seizures (CPS) of temporal lobe origin induced by kainic acid injection into the dorsal hippocampus (Griffin, Engel and Bandler, 1987). Cats showed a lasting period (up to 4 months) or recurrent, partial seizures of limbic origin with occasional secondary generalization. Enhanced defensive responsiveness was observed during CPS, which often only involved the amygdala. Interictal mood lability also appeared as an explosive defensive reaction to trivial provocation such as sudden movement or mild skin pinch, though gentle handling provoked no defensive response. In these periods, the cats showed interictal amygdala spiking and reduced electrical thresholds to elicit defense from the medial hypothalamus (MH).

Effects of seizures on cat anxiety — following massed seizures

Interictal enhancement of feline defensiveness has also been demonstrated following repeated electrically evoked amygdala seizures (Siegel, 1984). Seizures were closely timed in a massed stimulation paradigm. Siegel (1984) showed that seizures of amygdala origin potentiate defensive behavior elicited by electrical stimulation of MH by reducing thresholds and latencies. These changes were observed post ictally and for 2–6 weeks following electrically evoked amygdala seizures. The interictal changes eventually returned to baseline. Siegel's data complement Griffin, Engel and Bandler's (1987). Together, the two studies point to the importance of the amygdala and its projections to the MH in seizure effects on defense (see Adamec, 1989a for detailed review of these studies).

Cat personality — limbic excitability and limbic epilepsy

The above findings are consistent with the hypothesis that limbic seizures which invade the basal amygdala (Abm) potentiate its normal biasing function in defensive behavior (Adamec, 1978). A variety of data indicate that the Abm exerts a lasting, facilitatory effect on defense behavior, and a lasting inhibitory effect on predatory attack (see Adamec and Stark-Adamec, 1983d for review). The generalized or nomothetic quality and temporal stability of defensive bias suggests the existence of a defensive personality trait (Adamec, Stark-Adamec and Livingston, 1983, Adamec and Stark-Adamec, 1984).

The behavioral biasing function of the amygdala seems to involve at least two components. First, biasing is achieved by an enhanced response of amygdala cells tuned to species characteristic threats (O'Keefe and Bouma, 1969; Adamec, 1978; Adamec, 1989d). Second, there is an enhanced transsynaptic output of these cells associated with naturally occurring enhanced defensiveness (Adamec and Stark-Adamec, 1983d, 1984).

Repeated limbic seizures, without motor seizure (partial limbic kindling) produce long lasting and interictal increases in spontaneous defensive responses to species characteristic threat (Adamec, 1978; Adamec and Stark-Adamec, 1983b, c). The seizures appear to do so by enhancing naturally occurring processes which involve long-term potentiation (LTP) and possibly the benzodiazepine receptor (BZR) (Adamec, 1989b, c). It is the BZR involvement which suggests that there is an 'anxious' personality in the cat, and that limbic kindling alters this personality by enhancing anxious response to environmental threat.

In discussing these concepts, two lines of evidence will be examined. First, work will be described which indicates how the amygdala and its outputs contribute to individual differences in defensiveness. This is important in understanding how seizures modify amgydala function and behavior. Then how changes in these outputs contribute to lasting interictal changes in defensiveness will be discussed.

Cat personality and individual differences in behavior

Adult cats are separable into more- and less-defensive animals. More-defensive animals avoid threatening species characteristic stimuli such as rats, conspecific threat howls and novel environments. Less-defensive cats are predatory. Measures of defensive sensitivity to threat correlate highly across test situations, suggesting the existence of a defensive disposition or a nomothetic defensive trait (Adamec, 1978; Adamec, Stark-Adamec and Livingston, 1983). This appears to be a trait since defensiveness is stable over retest periods of up to one year (Adamec, 1978; Adamec, Stark-Adamec and Livingston, 1980c). It is of great interest that analogous findings of a defensive disposition have been reported in primates (Soumi *et al.*, 1981) and in human children (Kagan, Reznick and Snidman, 1988). Finally, feline defensive response is reduced by benzodiazepine receptor (BZR) agonists (Maeda, 1976; Wolgin and Servidio, 1979), and exacerbated by a BZR inverse agonist (FG-7142) (Adamec, 1989b), which produces anxiety in humans (Dorrow *et al.*, 1983). Moreover, the effects of FG-7142 are blocked by the specific BZR antagonist RO-15-1788 (Adamec, 1989b). These data suggest that the BZR is involved in feline defensiveness.

Cat personality and individual differences in limbic function

Naturally threatening stimuli produce large increases in cell firing in the amygdala and MH of defensive cats, whereas smaller responses are observed in less-defensive cats (Adamec, 1978, 1989d). In addition, the excitatory outputs of the amygdala differ between more- and less-defensive felines. Relative to less defensive cats, defensive animals show larger trans-synaptic excitatory evoked activity in the MH, and attenuated evoked activity in the ventral hippocampus (VH) when the amygdala is stimulated with single pulses (Adamec and Stark-Adamec, 1984). Moreover, the BZR inverse agonist, FG-7142, which enhances feline defensive response as well as human anxiety, increases evoked activity in the MH (Adamec, 1989b). Finally flow of information through the VH of defensive cats is attenuated because recurrent inhibition is enhanced (Adamec and Stark-Adamec, 1984). These differences in hippocampal excitability are of interest, since the VH in the cat functions to facilitate predatory attack and attenuate defensiveness (Adamec and Stark-Adamec, 1983a, d for review).

Taken together, naturally enhanced defensiveness seems to be mediated by:

(1) increased responses of amygdala cells to naturally threatening stimuli;
(2) a preferential routing of flow of amygdala response to stimuli into the MH, an area involved in production of defensive responses;
(3) an attenuation of the impact of amygdala excitation on the VH, an area involved in attenuating defensiveness and facilitating attack.

Preliminary data also suggest that flow of information to the MH is modulated by the BZR.

Ontogeny of cat personality

Cats may be born with their defensive dispositions. Experientially resistant individual differences in defensiveness emerge very early in development and persist into adulthood (Adamec, Stark-Adamec and Livingston, 1980a, b, c). Again, it is of great interest that analogous findings have been reported in primates (Soumi et al., 1981) and human children (Kagan, Reznick and Snidman, 1988).

Effects of partial limbic kindling on cat personality

Partial limbic kindling of the basal amygdala or VH (directly or via the perforant path) of defensive cats increases defensive response to several natural threats. Partial kindling is accomplished by repeatedly evoking electrical electrographic seizures (afterdischarges or AD) without motor seizure. Behavioral changes are interictal and very long lasting (up to 4 months, Adamec, 1975, 1978; Adamec and Stark-Adamec, 1983b, c). Except for a reduction of AD threshold, little kindling is produced (Adamec and Stark-Adamec, 1983c). Behavioral changes are, therefore, independent of mechanisms mediating motor convulsive epileptogenesis. This finding is consistent with other studies of the effects of kindling on behavior (Adamec, 1989a for review).

Interictal behavioral changes are associated with several equally long lasting changes in limbic excitability. First, excitatory transmission between the amygdala and MH is increased (Adamec and Stark-Adamec, 1983b, c), but returns to baseline in those cats whose behavior returns to baseline (Adamec, 1989e). Recurrent inhibition in the VH is increased in both the dentate (Adamec and Stark-Adamec, 1983c) and area CA3 (Adamec, 1989f). Excitatory transmission between Abm and VH is enhanced as well, but only in some cats. Such cats show less of an increase in defensiveness than those cats in whom Abm–VH transmission is not potentiated (Adamec and Stark-Adamec, 1986).

All of these changes depend on alterations of amygdala functioning. Several lines of evidence indicate that in cats partially kindled in the VH, it is spread of seizure activity into the Abm which is important for behavioral changes (Adamec and Stark-Adamec, 1983b, c; Adamec, 1989e).

Personality of the cat prior to kindling interacts with the site of kindling to influence the nature of interictal behavioral changes. If one partially kindles the amygdala of predatory cats, who are not very defensive, lasting increases in defensiveness are seen and the cats become less predatory. Abm–MH transmission is also potentiated (Adamec, 1978). However, if the VH of predatory cats is partially kindled, they become *less* defensive and more predatory, and no changes in Abm–MH transmission are seen (Adamec, 1975, 1978).

Taken together, the data indicate that repeated spread of seizures into the amygdala produces a lasting enhancement of excitability and behavioral functioning of circuits which normally participate in spontaneous response to threat. At the same time there is an attenuation of functioning in hippocampal circuits which antagonize response to threat. Increases in Abm–MH transmission are at least necessary for behavioral changes, though their sufficiency has not been demonstrated.

The mechanisms of these changes are unknown. There are some clues, however. LTP is produced by limbic kindling (Racine, 1978). In some circuits in the hippocampus, LTP is dependent on N-methyl-D-aspartate (NMDA) receptors (Collingridge and Bliss, 1987). Potentiation of Abm–MH transmission resembles LTP, and could involve NMDA receptors, though this possibility remains to be investigated. Kindling also produces interictal increases of recurrent inhibition in rodent hippocampus (Tuff, Racine and Adamec, 1983). The change in inhibition is accompanied by increases in numbers of BZR receptors, but not in GABA receptors (Tuff, Racine and Mishra, 1983). A similar mechanism may underlie changes in cat VH.

A different kind of change in BZR receptor function may be involved in enhanced defensiveness. Preliminary studies (Adamec, 1989b) indicate that increases in defensiveness produced by partial kindling of the VH are reversibly blocked by the BZR antagonist, RO-15-1788. RO-15-1788 normally has no anxiolytic action on cat defensive behavior, however. Its anxiolytic effects appear only after partial kindling. These findings are consistent with the view that a lasting change in preferred conformation of the BZR to an inverse agonist conformation has occurred. Other interpretations are possible, including enhancement of the functioning of an endogenous anxiogenic ligand, but the existing data do not favor this view (see Adamec, 1989b, c for a discussion).

Taken together, the data suggest that both modification of BZR function, and possibly NMDA-dependent LTP, are involved in interictal behavioral changes produced by partial limbic kindling. These receptor-based changes are likely anatomically specific. Upregulation of BZR receptors in VH contributes to interictally enhanced defensiveness by reducing VH excitability. On the other hand, an inverse agonist function of the BZR in other circuitry likely contributes to interictally enhanced defensiveness.

CONCLUSIONS

The behavioral, ontogenetic, neuropharmacological and neuroendocrine parallels between cat defensiveness and human anxiety support the view that defensive response to threat in the cat models some aspects of human anxiety. These data, combined with the evidence of the involvement of the BZR in interictal changes in behavior, also suggest that enhanced defensiveness produced by partial limbic kindling in the cat models some aspects of the effects of limbic epilepsy on human anxiety.

In addition to the pharmacological and behavioral parallels, there are two other similarities between cats and humans. First, emotional change produced by partial kindling in the cat is unrelated to generalized seizure expression. This is also the case in humans (Adamec, 1989a; Adamec, Perry and Stark-Adamec, 1989). Second the degree of emotional change and bias is related to the frequency and intensity of limbic seizure activity in the cat (Adamec, 1978). If intensity of aura experience reflects degree of excitation of limbic tissue, then a similar relationship exists in the human.

There is evidence that the premorbid 'anxious' personality of the cat interacts with the focus of the experimental seizure disorder to influence interictal behavioral outcome. It might be of use to investigate if such an interaction exists in humans. The developmental data in humans suggest that such an approach is feasible. Parental interview regarding childhood behaviors of adult epileptics could provide useful data regarding premorbid 'anxious' personality characteristics that are predictive of adult personality.

While there is a growing literature regarding the behavioral impact of limbic kindling on animal behavior (Adamec and Stark-Adamec, 1983; Adamec, 1989a for reviews), few of the behaviors investigated can be said to model clinically relevant phenomena in humans. The findings considered in this paper, on the other hand, suggest that the effect of limbic seizures on defensive behavior in the cat is a viable and clinically relevant model of anxiety disorder associated with limbic epilepsy in humans.

Taken together, the human and kindling data lend support to the view that limbic epilepsy alters a robust personality trait, namely neuroticism. The animal data are also consistent with the hypothesis that sensory–limbic hyperconnection is part of the pathophysiology of interictal emotional change in humans. Partial limbic kindling in the cat, therefore, should prove useful in furthering our understanding of the nature of molecular changes underlying interictal emotional change.

ACKNOWLEDGEMENTS

The work of the author which is reviewed in this chapter was supported by a grant to R. Adamec from the Medical Research Council of Canada (MRC MT-7022), and by a previous grant to R. Adamec from the National Institutes of Health, Bethesda, Maryland. The invaluable technical assistance of Raj Riar, Barbara Vari, Martin Graham, Naida Graham, Ann Marie Madden and Andrea Brown is gratefully acknowledged.

REFERENCES

Adamec, R. (1975). Behavioural and epileptic determinants of predatory attack behavior in the cat. *Can. J. Neurol. Sci.*, (**Nov.**), 457–466.

Adamec, R. (1978). Normal and abnormal limbic system mechanisms of emotive biasing. In: *Limbic Mechanisms* (eds K. E. Livingston and O. Hornykiewcz), pp. 405–455. Plenum Press, New York.

Adamec, R. (1989a). Does kindling model anything clinically relevant? *Biol.Psychiat.* (in press).

Adamec, R. (1989b). FG-7142 and 'anxiety' in the cat. Acute and lasting after effects on approach–attack behavior — implications for animal models of anxiety which use response suppression. *Eur. J. Pharmacol.* (in press).

Adamec, R. (1989c). FG-7142 and 'anxiety' in the cat II: acute and lasting after effects on approach-attack behavior — implications for animal models of anxiety which use response suppression. *Eur. J. Pharmacol* (submitted for publication).

Adamec, R. (1989d). Developmentally determined individual differences in multiunit response of the limbic system of cats to species characteristic threatening stimuli. *Behavioral Neuroscience* (submitted for publication).

Adamec, R. (1989e). The role of the amygdala and ventromedial hypothalamus in partial kindling induced increases in defensiveness in the cat. *Aggressive Behavior* (in press).

Adamec, R. (1989f). The effect of partial kindling on inhibition in the ventral hippocampus of the cat. *Behav. Neur. Biol.* (submitted for publication).

Adamec, R. and Stark-Adamec, C. (1983a). Limbic control of aggression in the cat. *Prog. Neuro-Psychopharmacol. Biol. Psychiat.*, **7**, 505–512.

Adamec, R. and Stark-Adamec, C. (1983b). Partial kindling and emotional bias in the cat: Lasting after effects of partial kindling of the ventral hippocampus. I. Behavioral Changes. *Behav. Neur. Biol.*, **38**, 205–222.

Adamec, R. and Stark-Adamec, C. (1983c). Partial kindling and emotional bias in the cat: Lasting after effects of partial kindling of the ventral hippocampus. II. Physiological changes. *Behav. Neur. Biol.*, **38**, 223–239.

Adamec, R. E. and Stark-Adamec, C. (1983d). Limbic kindling and animal behaviour — implications for human psychopathology associated with complex partial seizures. *Biol. Psychiat.*, **18** (2), 269–293.

Adamec, R. E. and Stark-Adamec, C. (1984). The contribution of limbic connectivity to stable behavioural characteristics of aggressive and defensive cats. In: *Modulation of Sensorimotor Activity During Alterations in Behavioral States* (ed. R. Bandler), pp. 325–339. Allan R. Liss, New York.

Adamec, R. E. and Stark-Adamec, C. (1986). Partial kindling and behavioural change — Some rules governing behavioural outcome of repeated limbic seizures. In: *Kindling 3* (ed. J. A. Wada), pp. 195–211. Raven Press, New York.

Adamec, R., Perry, D. and Stark-Adamec, C. (1989). Epilepsy and psychopathology: the contribution of auras to our understanding of the nature and pathophysiological basis of psychopathology associated with epilepsy in humans. *Epilepsia* (submitted for publication).

Adamec, R. E., Stark-Adamec, C. and Livingston, K. E. (1980a). The development of predatory aggression and defense in the domestic cat (*Felis catus*) I. Effects of early experience on adult patterns of aggression and defense. *Behav. Neur. Biol.*, **30**, 389–409.

Adamec, R. E., Stark-Adamec, C. and Livingston, K. E. (1980b). The development of predatory aggression and defense in the domestic cat (*Felis catus*) II. Development of aggression and defense in the first 164 days of life. *Behav. Neur. Biol.*, **30**, 410–434.

Adamec, R. E., Stark-Adamec, C. and Livingston, K. E. (1980c). The development of predatory aggression and defense in the domestic cat (*Felis catus*) III. Effects on development of hunger between 180 and 365 days of age. *Behav. Neur. Biol.*, **30**, 435–447.

Adamec, R. E., Stark-Adamec, C. and Livingston, K. E. (1983). The expression of an early developmentally emergent defensive bias in the adult domestic cat (*Felis catus*) in non-predatory situations. *Appl. Anim. Ethol.*, **10**, 89–108.

Brand, C. (1984). Personality dimensions: An overview of modern trait psychology. In: *Psychological Survey 5* (eds J. Nicholson and H. Beloff), pp. 30–40. British Psychological Society, Leicester, England.

Bear, D. M. (1979). Temporal lobe epilepsy: a syndrome of sensory-limbic hyperconnection. *Cortex*, **15**, 357–384.

Bear, D. M. and Fedio, P. (1977). Quantitative analysis of interictal behavior in temporal lobe epilepsy. *Arch. Neurol.*, **34**, 454–467.

Betts, T. A. (1974). A follow-up study of a cohort of patients with epilepsy admitted to psychiatric care in an English city. In: *Epilepsy: Proceedings of the Hans Berger Centenary Symposium* (eds P. Harris and C. Mawdsley), pp. 326–336. Churchill Livingston, Edinburgh.

Collingridge, G. L. and Bliss, T. V. P. (1987). NMDA receptors — their role in long-term potentiation. *TINS*, **10**(7), 288–293.

Dana-Haeri, J. and Trimble, M. R. (1984). Prolactin and gonadotropin changes following partial seizures in epileptic patients with and without psychopathology. *Biol. Psychiat.*, **19**, 329–336.

Digman, J. and Inouye, J. (1986). Further specification of the five robust factors of personality. *J. Pers. Soc. Psychol.*, **50**, 116–123.

Dorrow, R., Horowski, R., Paschelke, G., Amin, M. and Braestrup, C. (1983). Severe anxiety induced by FG-7142, a beta-carboline ligand for benzodiazepine receptors. *Lancet*, **ii**, 98–99.

Gloor, P., Olivier, O., Quesney, L. F., Andermann, F. and Horowitz (1982). The role of the limbic system in experiential phenomena of temporal lobe epilepsy. *Ann. Neurol.*, **12**, 129–144.

Graham, P. and Rutter, M. (1968). Organic brain dysfunction and child psychiatric disorder. *Br. Med. J.*, **3**, 695–700.

Griffin, N., Engel, J. and Bandler, R. (1987). Ictal and enduring interictal disturbances in emotional behavior in an animal model of temporal lobe epilepsy. *Brain Res.*, **400**, 360–364.

Halgren, E., Walter, R. D., Cherlow, D. G. and Crandall, P. H. (1978). Mental phenomena evoked by electrical stimulation of the human hippocampal formation and amygdala. *Brain*, **101**, 83–117.

Harper, M. and Roth, M. (1962). Temporal lobe epilepsy and the phobic anxiety-depersonalization syndrome. Part 1: a comparative study. *Compl. Psychiat.*, **3**(3), 129–151.

Hermann, B. P. and Whitman, S. (1984). Behavioral and personality correlates of epilepsy: a review, methodological critique, and conceptual model. *Psych. Bull.*, **95**, 451–497.

Hermann, B. P., Dikmen, S., Schwartz, M. S. and Karnes, W. E. (1982). Interictal psychopathology in patients with ictal fear: A quantitative investigation. *Arch. Neurol.*, **32**, 7–11.

Kagan, J., Reznick, J. S. and Snidman, N. (1988). Biological bases of childhood shyness. *Science*, **240**, 167–171.

Kling, M. A., Kellner, C. H., Post, R. M., Cowdry, R. W., Gardner, D. L., Coppola, R., Putnam, F. W. and Gold, P. W. (1987). Neuroendocrine effects of limbic activation by electrical, spontaneous, and pharmacological modes: Relevance to the pathophysiology of affective dysregulation in psychiatric disorders. *Prog. Neuropsychopharmacol. Biol. Psychiat.*, **11**, 459–481.

Maeda, H. (1976). Effects of psychotropic drugs upon the hypothalamic rage responses in cats. *Folia Psychiatr. Neurol. Jpn.*, **30**(4), 539–546.

Mark, V. H., Erwin, F. R. and Sweet, W. H. (1972). Deep temporal lobe stimulation in man. In: *Advances in Behavioral Biology*, Vol. 2 (ed. B. E. Eleftheriou), pp. 485–507. Plenum Press, New York.

Mittan, R. J. and Locke, G. E. (1982a). The other half of epilepsy: psychosocial problems. *Urban Health*, (**Jan-Feb**), 38–39.

Mittan, R. J. and Locke, G. E. (1982b). Fear of seizures: Epilepsies forgotten problem. *Urban Health*, (**Jan-Feb**), 40–41.

O'Keefe, J. and Bouma, H. (1969). Complex sensory properties of certain amygdala units in freely moving cat. *Exp. Neurol.*, **23**, 384–394.

Paykel, E. S. (1979). Recent life events in the development of the depressive disorder. In: *The Psychobiology of the Depressive Disorders: Implications for the Effects of Stress*, pp. 245–262. Academic Press, New York.

Pond, D. and Bidwell, B. H. (1960). A survey of epilepsy in 14 general practices 2. Social and psychological aspects. *Epilepsia*, **1**, 285–299.

Racine, R. J. (1978). Kindling: The first decade. *Neurosurgery*, **3**(2), 234–252.

Reynolds, E. H. (1981). Biological factors in psychological disorders associated with epilepsy. In: *Epilepsy and Psychiatry* (eds E. H. Reynolds and M. R. Trimble), pp. 264–290. Churchill Livingstone, Edinburgh.

Reynolds, E. H. and Travers, R. D. (1974). Serum anticonvulsant concentrations in epileptic patients with mental symptoms, a preliminary report. *Br. J. Psychiat.*, **124**, 440–445.

Robertson, M. M., Trimble, M. R. and Townsend, H. R. A. (1987). Phenomenology of depression in epilepsy. *Epilepsia*, **28**(4), 364–372.

Silberman, E. K., Post, R. M., Nurnberger, J., Theodore, W. and Boulenger, J. P. (1985). Transient sensory, cognitive and affective phenomena in affective illness — A comparison with complex partial epilepsy. *Br. J. Psychiat.*, **146**, 81–89.

Siegel, A. (1984). Anatomical and functional differentiation within the amygdala — Behavioral state modulation. In: *Modulation of Sensorimotor Activity During Alterations in Behavioral States* (ed. R. Bandler), pp. 229–324. Alan R. Liss, New York.

Skolnick, P. and Paul, S. M. (1983). New concepts in the neurobiology of anxiety. *J. Clin. Psychiat.*, **44** (2), 12–19.

Soumi, S. J., Kraemer, G. W., Baysinger, C. M. and De Lizio, R. D. (1981). Inherited and experiential factors associated with individual differences in anxious behavior displayed by rhesus monkeys. In: *Anxiety: New Research and Changing Concepts* (eds D. F. Klein and J. Rabkin), pp. 179–197. Raven Press, New York.

Spielberger, C. D., Gorsuch, R. L. and Lushere, R. E. (1971). *State-Trait Anxiety Inventory*. Consulting Psychologists Press, Palo Alto, California.

Stark-Adamec, C. and Adamec, R. E. (1986). Psychological methodology versus clinical impressions: Different perspectives on psychopathology and seizures. In: *The Limbic System: Functional Organization and Clinical Disorders* (eds B. K. Doane and K. E. Livingston), pp. 217–227. Raven Press, New York.

Stark-Adamec, C., Adamec, R. E., Graham, J. M., Hicks, R. C. and Bruun-Meyer, S. E. (1982). Analysis of facial displays and verbal report to assess subjective state in the non-invasive detection of limbic system activation by procaine hydrochloride. *Behav. Brain Res.*, **4**, 77–94.

Stoddard, S. L., Bergdall, V. K., Towsend, D. W. and Levin, B. E. (1986a). Plasma catecholamine associate with hypothalamically-elicited defense behavior. *Physiol. Behav.*, **36**, 867–873.

Stoddard, S. L., Bergdall, V. K., Towsend, D. W. and Levin, B. E. (1986b). Plasma catecholamine associate with hypothalamically-elicited flight behavior. *Physiol. Behav.*, **37**, 709–715.

Stoddard, S. L., Bergdall, V. K., Conn, P. S. and Levin, B. E. (1987). Increases in plasma catecholamines during naturally elicited defensive behavior in the cat. *J. Autonom. Nerv. Syst.*, **19**, 189–197.

Stoddard-Apter, S. and MacDonnell, M. F. (1980). Septal and amygdalar efferents to the hypothalamus which facilitate hypothalamically elicited intraspecific aggression and associated hissing in the cat. An autoradiographic study. *Brain Res.*, **193**, 19–32.

Stoddard-Apter, Siegel, A. and Levin, B. E. (1983). Plasma catecholamines and cardiovascular responses following hypothalamic stimulation in the awake cat. *J. Auton. Nerv. Syst.*, **8**, 343–360.

Strauss, E. (1988). Ictal and interictal manifestations of emotions in epilepsy. In: *Handbook of Neuropsychology* (eds F. Boller and J. Grafman). Elsevier/North-Holland (in press).

Takeuchi, T., Takahashi, T., Kotsuki, H., Aizawa, S., Maruyama, S. and Kodama, K. (1986). Life events related to the inception of anxiety neurosis. *Jpn. J. Psychiat. Neurol.*, **40**(2), 137–142.

Trimble, M. R. and Perez, M. M. (1980). Quantification of psychopathology in adult patients with epilepsy. In: *Epilepsy and Behavior '79* (eds B. M. Kulig, H. Meinardi and G. Stores), pp. 118–126. Swets and Zeitlinger, Lisse.

Tuff, L. P., Racine, R. J. and Adamec, R. (1983). The effects of kindling on GABA-mediated inhibition in the dentate gyrus of the rat: I. Paired pulse depression. *Brain Res.*, **277**, 79–90.

Tuff, L. P., Racine, R. J. and Mishra, R. K. (1983). The effects of kindling on GABA-mediated inhibition in the dentate gyrus of the rat: II. Receptor binding. *Brain Res.*, **277**, 91–98.

Wieser, H. G. (1983). Depth recorded limbic seizures and psychopathology. *Neurosci. Behav. Rev.*, **7**, 427–440.

Wolgin, L. and Servidio, S. (1979). Disinhibition of predatory attack in kittens by oxazepam. *Soc. Neurosci. Abstr.*, **5**, #2282.

9

Kindling, psychopathology and cerebral mechanisms in ethanol withdrawal

RALF HEMMINGSEN
Department of Psychiatry, Bispebjerg Hospital, University of Copenhagen, DK-2400 Copenhagen, Denmark

The purpose of the present paper is to summarize some evidence relating kindling to the mechanisms of ethanol intoxication and withdrawal. The studies from our own group have been performed in the Department of Psychiatry, Rigshospitalet, Copenhagen, Denmark. An essential point characterizing kindling is the progression of electrophysiological and behavioural changes occurring when the *same* stimulus is applied repeatedly with an interval of one or a few days (Goddard, McIntyre and Leech, 1969; Racine, 1972). Clinically there is decisive evidence that withdrawal from an episode of physical ethanol dependence (a drinking bout) is accompanied by more severe symptoms over the years of an alcohol career. This was empirically documented in a retrospective study (Ballenger and Post, 1978, Chapter 15), which confirmed that it takes 10–15 years to develop delirium tremens or withdrawal seizures whereas non-psychotic/non-convulsive withdrawal signs may occur after a much briefer alcohol career. Recently Brown *et al.* (1988) have confirmed that a group of patients experiencing withdrawal seizures have a significantly higher number of previous detoxification periods as compared to a group of alcoholics without seizures. Thus the number of prior detoxifications appeared to be a critical variable in the predisposition to alcohol withdrawal seizures. It thus seems as if an effect comprising cumulative central nervous system (CNS) dysfunction is at play. This effect may be due to actions of intoxification, the influence of repeated withdrawal, or both.

Kindling essentially comprises irreversible hyperexcitability of the CNS and hence it is necessary to consider whether the same is actually prevailing during clinical withdrawal from alcohol.

CLINICAL SIGNS OF ETHANOL WITHDRAWAL

Withdrawal seizures obviously reflect a state of CNS-hyperreactivity. Delirium tremens and acute withdrawal hallucinosis (impending delirium tremens) are clinically characterized by fluctuating hypervigilance where arbitrary sensory input may elicit vivid illusionary misinterpretations. This may progress into a state of rapidly changing attentional focus, a state where any event in the field of perception may cause hallucinations and unstructured delusions accompanied by excitement or even panic. Ultimately the mere state of being awake elicits an overwhelming activity of hallucinations and panic with delusional excitement. The main goal for the treatment of delirium tremens and related clinical states is to induce sleep in order to prevent psychomotor agitation from progressing into life-threatening physical exhaustion. The psychopathology and physical agitation in severe ethanol withdrawal is paralleled by an increase in cerebral blood flow (CBF) and by hyperventilation (Victor, 1973; Hemmingsen et al., 1988). The hallucinations during ethanol withdrawal mainly involve visual phenomena, but auditory hallucinations may also prevail (Victor and Adams, 1953; Surawicz, 1980).

It is important to know whether the whole withdrawal reaction or only a part of it is increased during the course of repeated withdrawal episodes. We have done a retrospective clinical review comparing the severity of the non-psychotic/non-seizure component of withdrawal in cases of acute withdrawal hallucinosis and of fully developed delirium tremens (Hemmingsen and Kramp, 1988). Applying our delirium tremens rating scale (comprising the items of perspiration, tremor, sleep, agitation, rectal temperature, hallucinations, orientation and level of consciousness) we found that fully developed cases of delirium tremens ($n = 9$) had a median total rating of 19 (13–26; quartiles) at admission compared to 12 (9–15) in cases of acute hallucinosis ($n = 11$)). This difference was due to the items agitation, hallucinations, orientation and level of consciousness, whereas the other items (covering physical withdrawal symptoms) were equal in the two groups as was blood pressure and pulse rate at admission. Furthermore the total amount of sedative (barbital) necessary to treat the two conditions was approximately the same (5 g).

In another study it has been reported that there were no statistically significant differences between patients with physical withdrawal, acute hallucinosis and fully developed delirum tremens as far as plasma concentrations of barbital needed for treatment were concerned (Kramp and Rafaelsen, 1978). From these clinical findings it may be tentatively suggested that psychotic signs of withdrawal develop by a mechanism that is qualitatively different from the physical signs. The two clusters of withdrawal phenomena do not seem to increase proportionally. We have suggested (Hemmingsen and Kramp, 1988) that the physical withdrawal signs are determined by the most recent episode of physical dependence, whereas the psychotic signs and the seizures are determined by a cumulative component increasing its influence during the progression of the life-time drinking career. Such a hypothesis may be the subject of clinical investigation. At present, however, we have to turn to the findings from animal studies in order to further explore the issue.

ANIMAL MODELS FOR THE STUDY OF PROGRESSING SIGNS OF ETHANOL WITHDRAWAL

A method for studying multiple successive episodes of ethanol intoxication and withdrawal in the rat was first developed in 1984 (Clemmesen and Hemmingsen, 1984). Before that only a small number of repeated episodes had been studied and the results were not conclusive (Clemmesen and Hemmingsen, 1984). The new method is a modification of Majchrowicz's intragastric intubation technique for the study of single intoxication and withdrawal episodes. The technique comprises weekly treatment cycles with 2 days of severe intoxication followed by 5 days without ethanol. These cycles can be repeated for at least 15 weeks still enabling the animals to increase their body weight. The severity of intoxication and of the non-convulsive withdrawal signs are rated by standardized rating scales (see Clemmesen *et al.*, 1988). Convulsive behaviour is evaluated by video-recordings obtained during the repeated withdrawal phases.

Table 1 summarizes the ratings of the non-convulsive withdrawal component during three experimental series (Clemmesen and Hemmingsen, 1984; Clemmesen *et al.*, 1988; Ulrichsen *et al.*, 1988). All the experimental series were performed using the technique described above. The minor differences concerning the number of episodes, number of items rated, calculation of ethanol dose and number of episodes are apparent from the table. In experiment I the same animals were evaluated at the 1st, the 10th and the 17th episode; this comparison indicated that no change occurred between the episodes as far as severity of the non-convulsive component of the withdrawal reaction was concerned. In experiment II the severity of the withdrawal reaction was the same in the single episode group and in a multiple episode group. An increase occurred in the severity of the withdrawal reaction in a single 4-day intoxication group that was compared with the single 2-day intoxication group. This finding is in accordance with the previous report of Majchrowicz and Hunt (1976). In experiment III there was a non-significant trend towards a more pronounced withdrawal reaction in the multiple episode groups.

Table 1. Ethanol consumption, intoxication score and withdrawal sum score in three experimental series comprising single and multiple weekly intoxication–withdrawal cycles in rats

Group	Ethanol dose (g/kg/d)	Intoxication score (0–6)	Withdrawal sum score
Experiment I			
First episode $(n = 20)$	15.6 ± 2.2	2.7 ± 0.5	5.3 ± 1.6
10th episode $(n = 19)$	15.2 ± 1.9	3.0 ± 0.2	4.5 ± 1.3
17th episode $(n = 15)$	13.3 ± 3.7	3.0 ± 0.2	5.3 ± 1.1 (0–12)
(Clemmesen and Hemmingsen, 1984)			
Experiment II			
Single episode $(n = 6)$	16.1 ± 1.1	2.7 ± 0.2	3.0 ± 0.0
11 episodes $(n = 6)$	16.9 ± 2.9	2.7 ± 0.3	3.5 ± 0.5
Single episode $(n = 6)$ (4 days)	11.1 ± 0.9	3.1 ± 0.1	5.5 ± 0.8 (0–9)
(Clemmesen *et al.*, 1988)			
Experiment III			
Single episode $(n = 6)$	25.0 ± 2.9	2.5 ± 0.2	2.8 ± 0.8
15 episodes $(n = 4)$ (+seizures)	20.5 ± 3.8	2.6 ± 0.2	4.0 ± 0.8
15 episodes $(n = 8)$ (−seizures)	20.1 ± 2.0	2.8 ± 0.1	4.1 ± 1.5 (0–9)
(Ulrichsen *et al.*, 1988)			

The withdrawal sum score includes the non-convulsive signs tremor, rigidity, hyperactivity and hypoactivity; in experiments II and III only the three first items were included (see Clemmesen *et al.*, 1988). In experiment series II a group subjected to a single 4-day intoxication period was also included. Means and standard deviations are indicated.

In conclusion these results from various independent series of repeated intoxication and withdrawal episodes in the rat indicate that the non-convulsive component of the withdrawal reaction is not — or is only slightly — influenced by the number of intoxication and withdrawal episodes, i.e. there is no carry over of dependence. On the contrary, the duration of the single intoxication episode is a strong determinant as far as the severity of the subsequent non-convulsive withdrawal reaction is concerned. Thus in each single episode the severity of the non-convulsive withdrawal reaction is determined by the duration of the episode and the severity of the intoxication during that specific episode.

Table 2 summarizes the findings concerning the convulsive component of the withdrawal reaction in the rat. Spontaneous convulsive seizures never occurred during withdrawal from a single 2-day intoxication episode. Actually, a spontaneous seizure before the 6th episode was never recorded in a series of weekly repeated intoxication–withdrawal cycles. In all experimental series spontaneous seizures developed after the 6th episode, the percentage of animals developing seizures varying between 16 and 30% of the animal group subjected to multiple cycles. When the experimental series are considered together 25% of all animals developed spontaneous seizures. The

Table 2. Number of animals and percentage with spontaneous partial clonic seizures during single and multiple weekly cycles comprising 2 days of severe ethanol intoxication and 5 days without alcohol

Group		Number of animals and % with spontaneous partial clonic withdrawal seizures	
Experiment I			
Single episodes	(n = 20)	0	—
10 episodes	(n = 19)	3	15.8%
(Clemmesen and Hemmingsen, 1984)			
Experiment II			
Single episodes	(n = 6)	0	—
11 episodes	(n = 18)	5	27.8%
Single 4 days episode	(n = 6)	0	—
(Clemmesen et al., 1988)			
Experiment III			
Single episode	(n = 6)	0	—
15 episodes	(n = 12)	4	33.3%
(Ulrichsen et al., 1988)			
Total			
Single episode	(n = 32)	0	—
Multiple episodes	(n = 49)	12	24.5%

In experiment series II a group subjected to a single 4-day intoxication period was also included.

seizures were incomplete clonic seizures involving facial, forelimb and axial musculature, rearing but only sometimes falling. These spontaneous seizures strongly resembled the stage 3–5 kindling response obtained by electrical amygdala kindling in the rat (Racine, 1972). The seizures did not bear any resemblance to the generalized tonic–clonic seizures elicited by electroconvulsive stimulation or chemically induced seizures.

Apart from the behavioural similarities between kindled seizures and seizures elicited during repeated episodes of ethanol intoxication–withdrawal, there is some evidence to suggest that cross-sensitization exists between the two categories of cyclic CNS excitation. Several studies have indicated that repeated electrical stimulation (kindling) of the brain potentiates the effect of subsequent alcohol withdrawal and increases seizure frequency; similarly ethanol exposure has been suggested to accelerate the rate of electrical kindling (see discussion by Brown et al., 1988). We have obtained confirmatory evidence (unpublished data) that fewer kindling stimuli are necessary to induce stage 5 kindled seizures in animals that have previously been subjected to multiple episodes of ethanol intoxication–withdrawal as compared with animals subjected to a single intoxication–withdrawal episode. In a group of six animals that had developed spontaneous seizures during multiple episodes of intoxication and withdrawal fully kindled seizures were established by six or fewer kindling stimuli (amygdala) in four of the animals. Such a rapid kindling effect has not been reported in normal rats.

Recently we have studied the possible relationship between withdrawal seizures and regional changes in cerebral glucose metabolism measured during a subsequent withdrawal phase (Clemmesen *et al.*, 1988). By means of the [^{14}C]2-deoxyglucose method, regional glucose consumption was determined in rat brains during withdrawal from a single 2-day intoxication episode as compared to withdrawal from 10 previous episodes. The regional glucose consumption was reduced by 18–31% in the cortical and most limbic regions during withdrawal, this being independent of the number of previous episodes. Two weeks after withdrawal from the 10th episode, the regional glucose consumption did not differ from control values, i.e. the suppression recorded during withdrawal was completely reversible. When the animals were grouped according to the occurrence of spontaneous and audiogenic seizures during previous ethanol intoxication–withdrawal episodes, we found that animals with previous spontaneous withdrawal seizures had a significantly more pronounced suppression of glucose metabolism in the amygdala as compared with other regions of the brain. Animals experiencing audiogenic seizures had a significantly more pronounced suppression of glucose consumption in auditory cortex, medial geniculate body, inferior colliculus, temporal cortex and cingulate cortex. Even though in this study the number of animals was small ($n = 4$ in each group), the result is remarkable because the amygdala is the most sensitive region of the brain as far as electrical kindling is concerned and it is assumed to play an essential role in the development of seizures. In addition, the regions with the lowest glucose metabolism in animals with previous audiogenic seizures represent part of the auditory system of the CNS (auditory cortex, medial geniculate body, inferior colliculus). Thus animals with cumulated CNS dysfunction expressed as seizures have significant and regionally specific physiological changes in addition to the general metabolic suppression occurring during the withdrawal reaction in the rat. The explanation for the stronger suppression in the regions relating to seizures can only be hypothetical: it may be analogous to the regional interictal suppression seen in patients with a focus in temporal lobe epilepsy.

The results from the animal studies described are reconcilable with the two-component hypothesis for the clinical withdrawal reaction suggested above: the non-convulsive/non-psychotic components of withdrawal may be determined by the most recent episode of physical dependence, whereas the convulsive component (and possibly the psychotic component) may be due to a longstanding or irreversible cumulative component, where the most recent intoxication–withdrawal episode just serves as an eliciting factor.

It is tempting to compare these data with the various types of severe withdrawal phenomena seen in patients. Except for reference to a general predisposition, it is not possible to explain why some patients experience seizures, some patients experience visual hallucinosis, some patients experience delirium tremens, and some patients experience auditory hallucinosis as the main feature of withdrawal. Hypothetically, it may be suggested that regional variation of CNS sensitivity to the effect of repeated withdrawal–excitation, combined with external stimuli may determine which part of the central nervous system will ultimately be responsible for the dominant clinical features of withdrawal in each single patient. Combining the clinical and experimental data one might suggest that individuals experiencing withdrawal seizures have an involvement of the amygdala as a main component in the mechanism of disease whereas, for example, withdrawal with acute auditory hallucinosis may involve mainly the auditory system. It may be possible to perform new experiments to test whether stimulation of various neuronal pathways during withdrawal reactions may lead to dominance of that specific pathway in the cerebral dysfunction noted during episodes of ethanol intoxication and withdrawal.

It should be underlined that even though the evidence favours the withdrawal reaction as the main determinant in the development of longstanding CNS dysfunction, a role of the repeated intoxication episodes cannot be ruled out at the present time.

Table 3 summarizes the relationship between electrical kindling and repeated episodes of ethanol intoxication and withdrawal. In both conditions the amygdala is involved as a highly sensitive region. Behaviourally, the spontaneous seizures which develop bear strong resemblances. The most 'effective' stimulus interval is within the same limits, and there is some evidence to suggest that cross-sensitization exists between electrical kindling and repeated episodes of ethanol intoxication and withdrawal (Bolwig,

Table 3. List of characteristics concerning electrical amygdala kindling and multiple episodes of ethanol intoxication and withdrawal

	Electrical amygdala kindling	Multiple episodes of ethanol intoxication and withdrawal
1. Amygdala highly sensitive	+	(+)
2. Seizures of partial clonic type (Racine, 1972; grade 3–5)	+	+
3. Stimulus interval 1–7 days	+	+
4. Cross-sensitization	+	+
5. Neuronal damage	(−)	(−)
6. Irreversible	+	?
7. Neurobiological mechanism	?	?

Parallels and unclarified issues are summarized. Discussion is given in the text.

personal communication). Neither condition is accompanied by marked neuronal damage although it must be stressed that our (unpublished) data concerning neuropathological changes after multiple intoxication and withdrawal episodes are quantitatively limited. Electrical kindling causes irreversible changes of CNS excitability. The issue of reversibility has not been settled as far as ethanol withdrawal is concerned.

Several antiepileptic drugs, i.e. diazepam, carbamazepine and barbiturates, are able to suppress electrical amygdala kindling (see Weiss *et al.*, 1985). It is less clear whether pharmacological interference is able to prevent the progression of CNS dysfunction during repeated ethanol intoxication and withdrawal episodes. Recently Brown *et al.* (1988) have suggested that although benzodiazepines may be effective inhibiting the acute withdrawal reaction it does not necessarily mean that benzodiazepines are able to prevent the 'repetition effect'. Hypothetically it may be suggested that some types of pharmacological interference (e.g. receptor-specific drug actions) may modify only parts of the withdrawal reaction that relate to that specific receptor or neurotransmitter system. Hence the possibility remains that complete inhibition of the progressive 'repetition effect' demands treatment with general CNS suppressants that exhibit complete cross-dependence with ethanol i.e. the barbiturates.

In conclusion, the concept of kindling has been a fruitful instrument in studying the progression of the ethanol withdrawal reaction over time. Furthermore, specific knowledge about kindling mechanisms may be helpful in future studies concerning prevention and treatment of the progressive and longstanding effects of repeated ethanol intoxication and withdrawal.

REFERENCES

Ballenger, J. C. and Post, R. M. (1978). Kindling as a model for alcohol withdrawal syndomes. *Br. J. Psychiat.*, **133**, 1–14.

Brown, M. E., Anton, R. F., Malcolm, R. and Ballenger, J. C. (1988). Alcohol detoxification and withdrawal seizures: clinical support for a kindling hypothesis. *Biol. Psychiat.*, **23**, 507–514.

Clemmesen, L. and Hemmingsen, R. (1984). Physical dependence on ethanol during multiple intoxication and withdrawal episodes in the rat: evidence of a potentiation. *Acta Pharmacol. Toxicol.*, **55**, 345–350.

Clemmesen, L., Ingvar, M., Hemmingsen, R. and Bolwig, T. G. (1988). Local cerebral glucose consumption during ethanol withdrawal in the rat: effects of single and multiple episodes and previous convulsive seizures. *Brain Res.*, **453**, 204–214.

Goddard, G. V., McIntyre, D. C. and Leech, C. K. (1969). A permanent change in brain function resulting from daily electrical stimulation. *Exp. Neurol.*, **25**, 295–350.

Hemmingsen, R. and Kramp, P. (1988). Delirium tremens and related clinical states: psychopathology, cerebral pathophysiology and psychochemistry: a two-component hypothesis concerning etiology and pathogenesis. *Acta Psychiat. Scand. Suppl.*, **345**, 94–107.

Hemmingsen, R., Vorstrup, S., Clemmesen, L., Holm, S., Tfelt-Hansen, P.,

Sørensen, A. G., Hansen, C., Sommer, W. and Bolwig, T. G. (1988). Cerebral blood flow during delirium tremens and related clinical states studied with Xenon–133 inhalation tomography. *Am. J. Psychiat.* (in press).

Kramp, P. and Rafaelsen, O. J. (1978). Delirium tremens: A double-blind comparison of diazepam and barbital treatment. *Acta Psychiat. Scand.*, **58**, 174–190.

Majchrowicz, E. and Hunt, W. A. (1976). Temporal relationship of the induction of tolerance and physical dependence after continuous intoxication with maximum tolerable doses of ethanol in rats. *Psychopharmacologia*, **50**, 107–112.

Racine, R. J. (1972). Modification of seizure activity by electrical stimulation II: motor seizure. *Electroencephalorg. Clin. Neurophysiol.*, **32**, 281–294.

Surawicz, F. G. (1980). Alcoholic hallucinosis: A missed diagnosis. *Canad. J. Psychiat.*, **25**, 57–63.

Ulrichsen, J., Clemmesen, L., Barry, D. and Hemmingsen, R. (1988). The GABA/benzodiazepine receptor chloride channel complex during repeated episodes of physical ethanol dependence in the rat. *Psychopharmacology*, **96**, 227–231.

Victor, M. (1973). The role of hypomagnesemia and respiratory alkalosis in the genesis of alcohol withdrawal symptoms. *Ann. N.Y. Acad. Sci.*, **215**, 235–248.

Victor, M. and Adams, R. D. (1953). The effect of alcohol on the nervous system. *Res. Publ. Assoc. Res. Nerv. Ment. Dis.*, **32**, 526–573.

Weiss, S. R. B., Post, R. M., Patel, J. and Marangos, P. J. (1985). Differential mediation of the anticonvulsant effects of carbamazepine and diazepam. *Life Sci.*, **36**, 2413–2419.

Storm, T., Caird, W. K. and Korbin, T. G. (1965) Short Term memory. ...

Tarter, R. E. ...

Wallgren, H. and Barry, H. (1970) Actions of Alcohol. Amsterdam, Elsevier ...

...

The Clinical Relevance of Kindling
Edited by T. G. Bolwig and M. R. Trimble
© 1989 John Wiley & Sons Ltd

Discussion — Session 3

KINDLING, AGGRESSION AND PERSONALITY

C. Wasterlain Dr Adamec, if the time course of acquisition of the behavioural changes is different from the time course of acquisition of kindling, what does that imply for the relationship between the two phenomena?

R. Adamec I do not think that much kindling is produced in my cats, in the sense of increasing epileptogenesis. I think what that suggests is that the behavioural changes are not dependent on those mechanisms that increase the epileptic disorder in the animal. My belief is LTP-like changes underlie the behavioural alterations. This is a secondary effect of the limbic disorder. I suspect that LTP is not involved in kindling, but some other mechanism is.

E. H. Reynolds Dr Edeh and Dr Toone did a community-based study of psychopathology in epilepsy, and they used the Clinical Interview Schedule. Your figure was rather similar to their figure for psychopathology in this community-based population of epileptic patients. Now, these were patients with what they called active, continuing epilepsy, and certainly, depression and anxiety figured very prominently in their findings; but they did have three groups of patients. One they classified as primarily generalized epilepsy. They had two groups of patients with partial epilepsy: one they called temporal lobe, and another group non-temporal lobe. They found much more psychopathology in both 'partial' groups. There were very few differences between the two 'partial' groups. Patients with partial epilepsy have more brain pathology, they have more frequent seizures, it is more difficult to control seizures and they take more drugs. These factors are all important in the development of the psychopathology.

R. Adamec Yes, they are contributing factors. We were intrigued by the 24.6%, because there are at least four different studies from 1960 until the present, which have listed between 25 and 35% of epileptics studied to be significantly disturbed.

E. Brodtkorb Dr Hemmingsen, can you tell me if repeated withdrawal seizures may kindle real epilepsy with spontaneous seizures in humans?

R. Hemmingsen I don't know.

L. Gram No, I don't think so. But Dr Hemmingsen you talked about spontaneous seizures. Were these seizures all occurring during the withdrawal period, or after?

R. Hemmingsen We videotaped the animals for a fixed time period, and this was at the peak of the withdrawal reaction. That means from the 10th to the 13th hour, around the 12th hour after last dose. They may have had other seizures which were unseen.

L. Gram In epileptology we would not call them spontaneous seizures.

M. Schmutz There is one point which strikes me as important; the fact that behaviour on one hand and seizures or EEG discharges on the other seem to be two quite different things. First of all, Dr Hemmingsen observed that when he kindled he had on one hand EEG and on the other the behaviour stages. Both events do not develop in parallel, and there are differences. Secondly, he observed that drugs affect both things differently. He also stated that with regard to behaviour, he did not find kindling with non-convulsive alcohol withdrawal behaviour, but he did find it with regard to the seizures. J. Mellanby told us that the EEG signs, or after-discharges, ceased much more rapidly in her model than the behavioural symptoms. Dr Adamec told us that the mechanisms responsible for the behavioural changes in his model are presumably not the same as those responsible for the seizures.

R. Hemmingsen When it comes to patients there is also not a very clear relationship between EEG changes and the non-convulsive component of the major withdrawal reactions.

The Clinical Relevance of Kindling
Edited by T. G. Bolwig and M. R. Trimble
© 1989 John Wiley & Sons Ltd

10

The process of epilepsy: is kindling relevant?

E. H. REYNOLDS
Maudsley and King's College Hospitals, London SE5, UK

INTRODUCTION

In this review I will develop a theme which has arisen from longitudinal studies of newly diagnosed epileptic patients by myself and my colleagues in the last 15 years, namely that epilepsy should be viewed as a process in which each seizure leaves its mark on the nervous system and influences subsequent prognosis (Reynolds, Elwes and Shorvon, 1983; Shorvon and Reynolds, 1986; Reynolds, 1987). This concept of epilepsy has potentially important implications for treatment and perhaps also for prevention (Reynolds, Elwes and Shorvon, 1983; Reynolds, 1988a). Although much that I will discuss is concerned with acceleration or escalation of epilepsy over time, there are two sides to the coin, as the brain generates inhibitory as well as excitataory processes. I will therefore also touch upon processes of remission of epilepsy.

The view of epilepsy which I will elaborate was in fact first hinted at by Gowers (1881) in his classic monograph on *Epilepsy and Other Chronic Convulsive Diseases*. Here he proposed that:

When one attack has occurred whether in apparent consequence of an immediate excitant or not, others usually follow without any immediate traceable course. The effect of a convulsion on the nerve centres is such as to render the occurrence of another more easy, to intensify the predisposition that already exists. Thus every fit may be said to be in part, the result of those which preceded it, the cause of those which follow it. The search for the causes of epilepsy must thus be chiefly an investigation into the conditions which precede the occurrence of the first fit.

Gowers' concept that seizures may beget more seizures was ignored or lost sight of until we came across it during the early part of our studies. The history of the drug treatment of epilepsy throughout this century confirms that his concept and its implications played no part in contemporary thinking. Indeed, until we began our studies of newly diagnosed patients in 1974, studies of the drug treatment of epilepsy had been conducted almost wholly in chronic patients (Shorvon, 1983).

I have called Gowers' concept 'The Gowers' Phenomenon' (Reynolds, 1981). Whether the process he envisaged has anything to do with kindling is not clear to me. Kindling is concerned with subclinical stimuli and the generation of the first seizure, whereas Gowers was concerned with the impact of seizures themselves and events after the first attack. He would however have seen, as we do, the analogies or parallels with kindling. He would probably have been intrigued by the concept and in his exhortation to search for the causes of epilepsy in events prior to the first seizure he may well have suspected, as we might, that the answers could be found in the kindling process.

THE NATURAL HISTORY OF UNTREATED EPILEPSY

Is there any evidence for 'The Gowers' Phenomenon'? One of the great difficulties in investigating this at the clinical level is that we remain ignorant about the natural history of untreated epilepsy, as standard practise for a century or more has dictated that treatment is initiated when a patient presents with two or more seizures, except in rare circumstances. My colleagues and I have attempted a limited study of the natural history of untreated epilepsy by retrospectively examining the time intervals between fits in patients presenting to the neurological department at King's College Hospital with between two and five untreated tonic–clonic seizures (Elwes, Johnson and Reynolds, 1988).

This sort of study, which depends on retrospective collection of data, can only be undertaken for tonic–clonic seizures, i.e. events of sufficient severity and emotional impact as to be reliably remembered by patients. Partial attacks, absences and myoclonic jerks, tend to occur much more frequently, may not be recalled and cannot be reliably dated, and were therefore excluded from the study. Partial attacks which were secondarily generalized, i.e. tonic–clonic, were included. Patients whose seizures were caused by drugs, alcohol, fever, acute metabolic disturbances or progressive neurological disease were excluded.

Table 1 summaries the 183 patients with two to five untreated tonic–clonic seizures included in the study. Table 2 summaries the time intervals between the first and second seizure in all 183 patients. In 31% the second attack occurred within 1 month of the first; in 51% within 3 months, and in 87% within 1 year. Table 3 illustrates the corresponding data for the time intervals

Table 1. Characteristics of 183 patients with two or more untreated tonic–clonic seizures

	n (%)
Male	99 (54)
Symptomatic Epilepsy	20 (11)
Neurological Handicap	18 (10)
Median age at first seizure years (range)	17 (2–65)
Pretreatment seizure number	
Two	101 (55)
Three	53 (29)
Four	18 (10)
Five	11 (6)
Median pretreatment interval months (range)	6 (1–132)
(95% confidence interval)	(5–8)
Median pretreatment seizure frequency, seizures per month (range)	0.5 (0.003–3)
(95%) confidence interval)	(0.33–0.56)

Elwes, Johnson and Reynolds (1988).

Table 2. Interval between first and second untreated tonic–clonic seizures in 183 patients

Interval between first two seizures	n (%)
Equal to or less than 1 month	56 (31)
Between 1 and 2 months	19 (10)
Between 2 and 3 months	18 (10)
Between 3 and 12 months	66 (36)
Between 1 and 2 years	14 (8)
Between 2 and 3 years	4 (20)
Greater than 3 years	6 (3)
Totals	183 (100)

Elwes, Johnson and Reynolds (1988).

Table 3. Interval between the first and second severe fit in 160 cases of epilepsy

Less than 1 week	18	} 55 cases under 1 month
1 week to 1 month	37	
1 month to 3 months	13	} 52 cases more than a month and less than a year
3 months to 6 months	21	
6 months to 1 year	18	
1 year to 2 years	18	} 53 cases more than a year
2 years to 3 years	6	
3 years to 5 years	7	
Over 5 years	22	

Gowers (1881).

between the first two seizures in Gowers' series of 160 patients. He too found that in one third the second attack occurred within one month; two thirds of his patients had the second seizure within one year.

Table 4 shows the median time intervals between successive seizures for our series of 183 patients as a whole, as well as for patients with three, four or five seizures separately. For all patients the median interval between successive seizures appeared to decrease with each seizure that occurred. The median interval between the first and second seizure was 12 weeks (95% confidence limit: 10 and 18 weeks), between the second and third it was 8 weeks (4 and 12 weeks), between the third and fourth it was 4 weeks (2 and 20 weeks) and between the fourth and fifth it was 3 weeks (1 and 4 weeks). When patients with three, four or five pretreatment seizures were considered separately similar results were obtained, but with wider 95% confidence limits.

Table 4. Median inter-seizure intervals (weeks) in untreated patients with tonic–clonic seizures

	All ($n = 183$)	Pretreatment seizure number			
		2 ($n = 101$)	3 ($n = 53$)	4 ($n = 18$)	5 ($n = 11$)
	Median inter-seizure interval weeks (25th to 75th centiles) (95% CL16)				
1st to 2nd seizure	12 (4–28)	12 (4–25)	12 (4–44)	22 (4–36)	24 (4–42)
2nd to 3rd seizure	8 (4–16)	–	8 (4–16)	16 (4–40)	4 (4–12)
3rd to 4th seizure	4 (2–23)	–	–	6 (2–24)	4 (2–20)
4th to 5th seizure	3 (2–4)	–	–	–	3 (2–4)

Elwes, Johnson and Reynolds (1988).

Eighty-two patients experienced at least three untreated seizures; in these patients the interval from the first to the second seizure was on average 18 weeks longer than the interval between the second and third, with 95% confidence limits at 5 and 31 weeks. In the 29 patients who experienced at least four untreated seizures the mean difference between the second interval (seizure 2–3) and the third interval (seizure 3–4) was 4 weeks with 95% confidence limits at 9 weeks and 17 weeks.

The majority of patients were treated following the second or third seizure. However it was possible to compare the interval between any two seizures with that between the subsequent two in 82 patients. The interval decreased in three fifths, remained the same in one fifth and increased in one fifth.

Within the limitations imposed on the study of untreated epilepsy by ethical and practical considerations our findings are in keeping with the observations and views of Gowers. Thus in many patients referred to a neurological clinic with tonic–clonic seizures an accelerating disease process may occur, at least in the early stages. It seems that once a major attack has occurred the brain may more readily undergo a further attack, as Gowers proposed. This is not an invariable phenomenon, nor does it go on *ad infinitum*. Gowers reported that in 680 patients with confirmed epilepsy, most of whom were untreated, the interval between seizures did not exceed 1 month in 80%. It is therefore of interest that in those few patients in our study who had had more than three seizures the median interval between them was roughly 1 month. As well as processes of acceleration of epilepsy the brain may generate processes of remission (*vide infra*).

THE PROGNOSIS OF NEWLY DIAGNOSED EPILEPSY

The picture described above of an accelerating disease process in many untreated patients with tonic–clonic seizures contrasts rather strikingly with the results of antiepileptic drug treatment, which for most newly diagnosed patients are very good.

My colleagues and I first reported the potential for carefully monitored monotherapy in newly referred patients in 1976 (Reynolds, Chadwick and Galbraith, 1986). Since then we have followed prospectively 108 patients newly referred with two or more untreated tonic–clonic and or partial seizures who were treated with either phenytoin or carbamazepine monotherapy (Elwes *et al.*, 1984). Figure 1 shows the 1- and 2-year remission curves for the whole series after a median duration of follow-up of 66 months (range 6–98 months). Seventy-three per cent were in 1-year remission by 2 years of follow-up, 88% by 4 years and 92% by 8 years; the pattern for 2-year remission rates was similar, with 73% in 2-year remission by 4 years of follow-up and 82% by 8 years. There were 79 patients in whom seizures were controlled for 2 years and subsequent follow-up data were available in 76; 51% remained completely seizure-free for the rest of follow-up; 25 had a recurrence of seizures, which consisted of only two attacks in 17 and was related to poor compliance in 16.

Other studies of shorter duration for periods of up to 2 years and utilizing various antiepileptic drugs have confirmed the good prognosis for newly diagnosed patients (Shorvon, 1984; Mattson *et al.*, 1985; Reynolds, 1987). Furthermore, there is no evidence that any one of the major antiepileptic drugs has superior efficacy to any other that is appropriate for the seizure type that is being treated (Mattson *et al.*, 1985; Chadwick and Turnbull, 1985; Reynolds, 1987). What is apparent, however, is the contrast between the generally good results of treatment in newly diagnosed patients and the uniformly poor outcome with the same drugs in chronic patients (Rodin, 1968; Reynolds, 1987). This poses questions about the evolution of chronic epilepsy (Reynolds, Elwes and Shorvon, 1983).

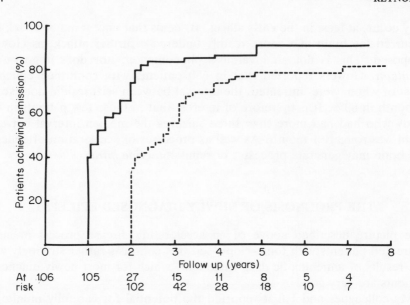

Figure 1. One- and 2-year remission rates in new referrals with epilepsy treated with monotherapy. Actuarial percentage of patients completely free of seizures for 1 year (——) and 2 years (----). [Reproduced with permission from Elwes *et al*. (1984)]

HOW DOES EPILEPSY BECOME CHRONIC?

There are two conflicting, but not necessarily mutually exclusive views about the development of chronic epilepsy (Reynolds, 1988a). The traditional view is that some patients are endowed with or acquire more 'severe' epilepsy from the start, the chronicity being the inevitable outcome of the inadequacy of the presently available treatment for such 'severe' epilepsy. However the concept of 'severe' epilepsy is a difficult one that has never been very clearly defined, perhaps because it would require the prolonged observation of untreated patients, which for obvious reasons has never been undertaken. Besides which it seems that some patients can at different times have either 'severe' or 'mild' epilepsy.

An alternative view is that epilepsy should be viewed as a process (Reynolds, Elwes and Shorvon, 1983; Shorvon and Reynolds, 1986; Reynolds, 1987). According to this view, epilepsy may escalate out of control and become chronic unless effectively treated at the onset, i.e. 'arrested' to use Gowers' (1881) much neglected word. It should be emphasized that according to this more dynamic view of epilepsy, it is possible for the disorder to remit spontaneously, as is well known to occur, for example, in petit mal or benign rolandic epilepsy of childhood.

In our prospective study of the treatment of newly diagnosed epilepsy described above (Elwes *et al.*, 1984), we confirmed that several factors, such as partial seizures compared to tonic–clonic seizures, and the presence of neurological, psychological and social handicaps, may contribute to a less satisfactory prognosis. Such factors had already been noted to adversely influence prognosis in studies of chronic patients (Rodin, 1968). However, we were also concerned to examine the influence of early treatment on prognosis, as it appeared that in the 21% of patients who failed to respond to treatment with optimum monotherapy nearly all went on to develop chronic epilepsy within the first 2 years of the treatment. Furthermore the most significant association with failure of monotherapy was poor compliance (Chesterman, Elwes and Reynolds, 1987). Figure 2 shows the 1-year remission curves for all our 106 patients and separately for these patients still having seizures after 1 and 2 years of treatment respectively (Elwes *et al.*, 1984). For patients still having seizures after 2 years of treatment the subsequent 1-year remission rate was approximately half that of the whole series.

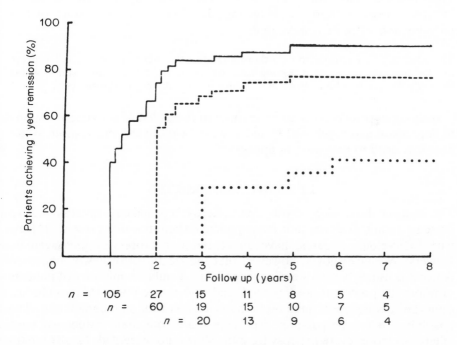

Figure 2. Influence of duration of seizures on 1-year remission rates in new referrals with epilepsy. All patients from start of treatment (——), patients with seizures in the first year of follow-up (----), and patients with seizures in the first 2 years of follow-up (· · ·). [Reproduced with permission from Elwes *et al.* (1984)]

REMISSION IN EPILEPSY

There seems little doubt that some forms of epilepsy, especially in childhood, may go into spontaneous remission. Petit mal and benign Rolandic epilepsy of childhood are classic examples. Perhaps maturational factors in the nervous system are important, but it is also plausible that in childhood and in the adult the brain may generate processes of inhibition as well as the putative excitatory mechanisms I have discussed.

An interesting experimental phenomenon is the resistance to seizures that can be demonstrated immediately following a convulsion (Herberg, Tress and Blundell, 1969; Green, Nutt and Cowan, 1981). Clinically it reminds one of those epileptic subjects who, following a seizure or bout of seizures, can be reasonably confident that they will not have another attack for a certain interval, which varies between patients, but is usually consistent in the individual. A variant which I have observed is the patient with frequent, perhaps daily complex partial seizures who, following a rare tonic–clonic seizure, may not have another complex partial seizure for a month or more. The tonic–clonic seizure seems to clear the system and prevent the minor attacks at least temporarily. Hughlings Jackson (1873) was aware of this phenomenon when he commented:

The other day I congratulated a mother on the fact that her son had not had a severe fit. She however regretted it, saying that the severe fit 'cleared the system', whilst the slight fits rendered him from their frequency unable to go to business.

Is this phenomenon related in any way to the action of convulsive therapy in depression and psychosis? Could any extension of this mechanism, whatever it is, lead to remission in epilepsy?

EPILEPSY AS A PROCESS

The concept developed here is that epilepsy is a dynamic process. I have presented some evidence that many patients when they first present, at least with tonic–clonic seizures, have an accelerating process as envisaged by Gowers. We have shown, however, that the treatment of newly diagnosed patients is usually very rewarding, except in a significant minority of patients in whom the process is not 'arrested' and who evolve into a state of chronic drug resistant epilepsy, quite often in association with poor compliance. The possibility that some patients, especially those with brain pathology, have inherently more severe epilepsy from the start is not excluded. Finally inhibitory processes may contribute to remission in some patients. This view of epilepsy has some important practical implications.

(1) The approach to and outcome of treatment will vary according to the

stage in the longitudinal evolution of the disorder that has been reached. The contrast between the good results of antiepileptic drug treatment in the newly diagnosed patient and the poor outcome with the same drugs in chronic patients is clear (Rodin, 1986; Reynolds, 1988a).

(2) The possibility arises that early effective treatment in the newly diagnosed patient may arrest the epilepsy and prevent the evolution of chronic epilepsy (Reynolds, Elwes and Shorvon, 1983; Reynolds, 1987, 1988a).

(3) In view of the potential importance of early treatment for epilepsy the question whether or not to treat a single seizure requires urgent and careful evaluation. The literature on the prognosis of a single unprovoked seizure has been controversial (Hauser, 1986; Elwes and Reynolds, 1988). I have discussed elsewhere the reasons for the controversy, which can to a large extent be explained by the varying time intervals between the single seizure and the entry into the several different single seizure studies (Reynolds, 1988b). Epidemiological studies in any case suggest that less than 25% of seizures remain single (Reynolds, 1988b). The management of a single seizure, however, remains uncertain for lack of any adequate treatment study.

(4) Finally an interesting question is whether antiepileptic drug therapy in addition to suppressing seizures enhances the prospects for natural remission of epilepsy?

THE RELEVANCE OF KINDLING

Is the process of accelerating epilepsy which I have discussed related in any way to the phenomenon of kindling? There must be some doubt about this if kindling is defined in terms of the experimental (and possibly clinical) effects of repeated subclinical stimuli which culminate in the occurrence of the first seizure. The events I have been concerned with occur after the first seizure. Is this an extension of kindling or a completely different phenomenon? Although recurrent spontaneous seizures have been described in the kindling model in some species this aspect seems to have received less attention. Furthermore, for the most part kindling studies are undertaken in animals which are not genetically predisposed to spontaneous seizures, whereas a genetic background of varying degree is widely suspected in clinical epilepsy.

For the time being it seems appropriate to consider the 'Gowers' Phenomenon' as separate and distinct from kindling even though the analogies between the two are readily apparent and probably would have fascinated Gowers. Both take a longitudinal view of seizure processes over time. In the case of kindling it is the impact of suitably spaced successive subclinical stimuli (SSSSS) that is the key. In the Gowers' Phenomenon we are concerned with the effect of suitably spaced successive seizures (SSSS). Exactly how each stimulus leaves its mark on the nervous system in kindling is unknown but if a subclinical stimulus can leave its unidentified but undoubted imprint is it not reasonable to suppose that a seizure itself can do something similar? (Reynolds, 1988a). Perhaps both phenomena have more in common with memory and learning. In the former the brain is 'learning' to develop a seizure, in the latter 'learning' to have more seizures. In both processes 'inhibitory' phenomena come into play which is why the spacing of the stimuli or the seizures is important.

If kindling can be viewed as a model at least for the development of the *first* seizure in epilepsy what could kindle a seizure in man? Presumably several different kinds of stimuli might operate, but one naturally occurring candidate, for example, is folic acid, or one of its derivatives. Following reports of the exacerbation of seizures by the vitamin in some patients with epilepsy (Reynolds, 1967) several studies in different species have confirmed the excitatory properties of folate derivatives, especially on circumventing the blood–brain barrier (Hommes *et al.*, 1979). Miller, Goff and Webster (1979) reported that folic acid enhances electrical kindling in the rat, and later O'Donnell, Leech and Miller (1983) showed that the vitamin itself can be used to kindle seizures. At the synaptic level folic acid appears to block GABA inhibition (Otis, Madison and Nicoll, 1985; Van Rijn *et al.*, 1988).

Finally, Post and I agree that there is a remarkable similarity between the clinical phenomena I have been describing above in epilepsy and that described by him and his colleagues in Chapter 14 for manic depressive illness. For seizures, substitute manic or depressive episodes. Post too takes the longitudinal view and observes in many patients increasingly rapid cycling as the intervals between episodes shorten. As in epilepsy the nature of the underlying disorder changes with each episode implying the need for different therapeutic strategies at different stages. Is this another example of a 'learning' phenomenon? Probably, for both disorders early treatment is important to prevent the development of the chronic more drug-resistant disease (Reynolds, Elwes and Shorvon, 1983; Reynolds, 1988a). Both disorders are examples of a dynamic neurology.

REFERENCES

Chadwick, D. and Turnbull, D. M. (1985). The comparative efficacy of antiepileptic drugs. *J. Neurol. Neuosurg. Psychiat.*, **48**, 1073.
Chesterman, P., Elwes, R. D. C. and Reynolds, E. H. (1987). Failure of monotherapy in newly diagnosed epilepsy. In: *The XVIth Epilepsy International Symposium. Advances in Epileptology*, Vol. 16 (eds P. Wolf, M. Dam, D. Janz and F. E. Dreifuss), pp. 461–464. Raven Press, New York.
Elwes, R. D. C. and Reynolds, E. H. (1988). Should people be treated after a first seizure? *Arch. Neurol.*, **45**, 490–491.

Elwes, R. D. C., Johnson, A. L., Reynolds, E. H. (1988). The course of untreated epilepsy. *Br. Med. J.*, **297**, 948–950.

Elwes, R. D. C., Johnson, A. L., Shorvon, S. D. and Reynolds, E. H. (1984). The prognosis for seizure control in newly diagnosed epilepsy. *N. Engl. J. Med.*, **311**, 944–947.

Gowers, W. R. (1881). *Epilepsy and Other Chronic Convulsive Diseases*. Churchill, London.

Green, A. R., Nutt, D. J. and Cowan, P. H. (1981). The increased seizure threshhold following convulsion. In: *The Psychopharmacology of Anticonvulsants* (ed. M. Sandler). Oxford University Press, Oxford.

Hauser, W. A. (1986). Should people be treated after a first seizure? *Arch. Neurol.*, **43**, 1287–1288.

Herberg, L. J., Tress, K. H. and Blundell, J. E. (1969). Raising the threshhold in experimental epilepsy by hypothalamic and septal stimulation and by audiogenic seizures. *Brain*, **92**, 313–328.

Hommes, O. R., Hollinger, J. L., Jansen, M. J. T., Schoofs, M., van der Weil, Th. and Kok, J. C. N. (1979). Convulsant properties of folate compounds: some considerations and speculations. In: *Folic Acid in Neurology, Psychiatry, and Internal Medicine* (eds M. I. Botez and E. H. Reynolds), pp. 285–316. Raven Press, New York.

Jackson, J. H. (1873). On the anatomical, physiological, and pathological investigation of epilepsies. *Rep. West Riding Lunatic Asylum*, **3**, 315–339.

Mattson, R. H., Cramer, J. A., Collins, J. F., Smith, D. B., Delgado-Escueta, A. V., Browne, T. R., Williamson, P. D., Treiman, D. M., McNamara, J. O., McCutchen, C. B., Homan, R. W., Crill, W. E., Lubozynski, M. F., Rosenthal, N. P. and Mayersdord, A. (1985). A comparison of carbamazepine, phenobarbital, phenytoin and primidone in partial and secondarily generalized tonic–clonic seizures. *N. Engl. J. Med.*, **313**, 145–151.

Miller, A. A., Goff, D. and Webster, R. A. (1979). Pre-disposition of laboratory animals to epileptogenic activity of Folic Acid. In: *Folic Acid in Neurology, Psychiatry, and Internal Medicine* (eds M. I. Botez and E. H. Reynolds), pp. 331–334. Raven Press, New York.

O'Donnell, R. A., Leach, M. J. and Miller, A. A. (1983). Folic acid induced kindling in rats: changes in brain amino acids. In: *Chemistry and Biology of Pteridines* (ed. J. A. Blair). Walter de Gruyter, Berlin.

Otis, L. C., Madison, D. V. and Nicoll, R. A. (1985). Folic acid has a disinhibitory action in the rat hippocampal slice preparation. *Brain*, **346**, 281–286.

Reynolds, E. H. (1967). Effects of folic acid on the mental state and fit frequency of drug-treated epileptic patients. *Lancet*, **i**, 1086–1088.

Reynolds, E. H. (1981). Biological factors in psychological disorders associated with epilepsy. In: *Epilepsy, Psychiatry* (eds E. H. Reynolds and M. R. Trimble), pp. 264–290. Churchill Livingstone, Edinburgh.

Reynolds, E. H. (1987). Early treatment and prognosis of epilepsy. *Epilepsia*, **28**(2), 97–106.

Reynolds, E. H. (1988a). The prevention of chronic epilepsy. *Epilepsia*, **29** (Suppl. 1), S25–S28.

Reynolds, E. H. (1988b). A single seizure. *Br. Med. J.*, **297**, 1422–1423.

Reynolds, E. H., Chadwick, D. and Galbraith, A. W. (1976). One drug (phenytoin) in the treatment of epilepsy. *Lancet*, **i**, 923–926.

Reynolds, E. H., Elwes, R. D. C. and Shorvon, S. D. (1983). Why does epilepsy become intractable? Prevention of chronic epilepsy. *Lancet*, **ii**, 952–954.

Rodin, E. A. (1968). *The Prognosis of Patients with Epilepsy*. Charles C. Thomas, Springfield, Illinois.

Shorvon, S. D. (1983). Aspects of the methodology of clinical anticonvulsant trial design and a bibliography of phenytoin and carbamazepine studies. In: *Research Progress in Epilepsy* (ed. F. Clifford Rose), pp. 384–401. Pitman, London.

Shorvon, S. D. (1984). The temporal aspects of prognosis in epilepsy. *J. Neurol. Neurosurg. Psychiat.*, **47**, 1157–1165.

Shorvon, S. D. and Reynolds, E. H. (1986). The nature of epilepsy: evidence from studies of epidemiology, temporal patterns of seizures, prognosis and treatment. In: *What is Epilepsy?* (eds M. R. Trimble and E. H. Reynolds), pp. 36–45. Churchill Livingstone, Edinburgh.

Van Rijn, C. M., Van der Velden, T. J. A. M., Rodrigues de Miranda, J. F., Feenstra, M. G. P. and Hommes, O. R. (1988). The influence of folic acid on the picrotoxin-sensitive site of the GABA-receptor complex. *Epilepsy Res.*, **2**, 215–218.

11

The prognosis of epilepsy

MOGENS DAM and ANNE SABERS
*University Clinic of Neurology, Hvidovre Hospital, DK-2650 Hvidovre,
Denmark*

INTRODUCTION

The prognosis of epilepsy is not a very well described topic. The reason for this is not any paucity of prognostic studies, but principally because of methodological problems. The major problems concern definition and ascertainment. The quality of case ascertainment varies widely. The inadequacies of hospital and clinical data are well known. Less apparent are the variations in the quality of community surveys. The adequacy of sample frames is difficult to assess. The quality of data obtained from questionnaires may vary considerably and be difficult to measure.

When reviewing the many papers dealing with the prognosis of epilepsy, the following questions arise:

(1) Is the recurrence rate of seizures 21% (Hauser, 1983) or is it 71% (Elwes, Chesterman and Reynolds, 1985)?
(2) Is it likely that 80% of all epilepsy patients have a chronic seizure disorder (Rodin, 1968), or is it that 70% will be in 5-year remission if followed for 20 years (Annegers, Hauser and Elveback, 1979)?
(3) Or, even better, will 92% be in 1-year remission by 8 years (Reynolds, 1987a)?

These are some essential questions which will be discussed in this review.

THE RISK OF RECURRENCE AFTER A SINGLE SEIZURE

It is often stated that only about 30% of adult patients who experience a single, unprovoked seizure will have more. This figure is derived from several studies which differed in their selection of patients and in the use of antiepileptic drugs. The critical interval between first seizure and entry into a study is often not defined. If this interval is 1–2 days the fraction of first-seizure patients who subsequently develop epilepsy will be greater than if this interval is 1–2 months, during which time the occurrence of further seizures will exclude many patients from initial consideration. Forty per cent of recurrent seizures occur within 2 months of the initial seizure (Elwes, Chesterman and Reynolds, 1985; Hirtz, Ellenberg and Nelson, 1984; Camfield, Camfield and Dooley, 1985). Any delay between the initial seizure and study entry will thus exclude many patients from consideration.

Cleland et al. (1981) found a recurrence rate of 39%, with a mean time from first seizure to study inclusion of 6.5 weeks. Similarly, Saunders and Marshall (1975) found a recurrence rate of 33%, with the interval between first seizure and study inclusion being 6 weeks. Hauser (1983) reported the lowest rate of seizure recurrence, namely 21%. The majority of the patients were, however, treated with antiepileptic drugs after the first seizure. This might also have been the case in other studies with a low recurrence rate.

Elwes, Chesterman and Reynolds (1985) investigated 133 patients, who were untreated. They were included in the trial 1 day after the initial seizure and the recurrence rate was 71%. Hauser (1983) also studied 435 newly diagnosed patients who had had two or more seizures by the time of their initial evaluation. If these patients had been examined sooner, before their second seizure, 71% of the entire group of newly diagnosed seizures would have experienced a second seizure by 24 months. Although there may be an overrepresentation of multiple-seizure patients, because multiple seizures may predispose to medical attention, it is probable that some of the patients would have been referred for their first seizure, but experienced a second seizure before evaluation. In a population-based study, Goodridge and Shorvon (1983) found that only 18% experienced a single seizure.

It seems thus, that epileptic patients outnumber patients who experience only a single seizure (Hart and Easton, 1986). It may be concluded therefore, that someone with a first seizure has a significant risk of recurrence, usually within the first 6 months.

THE DEVELOPMENT OF EPILEPTIC ACTIVITY

In a study of the course of untreated epilepsy, the time intervals between untreated tonic–clonic seizures were examined retrospectively in a series of 183 patients who had had between two and five seizures. The median interval between the first two seizures was 12 weeks, between the second and third, 8 weeks, between the third and fourth, 4 weeks, and between the fourth and fifth, 3 weeks.

These results suggest that in many patients there is an accelerating disease process in the early stages of epilepsy. Reynolds has termed this 'The Gowers' effect', as it is in keeping with the view first proposed by Gowers (1881) that seizures may beget seizures, which means that once a major attack has occurred the brain may more readily undergo a further attack (Elwes, Johnson and Reynolds, 1988). These data, and this theme are explained more fully in Chapter 10.

PROGNOSIS OF EPILEPTIC SYNDROMES

Convulsions in the neonatal period

Convulsions in the neonatal period are of various etiologies. Eighty per cent are due to two main causes, anoxic-ischemic encephalopathy and transient metabolic disorders. Other rare causes include infections, malformations, and inborn errors of metabolism. The long-term prognosis of all neonatal convulsions is relatively severe with an incidence of approximately 23% mortality and of 29% long-term sequelae.

Patients who suffer from benign familial neonatal convulsions are usually born at full term and their perinatal course is uneventful; only 3% are born prematurely. In 82% the onset of seizures is on the second or third day of life. The range of onset is between the first day and 2 years of age. Either partial or generalized seizures, or cyanotic spells may be observed in the same patient. The frequency may vary from 1–40 per day. In 70% the entire convulsion period lasts between 1 and 6 weeks. The EEG is normal in 50%, and the remainder show either epileptic activity or nonspecific disturbances. The outcome is excellent in the majority of cases, with normal motor and mental development. Only 11% will later develop epilepsy (Dobrescu and Larbrisseau, 1982).

Febrile seizures

Febrile convulsions in the first year of life have a better prognosis than afebrile convulsions, even though the effects of the former generally are more serious at that age than if they commence in later years (Lennox-Buchthal, 1973). They recur in more than 75% of cases. Factors which worsen the prognosis are previous encephalopathy, onset of convulsions in the first 6 months of life and recurrence within the first year (Cavazzuti, Ferrari and Lalla, 1984).

The incidence of subsequent epilepsy in those who have experienced febrile seizures is of the order of 2–4%. Features associated with the likely development of later epilepsy include prolonged febrile seizures, partial seizures, repeated seizures, onset of seizures in the first year of life, previous cerebral injury, associated mental handicap, female sex, and a family history of epilepsy (O'Donohoe, 1985).

Infantile spasms (West's syndrome)

In a study of 286 infants (Lambroso, 1983) with infantile spasms followed for 6 years there were no statistical clues as to etiology or prognosis provided by the analysis of either the prevailing seizure patterns or the frequency. Onset below 3 months old carried a more unfavorable prognosis. The presence of preceding neurological impairment resulted in a worse outcome. Typical hypsarrhythmic EEG at the onset of infantile spasms was associated with a better prognosis than those cases with an atypical EEG. Less than 25% developed Lennox–Gastaut's syndrome.

Cases in a cryptogenic group treated with adrenocorticotropic hormone (ACTH) had a better prognosis than those treated with antiepileptic drugs or with oral steroids alone. Infants treated with ACTH within a month of onset of infantile spasms had a better prognosis than those whose ACTH therapy was delayed (Lombroso, 1983). The significance of early treatment with ACTH has been confirmed in other studies (Riikonen, 1984), although a recent study did not confirm that short versus long treatment lag, or response to therapy, had any influence on the outcome (Glaze *et al.*, 1988). All patients with cryptogenic infantile spasms who have no relapse after ACTH therapy develop normally, while there is no correlation between the relapse and the outcome in symptomatic cases (Matsumoto *et al.*, 1981).

About 90% of patients with infantile spasms of less than 1 month duration, treated with ACTH daily for 2 weeks, followed by alternate-day therapy for 3 months, show an excellent response, whereas only about 60% of those who have had spasms for more than 1 month become seizure free. Relapse occurred in 3.7% of the first group and 21.4% of the second (Singer, Rabe and Haller, 1980). The prevailing view is that the earlier the treatment is instituted, the better the chance of a complete remission.

The relapse rate for all ACTH-treated patients is about 50%. A second course of treatment is then indicated, but the probability of a good response is less with the second than with the first attempt (Lacy and Penry, 1976).

In over 80%, mental and neurological development will be affected. This gloomy prognosis holds for all the symptomatic and for more than half the cryptogenic forms (Cavazzuti, Ferrari and Lalla, 1984). In the symptomatic group, as little as 5% have normal development or only mild impairment.

The overall prognosis for long-term outcome in patients with infantile spasms is poor (Glaze *et al.*, 1988).

Lennox–Gastaut's syndrome

Long-term follow-up studies of patients with Lennox–Gastaut's syndrome have shown that regardless of the type of treatment, the proportion of patients whose seizures stop is greater when there is late onset than when seizure onset is in the first 2 years of life (Blume, David and Gomez, 1973).

Other main indicators of a poor prognosis are: symptomatic character of the syndrome, particularly following West's syndrome (Ohtahara, Yamatogi and Ohtsuka, 1976); high frequency of seizures; long duration of aggravation periods; recurrence of status epilepticus; existence of constant slow EEG background activity, associated with localized abnormalities and diffuse slow spike and waves (Beaumanoir, 1985).

Benign focal epilepsy

Thirty-seven of 40 patients with centro-temporal EEG foci were reinvestigated from 13–27 years after their first seizure, at ages of 26–34 years. Thirty-six had been seizure free for 14–23 years and no epileptic discharges were seen on EEG (Blom and Heijbel, 1982). The earlier the onset, the longer the period with seizures. In another study of 168 patients, 165 were seizure free with a follow-up range from 7–30 years. Only 2% experienced generalized tonic–clonic seizures many years later (Loiseau et al., 1988). The long-term prognosis of this common seizure disorder in children is therefore good (Blom and Heijbel, 1982).

A similar good prognosis is found in infantile epilepsy with an occipital focus. The duration of the active phase is between 3 and 7 years. Most of them have a family history of epilepsy, and there are many similarities with Rolandic paroxysms (Beaumanoir, 1983).

Pyknoleptic petit mal

Pyknoleptic petit mal is a childhood epilepsy syndrome with a favorable prognosis. Differing criteria of patient selection and lengths of follow-up make for confusion in the literature. Sato, Dreifuss and Penry (1976) found 78% of 23 patients who had absence seizures only, to be seizure-free after a follow-up period of 6–8 years. Comparable rates were obtained by Dalby (1969) and Livingstone et al. (1965) of 79%, while Fois, Malandrini and Mostardini (1987) found 84% of patients with pure petit mal to be free of seizures with normalization of EEG. Where there had been inadequate therapy clinical and EEG normalization was only obtained in 22%. The shorter the duration of seizures, the greater the likelihood of seizure resolution.

Good prognostic indicators are the absence of any seizure activity before onset of petit mal (Sato, Dreifuss and Penry, 1976), onset between 4–8 years (Livingstone *et al.*, 1965; Currier, Kooi and Saidman, 1963; Roger, 1974), prompt response to treatment (Sato, Dreifuss and Penry, 1976; Loiseau *et al.*, 1983), and normal intelligence and normal neurological examination (Sato, Dreifuss and Penry, 1976; Roger, 1974). Despite normal intelligence and a favorable response to treatment in the majority of cases, Hertoft (1963) and Loiseau *et al.* (1983) have described poor social adaptation in up to one third of these patients. The prognosis seems mainly related to adequate therapy and not to the presence of other types of seizures before or after the absences (Fois, Malandrini and Mostardini, 1987).

Juvenile myoclonic epilepsy

Seventy-five per cent of patients receiving at least 3 years' treatment for this syndrome, will be free of seizures for at least 2 years. Effective treatment does not mean definitive recovery. Relapses occur in 91% of cases when dosage is reduced or medication withdrawn after at least 2 years' treatment. Complete recovery appears to be virtually impossible in cases of juvenile myoclonic epilepsy once generalized convulsions have started (Janz, 1985).

PHOTOSENSITIVITY

In the study of Jeavons, Bishop and Harding (1986), of 18 patients not receiving drugs, 10 were no longer photosensitive at the age of 25 years, whilst 31 patients who remained photosensitive were aged 22 years. This seems to indicate that photosensitivity is more likely to disappear at the later age.

In 10 patients receiving valproate, all photosensitivity had disappeared 1 year later, without there having been any alteration in their medication; at that time their mean age was 23 years. It may thus be possible that their photosensitivity had disappeared spontaneously by that age.

GRAND MAL EPILEPSIES

Of 103 patients with primary grand mal, focal grand mal and indeterminate grand mal, followed for from 2–10 years, 40% were free of seizures and 23% had fewer than one seizure per year, without differences between the three groups. The appearance of partial seizures or absences during follow-up did not change the prognosis of tonic–clonic seizures; 96% had a normal social adjustment. Grand mal epilepsies therefore appear to have a good prognosis (D'Alessandro *et al.*, 1986).

PARTIAL SEIZURES

Of 155 patients with complex partial seizures, 79% had secondary generalization within the first 3 years; seizure control was achieved in about 60%. The time of seizure onset did not influence the therapeutic outcome.

Seizure control was significantly lower (44%) in patients with a history of at least one convulsion per month, compared with those (79%) who had had less than six generalized convulsions in all. The frequency of secondary generalized seizures seems to be of predictive value for the seizure prognosis of patients with complex partial seizures (Schmidt, Tsai and Janz, 1983; Loiseau, Dartigues and Pestre, 1983).

In a study of 82 patients with chronic complex partial seizures, complete seizure control was achieved with high-dose drug therapy in 18. Those who became seizure free had experienced a significantly lower number in the year before the high-dose treatment (average three seizures), compared with 40 in patients with an increased or unchanged seizure frequency. Complex partial seizures without automatisms were found only in those patients with complete seizure control (22%).

Patients whose seizures remain uncontrolled frequently had a history of severe depression or psychotic episodes, clusters of complex partial seizures, two or more seizures per day, and a simple partial seizure preceding the complex partial seizure (Schmidt, 1984).

With regards to psychiatric outcome it has been shown that patients with a medio-basal temporal lobe focus demonstrate so-called 'epileptic' personality traits more often than patients with a lateral focus. Similarly, they tend to display schizoid–paranoid personalities (Nielsen and Kristensen, 1981). Patients with a left temporal lobe focus are emotionally labile compared with those who have a right temporal lobe focus. Patients with lateral right-sided temporal focus seem to have the most benign psychological prognosis (Nielsen and Kristensen, 1981).

EPILEPTIC SEIZURES IN THE ELDERLY

Only a relatively small number of elderly patients who are treated for repeated seizures obtain complete remission. About 18% are seizure free for 2 years and 8% for 5 years (Hauser and Kurland, 1975). Since most seizures in the elderly are caused by permanent structural brain damage, few can have their medication discontinued (Mahler, 1987).

However, Lühdorf, Jensen and Plesner (1986) found that 72% of those not previously treated entered remission during the first year of treatment. The first year seemed to be crucial in determining the long-term prognosis. It was concluded that patients with seizure onset after the age of 60 fare as well or even better than those in other age groups. About 6% suffer single or multiple seizures at onset. Seizures are evenly distributed among all pathological stroke subtypes, but seem to be restricted to lesions in the region of the carotid artery. Seizures are not of any help in discriminating cerebral haemorrhage from infarction but indicate a poorer prognosis if they occur during the first two days after the stroke (Shinton et al., 1988).

PROGNOSIS AFTER WITHDRAWAL OF ANTIEPILEPTIC DRUGS

In a study of 194 epileptic children reexamined 12 years later, 36% still had epilepsy and 60% were taking antiepileptic drugs. Three factors appeared to be especially important for seizure prognosis: abnormal neurological signs, mental retardation, and frequent seizures. The presence of all these factors indicated a bad prognosis with seizures persisting for 12 years in greater than 80% of cases. For those who were mentally and neurologically normal and had low seizure frequency, prognosis was excellent, only 11% still having active epilepsy after 12 years (Brorson and Wranne, 1987).

In a prospective study of 433 epileptic children (Todt, 1984), seizures recurred in 62% with a frequency of more than five per year, and in only 19% was the frequency less than five seizures per year. Relapses with a duration of more than 15 min were observed in 81% and in only 31% was the seizure duration less than 15 min. Fifty-four per cent of children with a seizure history longer than 2 years before complete control, had relapses, compared with 31% with a duration of less than 2 years. Withdrawal of therapy during puberty did not increase the risk of recurrence. Seizure-free periods of less than 3 years, and withdrawal periods of less than 6 months lead to highly significant increases in the rate of relapse ($P < 0.001$) (Todt, 1984).

In another study, 148 children were studied after prolonged control therapy had been withdrawn, and 85% had relapses within 5 years of withdrawal. Factors associated with an increased risk of relapse were a long duration of epilepsy before control, neurological dysfunction, and Jacksonian seizures or combinations of seizure types. There was no association between risk of recurrence and age of onset of epilepsy, total number of seizures before control, age at discontinuation of therapy, EEG abnormalities, or family history of epilepsy (Thurston et al., 1982).

Förster and Schmidberger (1982) followed 114 children with epilepsy after discontinuation of antiepileptic therapy. Seizures recurred in 30% of the patients. The relapse rate was high with complex partial seizures and with combinations of multiple seizure types. Only in complex partial seizures was seizure frequency related to relapse. Factors associated with an increased risk of relapse were mental and motor retardation, beginning of puberty, and onset of epilepsy between 3–7 years old.

Shinnar et al. (1985) discontinued antiepileptic medications in 88 children with epilepsy of varying etiology who had been seizure free for 2 to 4 years. The patients were followed for 6 months to 5 years, 75% remained seizure free. EEG characteristics, type of seizures, and age at onset were important in predicting outcome. A history of complex partial seizures that had been controlled for 2 years carried a relatively favorable prognosis, whereas a history of atypical febrile seizures carried a poor prognosis. Younger age at onset was also associated with a better outcome, but only if accompanied by EEG slowing.

In a study of 146 children with epilepsy from whom medication was withdrawn after a seizure-free period of at least 2 years, the cumulative probability of remaining seizure free was 74.5%.

In primary generalized epilepsy, no factor significantly increased the likelihood of a recurrence. In partial epilepsy, significant factors were the presence of neurological deficits, female sex, a positive family history of epilepsy, and the number of drugs necessary for the control of seizures (Arts et al., 1988).

In 92 patients who had been free of seizures during 2 years' treatment with a single drug, the antiepileptic therapy was withdrawn (Callaghan, Garrett and Goggin, 1988). The relapse rate was 34%. There was no significant difference between relapse rate of adults (35%) and that of children (31%). The relapse rate for generalized seizures was 37%; for complex or simple partial seizures 16%; whereas the relapse rate was significantly higher for complex partial seizures with secondary generalization (54%). Simple partial seizures carried less risk of relapse than generalized seizures or partial seizures with secondary generalization. Patients who had complex or simple partial seizures with secondary generalization thus had the worst prognosis (Callaghan, Garrett and Goggin, 1988). A similar recurrence rate (73%) was found by Janz et al. (1983) in a group of patients with partial seizures and secondary generalization. Patients whose seizures are controlled by the drug of first choice are less likely to relapse than those who receive a second drug, who in turn are less likely to relapse than patients receiving a third drug.

The number of seizures prior to establishment of control influences the risk of relapse. A high rate of relapse can be predicted among patients with abnormal EEG before treatment and persisting EEG abnormalities before withdrawal (Callaghan, Garrett and Goggin, 1988).

PROGNOSIS IN GENERAL

According to the early study by Rodin (1968) only approximately one-third of patients with epilepsy are likely to achieve a terminal remission of at least 2 years. The longer they were followed, the more likely was the recurrence of seizures; 80% of all patients with epilepsy were likely to have a chronic seizure disorder.

However, Rodin (1968) emphasized that his review was based on studies of chronic epileptics in institutions or attending special outpatient clinics. Most traditional studies show a generally poor prognosis for epilepsy. They have been hospital-based and inevitably overrepresent cases of chronic epilepsy.

Investigations (both hospital and community based) starting from the onset of seizures show a much better prognosis, and most patients suffer only a small total of seizures over a relatively short time and then remit (Shorvon, 1984). The longer the epilepsy is active, the less likely is eventual remission; chronic epilepsy develops in about 25% of cases. The pattern of chronicity is usually established relatively early in its course (Reynolds, Elwes and Shorvon, 1983). It is possible that early treatment may improve long-term prognosis (Shorvon, 1984).

The prevalance rates of active epilepsy vary from 4 to 10 per 1000, depending on definitions and methods of study (Zielinski, 1982). As 5% of the general population may at some time experience a nonfebrile seizure (Royal College of General Practitioners Research Committee, 1960), most of them do not develop chronic epilepsy.

In keeping with this, Goodridge and Shorvon (1983) found that the lifetime prevalence of epilepsy (excluding febrile convulsions but including single seizures) was 20.2 per 1000, whereas the prevalence of continuing 'active' epilepsy was 5.3 per 1000. Annegers, Hauser and Elveback (1979) retrospectively reviewed the prognosis of 475 patients who had an initial diagnosis of epilepsy. In contrast to Rodin's observations, remission rates improved relative to the length of follow-up: of those followed for 20 years, 70% were in 5-year remission and 50% had withdrawn medication. Goodridge and Shorvon (1983) reviewed the general practice records of a population of 6000. Of 122 patients identified with at least one nonfebrile seizure, 69% were in 4-year remission at 15-year follow-up.

Shorvon and Reynolds (1982) and Elwes et al. (1984) followed prospectively 106 adolescent or adult patients with newly diagnosed, previously untreated epilepsy. The overall prognosis for this population was very good: 73% were in 1-year remission at the second follow-up year; 88% by the fourth year, and 92% by eighth year. A number of factors had an adverse effect on remission rates: a high frequency of tonic–clonic seizures before treatment, a family history of seizures, and the presence of additional neurological, psychiatric, or social handicaps. Most of the patients responded to monotherapy. Two factors were clearly associated with failure of monotherapy, i.e. poor compliance and the presence of cerebral pathology (Reynolds, 1987a).

Another prospective study has shown that a large number of seizures before treatment, combined seizure types, earlier age at onset, and prolonged seizure duration seem to be associated with the development of moderate-to-severe epilepsy (Beghi and Tognoni, 1988).

The longer the seizures continue after onset of treatment, the less likely is it that the patient will go into remission (Reynolds, 1987a). The first 2 years of treatment thus seem to be very important in relation to longer-term prognosis.

CONCLUSION

It seems to be a fact that someone with a first seizure has a significant risk of recurrence, usually within the first 6 months. It seems to be a general trait that an early age of onset of seizures indicates a poor prognosis.

One may ask, why the prognosis of benign familial neonatal convulsions is so good, considering the high number of seizures. One may also ask, why the prognosis after febrile convulsions in the first year of life is better than that after afebrile convulsions. Why are the effects of febrile seizures in the first year of life more serious than if the febrile convulsions start later (Lennox-Buchthal, 1973)?

The proportion of Lennox–Gastaut cases whose seizures stop is greater when seizures begin late in childhood than when they begin during the first 2 years of life (Blume, David and Gomez, 1973). Is the tendency to develop chronic epilepsy attached to a certain age group? Has this propensity to develop seizures in a certain period of life a similarity to kindling?

Many factors seem to influence prognosis. The presence of preceding neurological, psychological, and social impairment results in a worse outcome. Such other factors as partial seizures as opposed to tonic–clonic seizures are related to a more adverse prognosis. Also the duration of the individual seizure is of importance to prognosis. Similarly, the duration of the epilepsy is an important factor: when duration of illness prior to complete control is more than 2 years, 54% of children relapse, compared with only 31% when the history is less than 2 years. Other factors of importance are neurological dysfunction, and Jacksonian seizures or combinations of seizure types.

Grand mal epilepsies appear to have a good prognosis. Why is this so, considering the poor prognosis of complex partial seizures? The onset of complex partial seizures does not influence the therapeutic outcome. Why is this in contrast to febrile seizures, infantile spasms and the seizures in Lennox–Gastaut's syndrome?

The frequency of secondary generalized seizures seems to have predictive value for the seizure prognosis of those with complex partial seizures. Complex or simple partial seizures with secondary generalization have the worst prognosis.

Has treatment any effect on prognosis, hindering the development of a neurophysiological process leading to chronic epilepsy? Infants started on ACTH within a month of onset of infantile spasms have a better prognosis than those in whom such therapy is delayed. The prevailing view is that the earlier the treatment is instituted, the better the chance of a complete remission.

The long-term prognosis of Rolandic epilepsy in children is good. Why is the prognosis so good for this syndrome with partial seizures, even though the patients may have suffered from many seizures?

It is a fact that with pyknoleptic petit mal the shorter the duration of seizures, the greater the likelihood of seizure resolution. The prognosis may be related mainly to adequate therapy and not to the presence of other types of seizures, before or after the absences.

In juvenile myoclonic epilepsy, relapse occurs in 91% of cases when dosage is reduced or medication withdrawn after at least 2 seizure-free years of treatment. According to Janz (1985) complete recovery is never seen when this syndrome is complicated with generalized convulsions. Juvenile myoclonic epilepsy is, like Rolandic epilepsy and pyknoleptic petit mal, cryptogenic; however, the prognosis is much worse, unless treatment is continued for many years, in all probability for the duration of the life.

Seizures controlled by the drug of first choice are less likely to recur than those which require a second drug, and, in turn, less likely again than those requiring a third drug.

Many patients may have an accelerating disease process in the early stages of epilepsy. The number of seizures that they have before control, influences the risk of relapse. Early effective treatment associated with good compliance may be important in the prevention of chronic epilepsy (Reynolds, 1987b).

Perhaps the kindling phenomenon, if it exists in man, may be relevant to some of the unanswered questions discussed in this chapter. At least it seems to be important to bring epileptic seizures under control as quickly as possible. If this is not achievable within 1 to 2 years, patients should be evaluated for possible surgical treatment.

REFERENCES

Annegers, J. F., Hauser, W. A., and Elveback, L. R. (1979). Remission of seizures and relapse in patients with epilepsy. *Epilepsia*, **20**, 729–737.

Arts, W. F. M., Visser, L. H., Loonen, M. C. B., Tjiam, A. T., Stroink, H., Stuurman, P. M. and Poortvliet, D. C. J. (1988). Follow-up of 146 children with epilepsy after withdrawal of antiepileptic therapy. *Epilepsia*, **29**, 244–250.

Beaumanoir, A. (1983). Infantile epilepsy with occipital focus and good prognosis. *Eur. Neurol.*, **22**, 43–52.

Beaumanoir, A. (1985). The Lennox–Gastaut syndrome. In: *Epileptic Syndromes in Infancy, Childhood and Adolescence* (eds J. Roger, C. Dravet, M. Bureau, F. E. Dreifuss and P. Wolf), pp. 89–99. John Libbey, London.

Beghi, E. and Tognoni, G. (Collaborative group for the study of epilepsy) (1988). Prognosis of epilepsy in newly referred patients: a multicenter prospective study. *Epilepsia*, **29**, 236–243.

Blom, S. and Heijbel, J. (1982). Benign epilepsy of children with centrotemporal EEG foci: a follow-up study in adulthood of patients initially studied as children. *Epilepsia*, **23**, 629–632.

Blume, W. T., David, R. B. and Gomez, M. R. (1973). Generalized sharp and slow wave complexes: associated clinical features and long-term follow-up. *Brain*, **96**, 289–306.

Brorson, L. O. and Wranne, L. (1987). Long-term prognosis in childhood epilepsy: survival and seizure prognosis. *Epilepsia*, **28**, 324–330.

Callaghan, N., Garrett, A. and Goggin, T. (1988). Withdrawal of anticonvulsant drugs in patients free of seizures for two years. *N. Engl. J. Med.*, **318**, 942–946.

Camfield, P. R., Camfield, C. S. and Dooley, J. M. (1985). Epilepsy after a first unprovoked seizure in children. *Neurology*, **35**, 1657–1660.

Cavazzuti, G. B., Ferrari, P. and Lalla, M. (1984). Follow-up study of 482 cases with convulsive disorders in the first year of life. *Dev. Med. Child Neurol.*, **26**, 425–437.

Cleland, P. G., Mosquera, I., Steward, W. P. et al. (1981). Prognosis of isolated seizures in adult life. *Br. Med. J.*, **283**, 1364.

Currier, R. D., Kooi, K. A. and Saidman, S. J. (1963). Prognosis of 'pure' petit mal. *Neurology*, **13**, 959–967.

Dalby, M. A. (1969). Epilepsy and three per second spike and wave rhythms. *Acta Neurol. Scand.*, **45**, suppl. 40.

D'Alessandro, R., Pazzaglia, P., Tinuper, P., Fabbri, R. and Lugaresi, E. (1986). Prognostic and electroclinical features of grand mal epilepsies. *Eur. Neurol.*, **25**, 339–345.

Dobrescu, O. and Larbrisseau, A. (1982). Benign familial neonatal convulsions. *Can. J. Neurol. Sci.*, **9.**, 345–347.

Elwes, R. D. C., Chesterman, P. and Reynolds, E. H. (1985). Prognosis after a first untreated tonic–clonic seizure. *Lancet*, **ii**, 752–753.

Elwes, R. D. C., Johnson, A. L. and Reynolds, E. H. (1988). The course of untreated epilepsy. *Br. Med. J.*, **297**, 948–950.

Elwes, R. D. C., Johnson, A. L., Shorvon, S. D. and Reynolds, E. H. (1984). The prognosis for seizure control in newly diagnosed epilepsy. *N Engl. J. Med.*, **311**, 944–947.

Fois, A., Malandrini, F. and Mostardini, R. (1987). Clinical experiences of petit mal. *Brain Dev.*, **9**, 54–59.

Förster, C. and Schmidberger, G. (1982). Prognose der Epilepsie im Kindesalter nach Absetzen der Medikation. *Monatsschr. Kinderheilkd.*, **130**, 225–228.

Glaze, D. G., Hrachovy, R. A., Frost, J. D., Kellaway, P. and Zion, T. E. (1988). Prospective study of outcome of infants with infantile spasms treated during controlled studies of ACTH and prednisone. *J. Pediatr.*, **112**, 389–396.

Goodridge, D. M. G. and Shorvon, S. D. (1983). Epilepsy in a population of 6000. 1. Demography, diagnosis and classification, and the role of the hospital services. 2. Treatment and prognosis. *Br. Med. J.*, **287**, 641–647.

Gowers, W. R. (1881). *Epilepsy and Other Chronic Convulsive Disorders: Their Causes, Symptoms, and Treatment*. Churchill, London.

Hart, R. G. and Easton, J. D. (1986). Seizure recurrence after a first unprovoked seizure. *Arch. Neurol.*, **43**, 1289–1290.

Hauser, W. A. (1983). Recurrence after a first seizure. *N. Engl. J. Med.*, **308**, 159.

Hauser, W. A. and Kurland, L. T. (1975). The epidemiology of epilepsy in Rochester, Minnesota, 1935 through 1967. *Epilepsia*, **16**, 1–66.

Hertoft, P. (1963). The clinical, electroencephalographic and social prognosis of petit mal epilepsy. *Epilepsia*, **4**, 298–314.

Hirtz, D. G., Ellenberg, J. H. and Nelson, K. B. (1984). The risk of recurrence of non-febrile seizures in children. *Neurology*, **34**, 637–641.

Janz, D. (1985). Epilepsy with impulsive petit mal (Juvenile myoclonic epilepsy). *Acta Neurol. Scand.*, **72**, 449–459.

Janz, D., Kern, A., Mössinger, H.-J. and Puhlmann, U. (1983). Rückfall-Prognose nach Reduktion der Medikamente bei Epilepsiebehandlung. *Nervenarzt*, **54**, 525–529.

Jeavons, P. M., Bishop, A. and Harding, G. F. A. (1986). The prognosis of photosensitivity. *Epilepsia*, **27**, 569–575.

Lacy, J. R. and Penry, J. K. (1976). *Infantile Spasms*. Raven, New York.

Lennox-Buchthal, M. A. (1973). Febrile convulsions. A reappraisal. *Electroencephalogr. Clin. Neurophysiol.*, **32** (Suppl.), 1–138.

Livingstone, S., Torres, I., Pauli, L. L. *et al.* (1965). Petit mal epilepsy. Result of a prolonged follow-up study of 117 patients. *J. Am. Med. Assoc.*, **194**, 113–118.

Loiseau, P., Dartigues, J. F. and Pestre, M. (1983). Prognosis of partial epileptic seizures in the adolescent. *Epilepsia*, **24**, 472–481.

Loiseau, P., Pestre, M., Dartigues, J. F., Commenges, D., Barberger-Gateau, C. and Cohadon, D. (1983). Long term prognosis in two forms of childhood epilepsy: typical absence seizures and epilepsy with rolandic (centrotemporal) EEG foci. *Ann. Neurol.*, **13**, 642–648.

Loiseau, P., Duché, B., Cordova, S., Dartigues, J. F. and Cohadon, S. (1988). Prognosis of benign childhood epilepsy with centrotemporal spikes: A follow-up study of 168 patients. *Epilepsia*, **29**, 229–235.

Lombroso, C. T. (1983). A prospective study of infantile spasms: clinical and therapeutic correlations. *Epilepsia*, **24**, 135–158.

Lühdorf, K., Jensen, L. K. and Plesner, A. M. (1986). Epilepsy in the elderly: prognosis. *Acta Neurol. Scand.*, **74**, 409–415.

Mahler, M. E. (1987). Seizures: Common causes and treatment in the elderly. *Geriatrics*, **42**, 73–78.

Matsumoto, A., Watanabe, K., Negoro, T., Sugiura, M., Hara, K. and Miyazaki, S. (1981). Prognostic factors of infantile spasms from the etiological viewpoint. *Brain Dev.*, **3**, 361–364.

Nielsen, H. and Kristensen, O. (1981). Personality correlates of sphenoidal EEG-foci in temporal lobe epilepsy. *Acta Neurol. Scand.*, **64**, 289–300.

O'Donohoe, N. V. (1985). Febrile convulsions. In: *Epileptic Syndromes in Infancy, Childhood and Adolescence* (eds J. Roger, C. Dravet, M. Bureau, F. E. Dreifuss and P. Wolf), pp. 34–38. John Libbey, London.

Ohtahara, S., Yamatogi, Y. and Ohtsuka, Y. (1976). Prognosis of the Lennox syndrome. *Folia Psychiat. Neurol. Jpn.*, **30**, 275–287.

Reynolds, E. H. (1987a). Early treatment and prognosis of epilepsy. *Epilepsia*, **28**, 97–106.

Reynolds, E. H. (1987b). The early treatment and prognosis of epilepsy. *Yale J. Biol. Med.*, **60**, 79–83.

Reynolds, E. H., Elwes, R. D. C. and Shorvon, S. D. (1983). Why does epilepsy become intractable? Prevention of chronic epilepsy. *Lancet*, **ii**, 952–954.

Riikonen, R. (1984). Infantile spasms: modern practical aspects. *Acta Paediatr. Scand.*, **73**, 1–12.

Rodin, E. A. (1968). *The Prognosis of Patients with Epilepsy*. Charles C. Thomas, Springfield, Illinois.

Roger, J. (1974). Prognostic features of petit mal absence. *Epilepsia*, **15**, 433.

Royal College of General Practitioners Research Committee. (1960). *Br. Med. J.*, **2**, 416–422.

Saunders, M. and Marshall, C. (1975). Isolated seizures: An EEG and clinical assessment. *Epilepsia*, **16**, 731–733.

Sato, S., Dreifuss, F. E. and Penry, J. K. (1976). Prognostic factors in absence seizures. *Neurology*, **26**, 788–796.

Schmidt, D. (1984). Prognosis of chronic epilepsy with complex partial seizures. *J. Neurol. Neurosurg. Psychiat.*, **47**, 1274–1278.

Schmidt, D., Tsai, J.-J. and Janz, D. (1983). Generalized tonic–clonic seizures in patients with complex-partial seizures: natural history and prognostic relevance. *Epilepsia*, **24**, 43–48.

Shinnar, S., Vining, E. P. G., Mellits, E. D., D'Souza, B. J., Holden, K., Baumgardner, R. A. and Freeman, J. M. (1985). Discontinuing antiepileptic medication in children with epilepsy after two years without seizures. *N Engl. J. Med.*, **313**, 976–980.

Shinton, R. A., Gill, J. S., Melnick, S. C., Gupta, A. K. and Beevers, D. G. (1988). The frequency, characteristics and prognosis of epileptic seizures at the onset of stroke. *J. Neurol. Neurosurg. Psychiat.*, **51**, 273–276.

Shorvon, S. D. (1984). The temporal aspects of prognosis in epilepsy. *J. Neurol. Neurosurg. Psychiat.*, **47**, 1157–1165.

Shorvon, S. D. and Reynolds, E. H. (1982). Early prognosis of epilepsy. *Br. Med. J.*, **285**, 1699–1701.

Singer, W. D., Rabe, E. F. and Haller, J. S. (1980). The effect of ACTH therapy upon infantile spasms. *J. Pediatr.*, **96**, 485–489.

Thurston, J. H., Thurston, D. L., Hixon, B. B. and Keller, A. J. (1982). Prognosis in childhood epilepsy. Additional follow-up of 148 children 15 to 23 years after withdrawal of anticonvulsant therapy. *N. Engl. J. Med.*, **306**, 831–836.

Todt, H. (1984). The late prognosis of epilepsy in childhood: results of a prospective follow-up study. *Epilepsia*, **25**, 137–144.

Zielinski, J. J. (1982). Epidemiology. In: *A Textbook of Epilepsy*, 2nd edn (eds J. Laidlaw and A. Richens), pp. 16–33. Churchill Livingstone, Edinburgh.

The Clinical Relevance of Kindling
Edited by T. G. Bolwig and M. R. Trimble
© 1989 John Wiley & Sons Ltd

12

Kindling, epilepsy and behaviour

M. R. TRIMBLE
Department of Psychological Medicine, National Hospital for Nervous Diseases, Queen Square, London WC1N 3BG, UK

INTRODUCTION

In examining the proposition that kindling may be a mechanism for the development of psychiatric symptoms in certain groups of patients, taking into account the obvious fact that kindling is a mechanism derived from experimental epilepsy, it might be expected that the mechanism would reveal itself most clearly in patients with epilepsy. If kindling from an epileptic focus leads to the development of psychopathology, then certain hypotheses need to be satisfied. It is the purpose of this chapter to view these, and to arrive at some conclusions on the relationship between kindling as a biological phenomenon and human cerebral processes.

BEHAVIOUR DISORDERS OF EPILEPSY

Hypothesis 1: Psychopathology is overrepresented in patients with epilepsy

The association between epilepsy and psychopathology has been discussed for many years, and over time there has generally been an agreement that psychopathology is overrepresented in epileptic populations. There are, nonetheless, a number of detractors from this viewpoint, their main objections being that the majority of quoted work derives from selected populations of chronically sick hospital patients, especially as seen in psychiatric clinics. Further, any increase in psychopathology may be unrelated to epilepsy *per se*, but to the secondary consequences of having epilepsy. These include the long-term administration of anticonvulsant drugs, the recurrent head injuries that occur in some patients with uncontrolled seizures, the social stigmatization with constant demoralization and rejection that patients with epilepsy suffer from, and the very fact that seizures themselves, if uncontrolled, may lead to bouts of anoxia with consequent changes of intellect and personality.

There are some epidemiological surveys of non-selected epileptic patients in which this question can be examined. Pond and Bidwell (1959), in a general practice survey, noted that 29% showed 'psychological difficulties', but pointed out that this was an underestimate since a number of the cases were not personally interviewed. Half the group showed neurotic symptoms, 5% the 'so-called epileptic personality', and 7% had been in a mental hospital before or during the survey years. Gudmundsson (1966) provided a valuable survey of the epileptic population of Iceland which he personally examined, and was also able to compare the prevalence rates of psychopathology in it with a general psychiatric survey of the same population carried out by Helgason (1964). Only 50% of epileptic patients were considered as having a normal personality, and 8% were regarded as psychotic. Zielinski (1974) provided data on nonselected epileptic patients from Poland. Fifty-eight per cent showed 'some mental abnormality' and approximately 3% had psychotic symptoms.

Edeh and Toone (1987) attempted a replication of Pond and Bidwell's 1959 study in 14 general practices from South London. They noted the prevalence rate of epilepsy to be 3.45/1000 and examined 88 of 103 identified practice patients (85%). Psychiatric morbidity was rated using the Clinic Interview Schedule (Goldberg et al., 1970). Thirty-one per cent had a history of psychiatric referral and only 52% were assessed as normal. Twenty-two per cent had depressive neurosis, while 4.5% had some form of psychosis. As with the Pond study, the prevalence of severe psychiatric disorder is likely to be underestimated here, taking into account the percentage of the sample who were not surveyed who may well have fallen into this spectrum, and the patients in institutional care who would have fallen out of the catchment of the study.

The most substantial study in children is that of Rutter and colleagues (1970). They used standardized and validated rating scales to quantify psychopathaloy in children resident on the Isle of Wight. They found the prevalence of psychiatric disorders to be 8% in the general population, nearly double in patients with chronic disability not involving the brain, and doubled again in those with uncomplicated epilepsy.

In summary, surveys of unselected populations reveal a considerable excess of psychopathology in patients with epilepsy, many patients showing an increase in neurotic disorders, but with an additional recognized excess of psychotic states.

Hypothesis 2: Patients with focal epilepsy, particularly deriving from the temporal lobes, show more psychopathology than those with a generalized seizure disorder

Since in animal models kindling is most readily elicited from medial temporal, limbic system structures, and since patients with temporal lobe epilepsy most usually have a focus of origin of seizure in the medial temporal lobe structures, if the mechanism of kindling were related to the development of psychopathology it would be more likely to be shown in the temporal lobe group.

This has been a considerable area of controversy. Notwithstanding the objections of authors such as Stevens and Hermann (1981), some evidence from the surveys already quoted may be presented. In Pond and Bidwell's 1959 survey, patients with temporal lobe epilepsy had a significantly higher rate of hospitalization in a mental hospital (nearly 20%), compared with others (7%). These patients had a higher rate of psychotic change and of severe personality disorder of the 'so-called epileptic type'. Gudmundsson (1966) reported 50% of patients with temporal lobe epilepsy to have psychological difficulties, and only 24% of those without temporal lobe epilepsy. Psychopathology was also overrepresented in patients with temporal lobe epilepsy in the studies of Zielinski (1974) and that of children by Rutter *et al.* (1970). Edeh and Toone (1987) compared patients with primary generalized epilepsy ($n = 41$) with focal non-temporal lobe epilepsy ($n = 22$) and temporal lobe epilepsy ($n = 25$). Significantly more patients with focal epilepsy had a history of psychiatric referral, although the difference between temporal lobe epilepsy and other non-focal patients was not significant. Patients with temporal lobe epilepsy rated more highly on anxiety than the non-temporal lobe group, and more highly on irritability, depression and impaired concentration than the primary generalized group. Further, on manifest psychiatric abnormalities, the temporal lobe group scored more highly on depressed affect than either of the other two groups. More patients with temporal lobe epilepsy were diagnosed as having depressive neurosis, but the number of psychotic patients was too small to make any generalizations. These data suggest that patients with focal epilepsy are more likely to manifest psychopathology, although they were not able to make many distinctions between a temporal and non-temporal site of focus. The question of the extent of limbic involvement from the frontal or extratemporal cortices was not discussed.

Some recent data of the prognosis of temporal lobe epilepsy has been published by Ounsted and colleagues (1981). In 1964, they examined a 'wholly unselected population' of children with temporal lobe epilepsy and obtained biographical and clinical information about them and their epilepsy.

These were followed up in 1977 and their outcome assessed. Thirty-three per cent were seizure-free and on no anticonvulsants, and five had died in childhood. In their original 1964 assessment, 85% were said to have some form of psychiatric difficulty. In 1977, of 95 survivors, eight were severely mentally handicapped, nine had developed a schizophreniform psychosis, and 12 had antisocial conduct problems. Neurotic illness was infrequent. In analysing the factors which were related to psychopathology they identified: failure of remission of epilepsy, frequent seizures, male sex, and left-sided temporal lobe lesions. Seven out of the nine cases who had a schizophrenia-like illness had a dominant hemisphere lesion. Disordered homes bore no relationship to the development of adult psychiatric disorder.

In conclusion, there is some evidence from these studies that patients with focal epilepsy are more susceptible to the development of psychopathology, especially severe psychopathology, than those with a generalized seizure disorder, and a number of studies specifically implicate the temporal lobes.

LIMBIC EPILEPSY

Although the concept of focal seizures arising from medial temporal structures is an old one, it was Fulton who first suggested that the term limbic should be applied to them (Glaser, 1967). He said 'temporal lobe seizures . . . might more properly be designated as seizures involving the limbic lobe . . .' (Fulton, 1953). The concept was more fully developed by Glaser (1967), who entitled a paper 'Limbic epilepsy in childhood', describing 120 children who had 'psychomotor seizures' with minimal secondary generalization. In common terminology, all would be described as suffering from complex partial seizures, and the majority of them suffered interictal behaviour disorders (mainly personality disturbances of varying degrees of intensity). Eight had psychotic reactions with schizophrenia-like disturbances, and the development of paranoid, delusional, and hallucinatory symptoms. Glaser pointed out the high incidence of susceptibility of limbic system structures to pathological processes, including ischaemia, encephalitis, and metabolic disturbances, and suggested that the term psychomotor, or temporal lobe, should give way to the designation 'limbic' when describing this form of epilepsy.

This idea represents the development of a concept elaborated many years previously, notably by Hughlings Jackson. Not only did he clarify the concept of focal epilepsy, delineating focal motor seizures which have since become referred to as Jacksonian, but in 1888 he described 'a peculiar variety of epilepsy', characterized by 'exceedingly complex and very purposive seeming actions during continuing consciousness' (Jackson, 1888). Such seizures could be accompanied by illusions and hallucinations, and, based on autopsy studies, Jackson related them to lesions in the temporal lobe, particularly in the uncinate gyrus and adjoining areas of the temporal pole (Jackson and Steward, 1899). Following Jackson, little seems to have been written about this form of epilepsy until Gibbs and colleagues (1937), using the newly introduced electoencephalogram (EEG), discovered a form of seizure disorder which they called psychomotor epilepsy which was found to be associated with observable abnormalities from the temporal lobes on the EEG. Jasper, Pertuiset and Flanigan (1951) introduced the term temporal lobe seizure to denote such focal seizures. This embraced a variety of focal seizure patterns from the uncinate seizures of Jackson to the psychomotor seizures of Gibbs and colleagues. Temporal lobe epilepsy became synonymous with psychomotor epilepsy which led to a considerable confusion, not the least because psychomotor seizures could arise from areas outside the temporal lobes, and patients with temporal lobe epilepsy presented with other seizure types than that classified as psychomotor.

The developing neuroanatomical and neurochemical techniques of the 1940s and 1950s, and the animal ablation and stimulation experiments, more sharply focused on differences with regards to both structure and function of the medial temporal lobe structures, and their associated limbic system circuits, in contrast to the neocortical temporal lobe with its extensive cortico-cortical connections. The idea that temporal lobe seizures could thus properly be subdivided into at least two categories, one being identified by a limbic system origin, was an obvious step. Girgis (1981) recommended the adoption of the term limbic epilepsy as a substitute for both psychomotor and temporal lobe, an idea formulated in the proposed ILAE Commission on Classification and Terminology International Classification of the Epilepsies (ILAE, 1985). The proposed classification shown in Table 1 includes the localization-related (focal, local, partial) epilepsies and syndromes. These are subdivided as shown in Table 2. Although in earlier discussions the term 'limbic epilepsy' was used, in this there is only the acknowledgement of seizures deriving from

Table 1. Classification of epilepsies (ILAE, 1985)

---

1. Localization related (focal, local, partial) epilepsies or syndromes
   Idiopathic with age-related onset (e.g. benign epilepsy of childhood)
   Symptomatic, e.g. frontal lobe, temporal lobe

2. Generalized epilepsies or syndromes
   Idiopathic
   Idiopathic and/or symptomatic (e.g. West's syndrome)
   Symptomatic

3. Epilepsies and syndromes undetermined as to whether they are focal or generalized

4. Special syndromes (e.g febrile convulsions)

Table 2. Varieties of symptomatic localization related epilepsies according to the anatomical localization

---

Frontal lobe epilepsies:
  Supplementary motor
  Cingulate
  Anterior (polar)
  Frontal region
  Orbito-frontal
  Dorso-lateral

Epilepsies of the motor cortex

Temporal lobe epilepsies
  hippocampal
  amygdala
  lateral posterior temporal
  opercular

Parietal lobe epilepsies

Occipital lobe epilepsies

---

specific limbic system structures. Nonetheless this classification supports the ideas laid down by Fulton and Glaser.

Hypothesis 3: Limbic epilepsy can be distiguished from localization-related epilepsies of non-limbic origin

A major problem with the ILAE classificaiton of epilepsies is that the subdivisions as given in Table 2 can only successfully be derived using implanted electrode studies. Nonetheless, there is reason to believe that limbic epilepsy is identifiable, and should be separated from other localization-related seizure disorders. The extensive anatomical and neurochemical distinctions between the medial and lateral temporal areas has already been mentioned, and will not be elaborated on here. However, more extensive reviews of this can be found (Trimble, 1988) in which both the neuroanatomy, the neurochemistry, and the afferent and efferent projections of the medial temporal structures can be distinguished, which have important biological significance. The hippocampus and amygdala integrate information derived from sensory input from the external world, via a cascading system of projections from primary sensory cortex to the entorrhinal cortex, and hence to the medial temporal structures, with knowledge of the internal state of the organism provided by connections to and from the limbic forebrain, hypothalamus, and descending and ascending brain stem pathways. The known role of the limbic structures in the modulation of emotion needs no elaboration, but the fact that such areas are the site of origin of seizures in many patients with temporal lobe epilepsy, provides an obvious anatomical and neurophysiological substrate for an understanding of psychopathology found associated with temporal lobe epilepsy, and as suggested below, with limbic system epilepsy in particular.

ON THE PROGNOSIS OF EPILEPSY

The clinical course and prognosis of epilepsy has been charted by a number of authors in recent years (e.g. Currie *et al.*, 1971). However, recently well-controlled prospective studies have been carried out which give more information on the kind of patients most susceptible to develop chronic problems. Reynolds (1987) prospectively followed 106 adolescents or adults with newly-diagnosed previously untreated epilepsy for a period up to 8 years. The overall prognosis was good, 73% being in 1-year remission by 2 years of follow up, 88% by 4 years and 92% by 8 years. The pattern of 2-year remission rates was similar. The factors which suggested a poor prognosis included partial as compared with tonic–clonic seizures, a high frequency of tonic–clonic seizures before treatment, a family history of seizures, and the presence of additional neurological, psychiatric or social handicap. When he examined the 1-year remission rates for patients still having seizures after 1 or 2 years of treatment, a progressive decline in remission was noted. In other words the longer the seizures continue after treatment the less likely it is the patient will go into remission.

Shorvon (1984), following a review of the literature of the prognosis of epilepsy, including some of his own studies, noted that the earlier gloomy prognosis given to epilepsy which was based largely on hospital- and institutional-based studies in the form of retrospective surveys (Rodin, 1968) was erroneous, and that epidemiological surveys revealed that most patients who develop seizures do not become 'chronic epileptics', and many enter long-term remission. In his own general practice epidemiological survey (Goodrich and Shorvon, 1983), he examined the prognosis of seizures after the first attack in 122 patients. In 82%, the seizures recurred but many had 10 or less seizures. The epilepsy remained active for only short periods of time in most patients, and once remission was achieved it was usually permanent. He distinguished between three patterns of seizures. The 'burst' pattern in which seizures were active only over a short period of time; the 'intermittent' pattern, observed in a minority of patients where the epilepsy took a relapsing and remitting course; and the 'continuous' category, in which seizures continue without remission. It is the latter that are likely to form chronic cases and 'in contra-distinction to the generality of patients with epilepsy, the longer a patient is followed the more likely is relapse'. In other words, patients with epilepsy have different seizure patterns, and only a minority go into the chronic condition.

Schmidt (1984) examined the clinical features associated with an unsuccessful response to anticonvulsant therapy in patients with complex partial seizures. Most of these patients had chronic epilepsy, psychiatric examination was abnormal in 56% and a suicide attempt was reported in 16%. Patients without seizure control had a significantly greater number of seizures per 12 months before the trial, had more automatisms, more depression or paranoid psychotic episodes, more clusters of seizures lasting more than two subsequent days, two or more complex partial seizures a day and an aura preceding the complex partial seizures.

In other words, data from these recent studies may be interpreted as suggesting that there are only some patients with epilepsy who develop a chronic disorder. This is most often associated with an identifiable seizure pattern, the presence of additional neurological psychiatric and social handicaps, and in complex partial seizures with severe psychopathology (depression or paranoid psychosis). Continuous seizures, poor prognosis, and psychopathology are thus interlinked, suggesting a subgroup of patients identifiable clinically. It is suggested that these patients are most likely to have limbic epilepsy, the latter being associated with the different seizures pattern, liability to psychopathology and poorer prognosis.

Hypothesis 4: In clinical studies, patients with limbic epilepsy are more likely to suffer from psychopathology

As already noted, identification of the precise site of origin of seizures without implanted electrodes is difficult. Nonetheless, several authors have examined the psychopathological profile of patients with lateral as opposed to mediobasal spikes or EEG changes, the latter being detected using such techniques as sphenoidal electrodes. Hermann *et al.* (1982) used the Minnesota Multiphasic Personality Inventory in patients with temporal lobe epilepsy, separating out a group with an aura of ictal fear. When compared with generalized seizure disorders, patients with temporal lobe epilepsy scored higher on many subscales, but the group that scored highest and most significantly differently were those with the aura of ictal fear. In particular, using Goldberg's sequential diagnostic system, patients with generalized epilepsy were classified as normal, patients with temporal lobe epilepsy without ictal fear as neurotic, and the group with ictal fear as psychotic. Since the aura of ictal fear arises in association with medial temporal discharges, it is most likely that the group with the most severe psychopathology had limbic epilepsy.

Nielsen and Kristensen (1981) gave the Bear–Fedio questionnaire to different groups of epileptic patients, and noted that those with a mediobasal temporal EEG focus had significantly more hypergraphia, elation, guilt and paranoia when compared with those with a lateral focus. In studies of epileptic psychosis, Kristensen and Sindrup (1979) noted that patients with psychosis were more likely to have automatisms and to show maximum spike activity in sphenoidal rather than lateral scalp electrodes compared with non-psychotic controls.

In conclusion, there is some evidence to suggest that patients with a limbic as opposed to a lateral neocortical origin for their seizures are more susceptible to severe psychopathology. It is therefore suggested that there is a subgroup of patients with epilepsy, who are least likely to go into remission, and whose seizures are more difficult to treat with conventional anticonvulsants. Such patients are more susceptible to develop severe psychopathology, and the latter appears to be linked to a medial temporal-limbic site for seizure generation. The suggestion is that limbic epilepsy represents a different form of epilepsy to treat, precisely on account of the site of origin of the seizures, namely in limbic system structures, which are known to have a low seizure threshold, and to be susceptible sites for kindling.

Hypothesis 5: Kindling is the relevant process involved in the development of psychopathology in epilepsy. Is there any evidence that the behaviour disturbance represents a seizure-related phenomena, and if so a kindled phenomena, or should the behaviour disturbance and the seizures be seen as both secondary to underlying pathological change?

The view that an underlying organic disorder is responsible for both manifestations was supported by Slater and colleagues (1963) on the grounds that a significant proportion of their psychotic patients had a defined organic basis for their epilepsy, and structural abnormalities were seen with radiological investigations. A similar view was taken by Kristensen and Sindrup (1979). Such a view is not supported by more recent neuro-imaging studies of patients with epilepsy and psychosis. Using Positron Emission Tomography and oxygen–15, Trimble and colleagues (Gallhofer *et al.*, 1985) have shown inter-ictal hypometabolism in patients with temporal lobe epilepsy. This is extensive, and is found in a wide distribution extending to basal ganglia structures and frontal cortex, maximally ipsilateral to the site of the focus. However, such metabolic changes are not accompanied by structural alterations. Conlon and Trimble (1988), using MRI, have noted highly localized areas of changed signal intensity in patients with a temporal lobe focus, corresponding to the side of the focus as detected on the EEG but not extending to the areas implicated by the metabolic studies. When patients with epileptic psychosis are compared to patients with epilepsy and no psychosis using MRI, no significant differences on quantitated T1 parameters are noted, suggesting that gross structural damage at least is not the significant variable related to the psychosis.

The view that the seizures are critical has been strongly argued by several authors. Flor-Henry (1969), criticizing the absence of control populations in some earlier studies, noted that in his series as well as in some others, an inverse relationship between the frequency of psychomotor seizures and the onset of the psychosis was recorded for some patients. Similarly, in a study of affective disorders in epilepsy, Robertson, Trimble and Townsend (1987), reported that 43% of patients had a decrease of seizure frequency prior to the onset of their depressive symptoms. Depth electrode studies have demonstrated that abnormal electrical abnormality in deep temporal structures may be associated with suppression of surface cortical activity, and that when patients display psychotic behaviour, abnormal spike wave activity may be detected in these structures, notably in the amygdala, hippocampus and septal regions, not identified by conventional surface electrodes (Heath, 1977). Lewis and colleagues (1982) studied 97 adolescent boys with behaviour disturbances and assessed them for psychomotor epileptic symptoms and signs. Irrespective of whether they had had a generalized convulsion, 78% had one or more symptoms characteristic of psychomotor epilepsy. A significant correlation was noted between the number of psychomotor epileptic signs and symptoms and psychotic phenomena such as auditory hallucinations, loose or rambling associations, paranoid ideation, and both visual and tactile hallucinations. Finally, the known association between seizures and psychosis in the setting of the ECT clinic provides a further link between psychopathology and seizure disorder, unrelated to structural alteration of the brain.

If some seizure-related factor is crucial for the development of psychopathology, and if kindling were involved, then the time between the onset of the seizures and the onset of the psychopathology would seem important. This has been studied mainly in relationship to psychosis, and reviewed by Toone (1981). It is clinical experience that most patients who present with a schizophrenia-like illness and who also have seizures develop the psychosis after the seizures. The psychosis usually follows between 12 and 23 years after the onset of the epilepsy, the seizure disorder developing in late childhood or early adolescence, with the onset of the psychosis in the mid–20s to mid–30s. In one study of Perez et al. (1985) it was patients with temporal lobe epilepsy and nuclear schizophrenia that had a significantly shorter interval between the length of the epilepsy and the length of the psychosis compared with patients presenting other patterns of a schizophrenia-like illness, and patients with generalized epilepsy and psychosis. This suggests that it may be a subgroup of patients who are identifiable and more susceptible to a kindling-like mechanism.

The evidence that kindling per se is the relevant mechanism for psychpathology of epilepsy, in particular epileptic psychosis, however, remains conjecture. There is animal data to suggest the possibility. Thus, kindling of the mesolimbic dopamine system has been shown to lead not to seizures, but to marked behaviour changes, which persist after the kindling has ceased

(Stevens and Livermore, 1978). Kindling from medial temporal structures such as the amygdala leads to activation of the entire limbic circuitry, supporting the vulnerability of limbic structures to epileptogenic conditions (Ben Ari, 1981). This is associated with behaviour changes which are maintained interictally but which are dependent upon the pre-kindled behavioural disposition of the animal stimulated (Adamec and Stark-Adamec, 1986). In some species, 'superkindling', in which additional stimulations are given following the development of kindled seizures, has been shown to lead to supersensitivity to the behavioural effects of apomorphine, and both kindled and superkindled animals have been shown to have increased H3 spiperone binding in limbic forebrain structures ipsilateral to the stimulating electrodes reflecting dopamine D2 receptor densities.

In that the higher in the phylogeny one progresses, the more difficult kindling becomes, the possibility therefore arises that in man similar mechanisms exist, and that chronic subictal activity leads to a slow kindling process within dopaminergic pathways, leading to dopaminergic supersensitivity and the development of abnormal behaviour patterns which include psychosis. The fact that in some animal models spontaneous remission of limbic seizures is rare, but those of neocortical origin may remit spontaneously is further support for the existence of at least two groups of patients with focal temporal seizures, one deriving from a limbic and the other a non-limbic source, with the latter having a good prognosis.

However, an argument against kindling being the relevant process derives from follow-up studies of patients with epilepsy and psychosis. Glithero and Slater (1963) followed 64 patients up a mean of 18 years (range 2–25 years) after the onset of their psychosis of epilepsy. Personality deterioration did not occur, but interestingly their epilepsy became less troublesome and better controlled; 16% became seizure free, although in half it was due to a temporal lobectomy. The authors however noted 'the excellent epileptic result was accompanied by a favourable development in the psychosis'. One third of this series had a complete remission of specifically schizophrenic symptoms, and in another third symptoms had improved. Kenwood and Betts (1988) have recently presented similar data on a group of hospitalized psychotic patients followed up after 20 years. In other words, with time, the psychosis and the seizures of many of these patients improves, not supporting the concept of kindling as the relevant process, at least from our current understanding from animal models.

CONCLUSIONS

It is suggested that psychopathology is overrepresented in patients with epilepsy, in particular severe psychopathology such as the psychoses, and that this is more likely to be associated with localization-related temporal lobe epilepsy. There is further evidence that it is patients with medial–basal as opposed to lateral neocortical sites of origin for seizures who are most susceptible, namely those with limbic seizures. It is suggested that they may represent a subgroup of epileptic patients who have a history of difficult-to-control attacks, and their identity rests in the discreteness and interconnectedness of the limbic structures, associated with the low seizure threshold, and the known associations between the limbic system and the modulation of emotion and affect.

One explanation for the development of psychopathology in such patients is that of kindling, but to date there are only hints and no direct evidence that it is the predominant mechanism associated with at least the psychoses related to epilepsy.

REFERENCES

Adamec, R. E. and Stark-Adamec, C. (1986). Limbic hyperfunction, limbic epilepsy and interictal behaviour. In: *The Limbic System, Functional Organisation and Clinical Disorders* (eds B. K. Doane and K. E. Livingston), pp. 129–145. Raven Press, New York.

Ben Ari, Y. (1981). Local injections of Kainic acid: a model of limbic seizures with local and distant pathology. In: *The Amygdaloid Complex* (ed. Y. Ben Ari), pp. 443–452. Elsevier/North-Holland.

Conlon, P. and Trimble, M. R. (1988). MRI in Epilepsy; a controlled study. *Epilepsy Res.*, **2**, 37–43.

Currie, S., Heathfield, K. W. G., Henson, R. A. and Scott, D. F. (1971). Clinical course and prognosis of temporal lobe epilepsy: a study of 666 patients. *Brain*, **94**, 173–190.

Edeh, J. and Toone, B. (1987). Relationship between interictal psychopathology and type of epilepsy. *Br. J. Psychiat.*, **151**, 95–101.

Flor-Henry, P. (1969). Psychosis and temporal lobe epilepsy. *Epilepsia*, **10**, 363–395.

Fulton, J. F. (1953). Discussion. *Epilepsia*, **2**, 77.

Gallhofer, B., Trimble, M. R., Frackowiak, R., Gibbs, J. and Jones, T. (1985). A study of cerebral blood flow and metabolism in epileptic psychosis using positron emission tomography and oxygen–15. *J. Neurol. Neurosurg. Psychiat.*, **48**, 201–206.

Gibbs, F. A., Gibbs, E. L. and Lennox, W. G. (1937). Epilepsy: a paroxysmal cerebral dysrhythmia. *Brain*, **60**, 377–388.

Girgis, M. (1981). *Neurol Substrates of Limbic Epilepsy*. Warren H. Green, Missouri.

Glaser, G. H. (1967). Limbic epilepsy in childhood. *J. Nerv. Ment. Dis.*, **144**, 391–397.

Glithero, E. N. and Slater, E. (1963). Follow up record and outcome. *Br. J. Psychiat.*, **109**, 134–142.

Goldberg, D. P., Cooper, B., Eastwood, M. R., Kedward, H. B. and Shepherd, M. A standardized psychiatric interview for use in community surveys. *Br. J. Prevent. Soc. Med.*, **24**, 18–23.

Goodridge, D. M. G. and Shorvon, S. D. (1983). Epileptic seizures in a population of 6000. *Br. Med. J.*, **287**, 641–644.

Gudmundsson, G. (1966). Epilepsy in Iceland. *Acta Neurol. Scand.*, **43** (Suppl. 25), 1–124.

Heath, R. G. (1977). Subcortical brain function correlates of psychopathology in epilepsy. In: *Psychopathology and Brain Dysfunction* (eds C. Shagass, S. Gershon, A. J. Friedhoff). Raven Press, New York.

Helgason, T. (1964). Epidemiology of mental disorders in Iceland. *Acta Psychiat. Scand.*, Suppl. 142.

Hermann, B. P., Dikmen, S., Schwartz, M. S. and Carnes, W. E. (1982). Interictal psychopathology in patients with ictal fear: a quantitative investigation. *Neurology*, **32**, 7–11.

ILAE (1985). Proposal for classification of epilepsies and epileptic syndromes. *Epilepsia*, **26**, 268–278.

Jackson, H. J. (1888). On a particular variety of epilepsy (intellectual aura). One case with symptoms of organic brain disease. *Brain*, **11**, 179–207.

Jackson, H. J. and Steward, P. (1899). Epileptic attacks with a warning of accrued sensation of smell and with the intellectual aura (dreamy state) in a patient who had symptoms pointing to gross organic disease of the right temporosphenoidal lobe. *Brain*, **22**, 534–549.

Jasper, H. H., Pertuiset, B. and Flanigan, H. (1951). EEG and cortical electrograms in patients with temporal lobe seizures. *Arch. Neurol. Psychiat.*, **65**, 272–290.

Kenwood, C. and Betts, T. (1988). 20 year follows up of epileptic psychosis. *British, Danish, Dutch Epilepsy Congress Abstracts*, p. 53. Heemstede, Netherlands.

Kristensen, O. and Sindrup, E. G. (1979). Psychomotor epilepsy and Prognosis. *Acta Neurol. Scand.*, **57**, 661–670.

Lewis, D. O., Pincus, J. H., Shanok, S. S. and Glaser, G. H. (1982). Psychomotor epilepsy and violence in a group of incarcarated adolescent boys. *Am. J. Psychiat.*, **139**, 882–887.

Nielsen, H. and Kristensen, O. (1981). Personality correlates of sphenoidal EEG foci in temporal lobe epilepsy. *Acta Neurol. Scand.*, **64**, 289–300.

Ounsted, C. and Lindsay, J. (1981). The long-term outcome of temporal lobe epilepsy in childhood. In: *Epilepsy and Psychiatry* (eds E. H. Reynolds and M. R. Trimble), pp. 185–215. Churchill Livingstone, Edinburgh.

Pond, D. A. and Bidwell, B. H. (1959). A survey of epilepsy in 14 general practices. *Epilepsia*, **1**, 285–299.

Perez, M. M., Trimble, M. R., Murray, N. M. S. and Reider, I. (1985). Epileptic psychosis and evaluation of PSE profiles. *Br. J. Psychiat.*, **146**, 155–163.

Reynolds, E. H. (1987). Early treatment and prognosis of epilepsy. *Epilepsia*, **28**, 97–106.

Robertson, M. M., Trimble, M. R. and Townsend, H. R. A. (1987). Phenomenology of depression in epilepsy. *Epilepsia*, **28**, 364–372.

Rodin, E. A. (1968). *The Prognosis of Patients with Epilepsy*. Charles Thomas, Springfield, 1968.

Rutter, M., Graham, P. and Yale, W. (1970). A neuropsychiatric study in childhood. *Clinics in Developmental Medicine*, **35**, Heinemann, London.

Schmidt, D. (1984). Prognosis of chronic epilepsy with complex partial seizures. *J. Neurol. Neurosurg. Psychiat.*, **47**, 1274–1278.

Shorvon, S. D. (1984). The temporal aspects of prognosis in epilepsy. *J. Neurol. Neurosurg. Psychiat.*, **471**, 1157–1165.

Slater, E. and Beard, A. W. (1963). The schizophrenia like psychosis of epilepsy. *Br. J. Psychiat.*, **109**, 95–112.

Stevens, J. R. and Hermann, B. P. (1981). Temporal lobe epilepsy, psychopathology and violence: the state of the evidence. *Neurology*, **31**, 1127–1132.

Stevens, J. R. and Livermore, A. (1978). Kindling in the mesolimbic dopamine system: animal model of psychosis. *Neurology*, **28**, 36–46.

Toone, B. (1981). Psychoses of epilepsy. In: *Epilepsy and Psychiatry* (eds E. H. Reynolds and M. R. Trimble), pp. 113–137. Churchill Livingstone, Edinburgh.

Trimble, M. R. (1988). *Biological Psychiatry*. Wiley, Chichester.

Zielinski, J. J. (1974). *Epidemiology and Medical-Social Problems of Epilepsy in Warsaw*. Warsaw Psychoneurological Institute, Warsaw.

Discussion — Session 4

DOES EPILEPSY IMPLY KINDLED SEIZURES?

R. Adamec Dr Reynolds, your data are very interesting, and certainly are consistent with a kindling process. I wonder whether you have any data on whether a similar kind of process seems to exist in the progression of seizure type. Is there progression from, for example, a partial seizure to a secondary generaliztion? Is that an inevitable end point, or are patients at risk for developing a secondary generalization, if partial seizures are allowed to persist without treatment.

E. H. Reynolds I cannot answer your question. It is difficult to answer retrospectively, because you are relying on patients' memories, and they just simply cannot recall all their partial seizures. Some of them are not aware of partial seizures. That could only be done prospectively and has not been done.

C. Wasterlain Is there any evidence that delaying the onset of treatment makes control more difficult?

E. H. Reynolds It has not been examined.

P. Vestergaard It was very fascinating to listen to your line of argument for a more vigorous treatment of the first seizure. If you substitute epileptic seizures with mania, you have the same line of argument. The first manic attack should be treated vigorously, for exactly the same reasons. But then you have another problem, and that is that patients do not accept their diagnoses of a serious illness after only one attack.

E. H. Reynolds I agree with you and what you said about mania may also apply to schizophrenia. My own views about early treatment for epilepsy have come to haunt me this very week, when an Indian doctor brought his

191

8-year-old daughter to see me, and all she had had was three auras over the period of about 9 months. These were subjective auras and they probably were of temporal lobe origin, because there was a family history of temporal lobe epilepsy. What really worried the doctor was that he had a sister who at the age of 30 had had some partial seizures which had gone on to generalize and had developed chronic epilepsy. I was confronted with an 8-year-old girl with three auras, and he said: 'I've read somewhere that it's important to treat epilepsy early.' I did not treat this 8-year-old girl, because I told him I did not really know what the prognosis was.

R. Post   To potentially complicate the recommendation to treat early — if some data we have in animals are at all relevant to man, we would have to say that if one treats early, one had better treat with a drug that is going to be effective, because if one treats with a drug that is not effective, early, you may lose the possibility of having that drug work later on. Schmutz showed that carbamazepine and some other drugs did not inhibit the development of kindling, even though they are excellent anticonvulsants for the established or completed stage. If one treats with these drugs in those early development stages, they won't work later on, in the kindling model.

M. Dam   I do not know whether this theory holds. We have many other drugs in the same category, and if we do not have any effect of carbamazepine, I would immediately proceed to oxcarbazepine, which is even better, with fewer side effects. I never treat after the first seizure. I would also always hesitate to make the diagnosis of epilepsy after the second seizure. There may be an interval between the first and second seizure of more than a year, and then whether or not the patient should be treated is a difficult question.

F. Schulsinger   What characterizes schizophrenia, what is specific for schizophrenia, are the 'negative' symptoms. What about hallucinations and delusions, the positive symptoms? — Yes, they appear in schizophrenics, but they also appear in epileptics, in amphetamine psychoses and a lot of other conditions. Be very cautious about dividing schizophrenia into positive and negative symptom groups. It may not be very fruitful.

M. R. Trimble   The importance of Schneiderian first rank symptoms for the diagnosis of schizophrenia has been held paramount by British psychiatry for years, but has not influenced American psychiatry very much until DSM III. It has not influenced Scandinavian psychiatry. However, this issue is *not* that those patients have what you might call schizophrenia, but that schizophrenic patients have neurological symptoms, and amongst those symptoms are hallucinations and delusions of a specific type that Schneider defined. My theme is that these symptoms are consequent on a temporal lobe abnormality. In other words: the first rank symptoms of Schneider for the psychiatrist are like a Babinski response for a neurologist. They tell us that something is going on in the brain of that patient. Their presence does not, in my opinion, mean that you have to make a diagnosis of schizophrenia, because, as you pointed out they can occur in many other conditions. However, if you look at the recent studies in schizophrenia, many are pointing to the fact that the temporal lobes are involved, both neurochemically and pathologically, in *some* schizophrenic patients. Now, the negative symptoms you define are probably not temporal lobe phenomena. They are much more likely to be frontal lobe phenomena. The lesson for psychiatry is that the temporal lobes are involved in the pathology of some schizophrenic patients, and it is up to us to define further the extent of that involvement and the relationship of that involvement to treatment and prognosis.

The Clinical Relevance of Kindling
Edited by T. G. Bolwig and M. R. Trimble
© 1989 John Wiley & Sons Ltd

13

Convulsive therapy and kindling

MAX FINK
*Department of Psychiatry and Behavioral Science, School of Medicine, State
University of New York at Stony Brook, New York 11794, and International
Association for Psychiatric Research, St James, New York 11780, USA*

Demonstrations that 'periodic bipolar stimulation of any number of sites
throughout the olfactory-limbic system can lead to the gradual development
and intensification of behavioral convulsions (kindling) in a variety of species
even at current intensities intially too low to produce any behavioral or
electrographic effects' excited researchers that a model of human epilepsy
had been found (Goddard, McIntyre and Leach, 1969; Pinel and Van Oot,
1975). Pinel and Van Oot go on:

For example, if the rat amygdala is periodically stimulated at a level which produces
neither electrographic nor behavioral effects, eventually the afterdischarge threshold
may be reduced to the point that subsequent stimulations reliably elicit an afterdischarge. If stimulations are then continued, mild motor automatisms may appear
which increase in severity with each successive stimulation until motor seizures,
characterized by facial and forelimb clonus, rearing, and a loss of equilibrium can be
reliably elicited.

'Kindling' is a phenomenon that occurs under the explicit circumstances
of intracerebral, spaced, discrete, repetitive stimulation in specific brain
regions in sensitive individuals (Goddard, 1967; Goddard, McIntyre and
Leach 1969; Racine, 1975; Adamec and Stark-Adamec, 1983). Species vary
as to susceptibility, so that relatively few stimulations in some rat strains
excite the phenomenon, but greater numbers of stimulations are needed in
other species.

The phenomenon would have remained an interesting laboratory exercise except that its students sought to relate their findings to clinical practice. Pinel and Van Oot (1975) argued:

'. . . we have tried to determine what implications the kindling phenomenon might have for the application of various forms of convulsive therapy in the treatment of psychpathology.'

And again,

The generality of the kindling phenomenon has two rather direct implications for the use of convulsive or potentially convulsive therapies. First, clinicans should be aware of the enduring changes in brain function which can be induced by such agents and weigh the hazards involved against possible therapeutic benefits. Second, if such therapeutic agents are employed, it is important that the subsequent exposure to potentially convulsive agents be carefully monitored.

In a later study, these authors reported that repeated ECS administered once every 3 days to rats at one of two current intensities led to progressive intensification of motor seizure patterns (Pinel and Van Oot, 1977). The incidence of convulsive symptoms elicited by subsequent alcohol exposure and withdrawal was greatly increased by prior exposure to repeated ECS. They concluded:

These results illustrate a treatment-drug interaction which could have hazardous consequences for patients undergoing electroconvulsive therapy.

In their discussion they argued:

Thus, one major feature of kindling . . . is that the increase in seizure susceptibility produced by the repeated administrations of one convulsive agent is not limited to seizures produced exclusively by that agent.

With this observation, they warned against the exposure of patients receiving ECT to psychotherapeutic agents, specifically antidepressant drugs.

Although all drug administrations are typically discontinued the morning before an ECS treatment, the potential hazard does not exist during the treatment session itself, but some time afterward when the patient is no longer under the immediate supervision of the doctor. It is during this period after the treatments that the convulsive reaction to an otherwise innocuous agent might be dangerously potentiated.

The apparent similarity of repeated electrical stimulations which excited a kindled focus to those which were used in electro-convulsive therapy (ECT) led Goddard (1967) and Pinel and Van Oot (1975, 1977) to suggest that kindling was a model both for the clinical efficacy and the risks inherent in a course of ECT. It is easy to see the apparent similarity in the repeated electrical inductions of ECT and the electrical stimulations in kindling. This belief, that the Goddard kindling paradigm bears a direct relationship to the clinical convulsive therapy process, has been a focus of concern and discussion for more than two decades. But the issues have become somewhat clouded by imprecision in the definition of 'kindling' and the diversity in its usage.

For some authors, the kindling paradigm remains a model for the development of elicited and spontaneous epileptic seizures or their behavioral equivalents. In this view, the repeated stimulation of specific brain areas with low currents will elicit longer and longer electrical discharges, which eventually develop to full motor seizures. For others, the term 'kindling' is applied to the intracerebral electrical phenomenon alone, such as the increase in duration of elicited electrical activity after a subthreshold stimulus of the same strength.

In most laboratory descriptions of kindling, the brain is impaled by stimulating and recording electrodes, and definite evidence of cellular damage about these sites is reported. The experimentalists studying the paradigm argue, however, that the placement of these electrodes is a matter of laboratory convenience, and is not essential to the kindling process, since similar increased electrical activity may be elicited by the repeated extra-cerebral (intraperitoneal) administration of pentylenetetrazol, lidocaine, and cocaine (Pinel and Van Oot, 1975). These authors also believe that the effects of kindling are permanent, and that the very permanence is evidence of brain damage.

It is of historical interest that the clinical cautions presented by Goddard (1967) and by Pinel and Van Oot (1975, 1977) occurred at a time when antigovernmental and anti-authoritarian feelings ran high in America as a result of excessive governmental zeal in the pursuit of the Vietnam War. Antimedical feelings led to legal proscription of intrusive treatments, notably leucotomy and ECT. In this climate, the suggestions that ECT was an analog of the kindling process with a caution that the process involved *permanent* changes in brain function, and evidence of *brain damage* were given a currency among the laity that was not earned. Despite disclaimers and arguments that the two processes are distinct (Fink, 1979; Small *et al.*, 1981), neuroscientists continue to harbor the nagging suspicion that Goddard kindling with its associated brain damage and development of a seizure focus is somehow a feature of ECT. This discussion will focus on the similarities and differences between clinically applied electroconvulsive therapy and Goddard kindling paradigms. In part, the focus will be on the differences in the two phenomena, to allow the reader to judge whether the cautions urged by the early workers justifies special concerns today.

SIMILARITIES IN GODDARD KINDLING AND ECT

The main similarity between Goddard kindling and ECT is that both use repeated electric currents for a behavioral effect. A second aspect, now of historical interest, are early reports of spontaneous ('tardive') seizures in patients during the course of ECT. This phenomenon was described in the first two decades of the use of ECT, but is not a feature of modern treatment.

Seizures induced chemically and electrically

The superficial similarity between Goddard kindling and ECT lies in the repeated administration of electrical stimulations. Yet, convulsive therapy may be as effective with the administration of intravenous pentylenetetrazol or the inhalation of flurothyl, as by the use of electric currents (Fink, 1979).

Meduna based his actions on both neuropathological and clinical evidence of an antagonism between seizures and dementia praecox (schizophrenia, today). As a neuropathologist, he had counted the concentration of glia cells in different brain areas. He reported a relative paucity of glia cells in patients with dementia praecox, a disease believed at that time to be inherited and genetic. In patients with severe forms of epilepsy, he reported a relative over-concentration of glia in the same areas. Contemporary clinical surveys reported that the symptoms of dementia praecox were relatively rare in populations of severe epileptics, and that epilepsy was a rarity among patients hospitalized with dementia praecox.

In 1918, Wagner-Jauregg demonstrated that patients with dementia paralytica (neurosyphilis) could be successfully treated with an experimental infection with malaria. This experience led to a general acceptance of a therapeutic model considered reasonable by many at the time, that one disease could be treated by another. Some scientists administered the blood of dementia praecox patients to those with epilepsy, a trial without success. Meduna sought to develop seizures in patients with dementia praecox. After pharmacologic trials, he found instramuscular camphor in oil successful in eliciting seizures, and he treated his first patient on 24 January 1934 (Meduna, 1985). Camphor was soon replaced by pentylenetetrazol (Metrazol) and this induction was the mainstay of the treatment until 1938.

The behavioral effects of convulsive therapy result from repeated inductions of grand mal epileptic seizures. Pharmacologically induced seizures, such as with pentylenetetrazol or flurothyl, have the same efficacy, require the same numbers of seizures, and exhibit the same effects on mood, neuropsychological tests, cognition, language, EEG, and biochemistry. From this experience we conclude that no aspect of the *electrical* induction is central to the therapeutic process in convulsive therapy. Insofar as kindling of seizure foci seem to depend so heavily on *electrical* stimulations, there is no basis for an association with the convulsive therapy process.

Tardive seizures

Perhaps the observation which most connects Goddard kindling to ECT are reports of tardive seizures occurring during a course of ECT. Such delayed seizures were thought to occur mainly in patients with a prior history of seizure disorder or brain injury. Until 1958, 71 cases had been reported, and in the next two decades, only one additional case has appeared (Fink, 1979). Most of the cases were reported in young adults. At the time of the American Psychiatric Association (APA) Task Force report and survey (1978), the respondents (10% of the APA membership randomly selected) were queried as to their experience with tardive seizures. Five cases were reported, with four occurring within the hour of treatment.

The rarity of tardive seizures today may result from changes in ECT practice. Present practice elicits seizures with stimuli that are just above the threshold for seizure induction. Alternating currents have been replaced by brief pulse stimulations, the latter delivering much less energy (30–80% less) to elicit a seizure. Awareness that cognitive deficits were related to the intensity of currents (while efficacy was related to the seizure itself), led to studies of the minimal currents necessary to induce a seizure. The use of minimal currents, just greater than seizure thresholds, is routine. This practice has been aided by our finding that seizure thresholds rise with age, so that modern manuals emphasize the use of lower energies in young adults and higher energies in older adults (Fink, 1988).

Monitoring of seizure duration by cuff and by EEG methods has become routine. In treatments modified by methohexital and succinylcholine it is customary to find the seizure duration in the cuffed limb shorter than the duration estimated from the tachycardia response, and both estimates are shorter than those based on the scalp EEG (Fink and Johnson, 1982). Dysrhythmic activity in the EEG usually ends abruptly and is followed by an isoelectric period. From time to time, the end-point is imprecise, with seizure activity recurring, or waxing and waning for many minutes. At such times, no overt motor activity may be manifest. On rare occasions, rhythmic motor activity accompanies irregular EEG seizure activity, and the seizure duration is seen as prolonged (Greenberg, 1985). These manifestations usually end abruptly, or are terminated by intravenous barbiturate or diazepam.

When tardive seizures have been observed, it is usually in the treatment or recovery room, and we now believe that these are prolonged seizures secondary to high intensity stimulation in young adults. The introduction of anesthesia in the 1950s shortened seizure durations and raised seizure thresholds, reducing the likelihood that the currents would be excessive (far

Table 1. Kindling and ECT

	Kindling	ECT
Aim	Induce seizures	Mood change
Stimulation	Electrical	Electrical, Pharmacologic
Locus	Intracerebral	Extracranial
Intensity	Low subthreshold	High suprathreshold
Number of stimulations	Repetitive (more than 50)	Repetitive (6–12)
Effect of ECS	Blocks	None
Seizure threshold	Lowered	Raised
Effect of barbiturate	Blocked	Not blocked
Duration of effect	'Permanent'	Transient
Class action	Convulsant	Anticonvulsant

above threshold) and lead to a prolonged seizure, and reducing the incidence of tardive seizures.

DIFFERENCES IN GODDARD KINDLING AND ECT

The two processes differ mainly in the strength of the currents used and the immediate effects of stimulation. They also differ in numbers of seizures, role of brain injury, barbiturate anesthesia, and effects on seizure threshold and the anticonvulsant activity of ECT. An additional point made about Goddard kindling is its permanence, while the ECT process (alas) is too often transient.

Current intensity

Kindling depends on the administration of low-energy subconvulsive currents which do not elicit a seizure, while convulsive therapy requires a grand mal seizure with each stimulation. Indeed, the induction of a grand mal seizure in the kindling process may prevent the kindling of spontaneous seizure activity (Babington and Wedeking, 1975; Post *et al.*, 1986).

Direct brain stimulation

Kindling currents must be applied to the brain directly. There is no evidence that a focus can be stimulated by the administration of low energy currents extra-cerebrally. Indeed, the use of subconvulsive currents, sufficient to elicit a hemi-seizure of the Jacksonian type, gives little clinical benefit. In a recent discussion of kindling, Schmutz (1987) notes in his abstract:

Human data: one case of human brain kindling and several cases of spontaneously recurrent seizures following electroconvulsive treatment are known. . .

In the case material present in the text, however, he notes that:

. . . one striking case of human brain kindling is published. . . The patient developed phantom pain after a hand injury. She underwent coagulation of part of the left nucleus ventralis posteromedialis of the thalamus and then daily electrical stimulation of the thalamus. In the third week of stimulation, she perceived spontaneous mild movements of the right half of her face, *etc.*

This human study is similar to animal models of kindling, insofar as brain injury was initially established, followed by repeated daily intracerebral, subthreshold, electrical stimulation. Neither direct brain damage, nor direct brain stimulation, nor subthreshold stimulations are features of the convulsive therapy process, clearly dissociating one from the other, and the association of the case with the tardive seizures of ECT in Schmutz' summary reflects a failure to separate the two phenomena.

Barbiturate anesthesia

Goddard kindling is inhibited by barbiturate anesthesia. ECT is now generally administered under barbiturate anesthesia, making the kindling process even less likely. Even if extra-cerebral stimulations of high energy currents (sufficient to elicit a seizure) were suggestive of Goddard type kindling, the process would be inhibited by our routine use of methohexital or Pentothal anesthesia.

Seizure threshold

Seizure thesholds fall in Goddard kindling, so much so that seizures may be elicited with subthreshold currents or even spontaneously. In contrast, seizure thresholds rise in ECT (Brockman *et al.*, 1956; Green, 1960). In treatments with pentylenetetrazol, it was routinely necessary to increase dosages with successive seizures to elicit a satisfactory treatment. This experience argued for a rise in seizure threshold (a lowered sensitivity to Metrazol) with successive treatments.

Early studies of ECT included explorations of different stimulation currents and different dosages to elicit seizures. A titration technique for dosage of currents was developed. Patients, while anesthetized, were first administered currents that failed to elicit a grand mal seizure. Dosage was increased until a seizure threshold was just exceeded and a satisfactory grand mal convulsion occurred. Seizure thresholds varied with age, being lower in younger patients than in the elderly, and rise with successive treatments. In one study in my laboratory, Green (1960) observed that seizure thresholds rose in 24/39 patients, and remained the same in 15. In no patient did seizure thresholds fall with successive treatments. These observations have been replicated in more elegant and better controlled studies by Small *et al.* (1981,

1988) and Sackeim *et al.* (1986). In parametric studies in which induction currents have been maintained constant, beginning above the threshold for the first seizure, seizure durations are shown to fall progressively, complementing the rise in seizure threshold.

A rise in seizure threshold is a regular feature of convulsive therapy. It is this physiologic phenomenon which contrasts so sharply with the progressive *fall* in seizure threshold in Goddard kindling that further differentiates ECT and kindling.

Numbers of inductions

The number of stimulations for the two processes differ. It usually requires hundreds of stimulations to induce a kindling focus, but only 6–20 stimulations for clinical ECT (Fink, 1988).

ECT as anticonvulsant

The rise in seizure threshold is the basis for the application of ECT in patients with intractable status epilepticus. While the reports are few, they do go back to the early trials with ECT (Kalinowsky and Kennedy, 1943), and have been invoked more recently (Sackeim *et al.*, 1983). The animal studies of Post *et al.* (1984, 1986) demonstrate the anticonvulsant (as well as the antikindling) effects of ECS. Such clinical and laboratory demonstrations argue that induced seizures are a potent and effective anticonvulsant.

KINDLING AS A MODEL FOR CLINICAL ACTIVITY OF ECT

Putting aside the arguments of Goddard kindling as a model of the ECT process, another application of kindling has been as a model for the pathophysiology of psychoses and as an explanation for the clinical efficacy of ECT.

Epilepsy and psychosis

'Kindling' theory has been invoked to suggest that epileptic foci are the basis for psychotic behavior. Post and his colleagues observe that anticonvulsant drugs (like carbamazepine), when used alone or in conjunction with lithium or antipsychotic drugs, reduce the clinical symptoms of mania (Post *et al.*, 1984, 1986; Post and Uhde, 1985). They look at the anticonvulsant action of carbamazepine and infer that manic behavior may result from subclinical seizure activity, from brain foci that have been 'kindled' by trauma or by genetic influences (see Post, Chapter 14). To support their views, they studied the effects of anticonvulsants and ECS in animals with amygdala-kindled seizures. Both seizures and carbamazepine prevent the kindling of seizures, and prevent the expression of kindled seizures (Post *et al.*, 1984). Kindling of an epileptic focus is seen as both a mechanism for the pathophysiology of the disorder and an explanation for the efficacy of carbamazepine and ECT.

Studies of temporal lobe epilepsy (TLE) provide another example. Some psychotic patients exhibit EEG seizure foci, often in temporal areas, in clinical recordings leading some authors to argue that the psychotic symptoms result from subclinical seizure activity and to label the syndrome 'temporal lobe epilepsy'. To relieve the psychotic symptoms, they recommend anticonvulsants. These threads lead to the conclusion that seizure activity may be a factor in manic behavior and some psychoses, and that in both instances, the abnormal brain activity is 'kindled' along lines described by Goddard.

An opposite view is presented by Meduna and others who argue for an antagonism between epilepsy and psychosis. It was this view that led Meduna to suggest that induced seizures would ameliorate the psychotic symptoms of dementia praecox. His success led to trials in other conditions and the demonstration that ECT is also effective in relieving other psychoses, for example, those associated with mood disorders. Formal psychoses are still rare today in patients with epilepsy, and patients with affective disorders rarely exhibit spontaneous seizures; when they do, it is more likely incidental to post-traumatic or post-infectious causes. In such instances, when spontaneous seizure activity is allowed expression (as by inadequate anticonvulsant drug therapy), there may be an amelioration of affective and psychotic symptoms. This phenomenon is described as 'forced normalization'. When clinical seizures occur, psychotic and affective symptoms are controlled, and EEG records show persistent dysrhythmic patterns; when seizures are controlled, psychotic and affective symptoms become clinically manifest, and EEG records show 'normal', non-dysrhythmic patterns (Pakalnis *et al.*, 1987; Pollack, 1987).

What effect does ECT have on these two conditions, manic behavior and psychoses associated with epilepsy? ECT is effective in treating the symptoms of mania. Indeed, ECT is often effective in patients in whom other antimanic therapies, including carbamazepine, have failed (Small, 1985; Alexander *et al.*, 1988). ECT is also an effective antipsychotic agent. This is documented in patients with depressive disorders with psychosis (delusional depression), manic delirium and psychosis, involutional and post-partum psychoses, positive symptom psychosis, schizo-affective disorders, *etc*. While no direct study comparing anticonvulsants and ECT in the treatment of patients with psychosis associated with TLE is known, there is little reason to question its antipsychotic activity in such conditions.

Kindling and a theory of the antidepressant efficacy of ECT

Some authors suggest that the antidepressant effects of ECT result from its anticonvulsant activity. The critical aspect of the ECT process is not the elicitation of the seizure, but the process which terminates the seizure. Termination of the seizure does not result from neuronal exhaustion or deficiency of oxygen or glucose, but from the potentiation of an active inhibitory process and enhanced inhibitory neurotransmission (Sackeim *et al.*, 1983).

The evidence has already been described: the antagonism of ECS for the development and expression of kindled seizures; the efficacy of ECT in cases of intractable epilepsy; the increase in seizure threshold and fall in seizure duration with successive treatments; and postictal reductions in regional cerebral blood flow and the development of EEG slow wave activity. An increase in the functional activity of inhibitory neurotransmitters, notably gamma-aminobutyric acid (GABA) and endogenous levels of monoamine oxidase inhibitors, are the operational step in the antidepressant activity of ECT.

We should be able to predict from this view that anticonvulsant drugs should be effective as antidepressant and antimanic treatments; and that antidepressant drugs should be active anticonvulsants. But such suggestions are clearly inconsistent with clinical experience. While anticonvulsant drugs, including carbamazepine, phenytoin, and valproic acid, exhibit antimanic activity, their role as antidepressant drugs is unimpressive. Established tricyclic antidepressant drugs (TCA) and monoamine oxidase inhibitors (MAOI) are hardly anticonvulsant. Whatever it is in the ECT process that makes for its antidepressant activity, it is not those features which are prominently shared by anticonvulsants, nor aspects reflected in the Goddard kindling phenomenon.

ASSUMPTIONS

The assumed association between kindling and the efficacy of convulsive therapy is symptomatic of an occasional flaw in pharmacologic research, particularly transmitter and receptor studies. Comparisons are made between the effects of TCA drugs and ECS on the assumption that the therapeutic action of drugs and ECS is the same; that the physiology and pharmacology of the normal rat are equal to that of the mentally ill human; and that species specificities in pharmacology are immaterial or incidental.

When one looks directly at such assumptions, they are difficult to justify. The range of clinical activity of TCA drugs and ECT is not similar. ECT is routinely effective in cases where TCA drugs are ineffective, the treatment of patients with delusional depression being a prominent example. The activity of TCA drugs is more restricted than that of ECT, and their potency is less. While TCA drugs may stimulate manic or psychotic behavior in patients with bipolar disorders and are contra-indicated in manic patients, ECT is as effective an antimanic agent as an antidepressant. The biochemical and physiologic effects of TCA and ECT are distinctive, whether measured in blood or CSF over a wide range of measures.

Results of studies of brain transmitters and receptors in the normal rat are often extrapolated to that of man, and further, to that of depressed man. But the physiology of man is distinctive from that of the rat, as is the physiology of depressed patients from that of normal man. Prominent examples include abnormal neuroendocrine regulation, differential sensitivity to CNS drugs (e.g. sedation threshold studies), and the presence of abnormal mood, cognition, vigilance, and vegetative symptoms in patients. These abnormalities normalize in treatment with ECT. It is difficult enough to justify and extrapolate information from studies of normal man to patients with depression; it is impossible to extrapolate from studies of the normal rat, a species not only different in pathophysiology since it lacks the depressive diathesis, but a nocturnal species with extensive differences in physiology and pharmacology. Since we do not know the salient pathophysiology of depressed man, is it not overtly optimistic to assume that the abnormal pathophysiology of patients is somehow similar to the brain functions of the normal rat, an extremely unlikely happenstance?

Our continued search among animal models for theories or clinical clues in psychiatric patients remains a Sisyphean endeavor. The misidentification of Goddard kindling with the ECT process is one small example in a long line of misapprehensions that have resulted from a superficial translation of the results of animal experiments to human endeavors. While Goddard kindling is a laboratory phenomenon of considerable interest in studies of the brain to external events (its 'plasticity') or as a model of 'learning', it clearly is not a model of clinical interest in convulsive therapy.

SUMMARY

Goddard's demonstration of the kindling of spontaneous seizure activity in rodents by repeated intracerebral stimulation with low intensity, subthreshold currents occurred at a time when ECT was reintroduced into clinical practice. The simplistic similarity between the repeated electrical stimulation in kindling and in ECT and the occasional reports of tardive seizures in ECT led to the suggestion that the two phenomena were functionally similar. But the two processes differ in many salient ways including the strength of currents, prerequisite brain injury, role of barbiturate anesthesia, seizure threshold, number of stimulations, anticonvulsant activity of ECT, and permanence. Indeed, ECT is clearly anticonvulsant in activity, and is arguably an effective 'anti-kindling' agent.

Kindling has also been suggested as the basis for manic activity and the psychoses of temporal lobe epilepsy, with the recommendation that the efficacy of carbamazepine, an anticonvulsant drug, may lie in its action on kindled foci. In this view, the efficacy of ECT in mania is based on its anticonvulsant activity. And, kindling has been proposed as a model for the antidepressant activity of ECT. The role of kindling in mania, in the anti-manic activity of carbamazepine, and in the anticonvulsant activity of ECT is poorly supported. Further, the merits of animal models for hypotheses about ECT or antidepressant drugs is challenged, as poorly justified in theory and in practice.

REFERENCES

Adamec, R. E. and Stark-Adamec, C. (1983). Limbic kindling and animal behavior: Implications for human psychopathology associated with complex partial seizures. *Biol. Psychiat.*, **18**, 269–294.

Alexander, R. C., Salomon, M., Ionescu-Pioggia, M. and Cole, J. O. (1988). Convulsive therapy in the treatment of mania. McLean Hospital 1973–1986. *Convulsive Ther.*, **4**, 115–125.

American Psychiatric Association (1978). *Electroconvulsive Therapy*. American Psychiatric Association Press, Washington, DC.

Babington, R. G. and Wedeking, P. W. (1975). Blockade of tardive seizures in rats by electroconvulsive shock. *Brain Res.*, **88**, 141–144.

Brockman, R. J., Brockman, J. C., Jacobson, U., Gleser, G. C. J. and Ulett, G. A. (1956). Changes in convulsive threshold as related to type of treatment. *Confin. Neurol.*, **16**, 97–104.

Fink, M. (1979). *Convulsive Therapy: Theory and Practice*. Raven Press, New York.

Fink, M. (1988). Convulsive therapy: A manual of practice. *Review of Psychiatry*, pp. 482–497. American Psychiatric Association Press, Washington, DC.

Fink, M. and Johnson, L. (1982). Monitoring duration of ECT seizures: 'cuff' and EEG methods compared. *Arch. Gen. Psychiat.*, **39**, 1189–1191.

Goddard, G. V. (1967). Development of epileptic seizures through brain stimulation at low intensity. *Nature*, **214**, 1020–1021.

Goddard, G. V., McIntyre, D. C. and Leech, C. K. (1969). A permanent change in brain function resulting from daily electrical stimulation. *Exp. Neurol.*, **25**, 295–330.

Green, M. A. (1960). Relation between threshold and duration of seizures and electrographic change during convulsive therapy. *J. Nerv. Ment. Dis.* 131: 117–120.

Greenberg, L. B. (1985). Detection of prolonged seizures during electroconvulsive therapy: A comparison of electroencephalogram and cuff monitoring. *Convulsive Ther.* 1: 32–37.

Kalinowsky, L. B. and Kennedy, F. (1943). Observations in electric shock therapy applied to problems of epilepsy. *J. Nerv. Ment. Dis.*, **98**, 56–67, 1943.

Meduna, L. (1985). Autobiography. *Convulsive Ther.*, **1**, 43–57, 121–135.

Pakalnis, A., Drake, M. E., John, K. and Kellum, J. B. (1987). Forced normalization. Acute psychosis after seizure control in seven patients. *Arch. Neurol.*, **44**, 289–292.

Pinel, J. P. J. and Van Oot, P. H. (1975). Generality of the kindling phenomenon: Some clinical implications. *Can. J. Neurol. Sci.*, **2**, 467–475.

Pinel, J. P. J. and Van Oot, P. H. (1977). Intensification of the alcohol withdrawal syndrome following periodic electroconvulsive shocks. *Biol. Psychiat.*, **12**, 479–486.

Pollack, D. C. (1987). Models for understanding the antagonism between seizures and psychosis. *Prog. Neuro-Psychopharmacol. Biol. Psychiat.*, **11**, 483–504.

Post, R. M. and Uhde, T. W. (1985). Are the psychotropic effects of carbamazepine in manic-depressive illness mediated through the limbic system? *Psychiat. J. Univ. Ottawa.*, **10**, 205–219.

Post, R. M., Putnam, F., Contel, N. R. and Goldman, B. (1984). Electroconvulsive seizures inhibit amygdala kindling: Implications for mechanisms of action in affective illness. *Epilepsia*, **25**, 234–239.

Post, R. M., Putnam, F., Uhde, T. W. and Weiss, S. R. B. (1986). Electroconvulsive therapy as an anticonvulsant: Implications for its mechanism of action in affective illness. *Ann. N.Y. Acad. Sci.*, **462**, 376–388.

Racine, R. (1975). Modification of seizure activity by electrical stimulation: Cortical areas. *Electrencephalogr. Clin. Neurophysiol.*, **38**, 1–12.

Sackeim, H. A., Prohovnik, I., Decina, P., Malitz, S. and Resor, S. (1983). Anticonvulsant and antidepressant properties of ECT: A proposed mechanism of action. *Biol. Psychiat.*, **18**, 1301–1310.

Sackeim, H. A., Decina, P., Prohovnik, I., Portnoy, S., Kanzler, M. and Malitz, S. (1986). Dosage, seizure threshold, and the antidepressant efficacy of electroconvulsive therapy. *Ann. N.Y. Acad. Sci.*, **462**, 398–410.

Schmutz, M. (1987). Relevance of kindling and related processes to human epileptogenesis. *Prog. Neuro-Psychopharmacol. Biol. Psychiat.*, **11**, 505–525.

Small, J. G. (1985). Efficacy of electroconvulsive theraphy in schizophrenia, mania, and other disorders. II. Mania and other disorders. *Convulsive Ther.*, **1**, 271–276.

Small, J. G., Milstein, V., Small, I. F. and Sharpley, P. H. (1981). Does ECT produce kindling? *Biol. Psychiat.*, **16**, 773–778.

Small, J. G., Milstein, V., Miller, M. J., Sharpley, P. H., Small, I. F., Malloy, F. W. and Klapper, M. H. (1988). Clinical, neuropsychological, and EEG evidence for mechanisms of action of ECT. *Convulsive Ther.*, **4**, 280–291.

Wagner-Jauregg, J. (1918–1919). Über die Einwirkung der Malaria auf die Progressive Paralyse. *Psychiat.-Neurol. Wochnschr.*, **20**, 132–141, 251–262.

The Clinical Relevance of Kindling
Edited by T. G. Bolwig and M. R. Trimble
© 1989 John Wiley & Sons Ltd

14

Kindling and manic-depressive illness

ROBERT M. POST and S. R. B. WEISS
Biological Psychiatry Branch, National Institute of Mental Health, Bethesda, Maryland, USA

INTRODUCTION

In discussing the relevance of the kindling concept for conceptualizing the course of manic-depressive illness, one must begin with a series of caveats. It is clear that the kindling process deals with alterations in thresholds for excitability, afterdischarges, and seizures. The emergence of seizures to a previously subconvulsant stimulation is the sine qua non of the kindling phenomenon. Clearly, manic-depressive illness is not a seizure disorder in any sense of the term clinically. Thus, from the outset, we must consider kindling at best a nonhomologous model for only some aspects of the longitudinal course of manic-depressive illness. Specifically, we are using the kindling analogy to focus on factors which might be influential in the initial emergence of affective illness as well as its progression to various stages. Elsewhere, we have discussed in detail (Post, 1988a) the usual requirements for an animal model of affective illness. These include similarities of inducing principles, common pathophysiologies, homologous behavioral abnormalities, and parallelism in response to pharmacologic interventions. Again, kindling does not meet most of these formal requirements; nonetheless, we hope to use the kindling analogy to help us focus on the longitudinal course of manic-depressive illness and raise a series of questions based on preclinical data that deserve careful clinical and theoretical investigation.

Throughout this chapter we will also attempt to distinguish the phenomenon of behavioral sensitization to psychomotor stimulants from that of electrophysiological kindling. In the former, a behavioral end-point such as hyperactivity or stereotypy is the outcome measure, while in electrical or pharmacological kindling, a seizure is the measure end-point. Repeated administration of low doses of the psychomotor stimulant cocaine is associated with behavioral sensitization, a phenomenon also observed with the nonlocal anesthetic psychomotor stimulants amphetamine and methylphenidate. Sensitization has been most closely associated with dopaminergic mechanisms. Repeated administration of higher doses of cocaine, in addition to behavioral sensitization, may also lead to the induction of seizures; i.e. the phenomena of pharmacological kindling. It is believed that the kindling effect is attributable to the local anesthetic rather than the psychomotor stimulant effects of cocaine. Even though behavioral sensitization and pharmacological kindling can be induced by the same pharmacological agent (i.e. cocaine), we think it is important to distinguish between these two phenomena, as their underlying mechanisms appear to be markedly different.

A final caveat is that the efficacy of anticonvulsants in the treatment of manic-depressive illness cannot be used to infer a kindling-like mechanism. As we will describe, the anticonvulsant carbamazepine is differentially effective in some stages of kindling and not others, and this differs according to the type of kindling — electrical versus pharmacological. Moreover, carbamazepine is clearly effective in a variety of neuropsychiatric syndromes that do not involve seizures or convulsive phenomena. Therefore, as intriguing as the kindling concept might be in helping to conceptualize the longitudinal course of manic-depressive illness, one cannot use response to a certain class of anticonvulsant agents to infer that a kindling-like process underlies aspects of the syndrome.

COCAINE-INDUCED BEHAVIORAL SENSITIZATION

Cocaine is a fascinating substance of great current interest because of the epidemic of use in the United States and related North and South American countries. Cocaine induces a variety of affective changes acutely, ranging from mood elevation to dysphoria (Post, 1976). As such, observations of cocaine's effects may provide an interesting potential model for manic and depressive illness, especially since a variety of the syndromes induced by cocaine use in man appear to parallel phenomena observed in the affective disorders. Moreover, with repeated cocaine administration, there appears to be an evolution in responsivity to cocaine. Positive effects of the drug become harder to maintain, and an increasing dysphoric response emerges in spite of adequate maintenance of cocaine-induced blood levels (Sherer et al., 1988). Similar to that reported with amphetamines, repeated use of cocaine can lead to the development of paranoid psychosis (Post, 1975; Manschreck, Allen and Neville, 1987; Sherer et al., 1988). These effects of cocaine are thought to be largely dependent on the psychomotor stimulant properties, with dopaminergic mechanisms, particularly in mesolimbic and mesocortical areas.

In 1975 we suggested that cocaine was a particularly interesting model stressor in light of its ability to potentiate catecholamines and indoleamines. Recent data support and extend this supposition (Post, 1975). Antelman and Chioco (1984) have documented that a variety of stressors show cross-sensitization to stimulant-induced behavioral sensitization and vice versa. In addition, recent evidence of Rivier and Vale (1987) and Calogero and colleagues (1988) have suggested that cocaine may also release the paradigmatic stress hormone, corticotropin releasing factor (CRF). Thus, cocaine appears to activate or potentiate a variety of neurotransmitter and neuropeptide systems intimately involved in the stress response. While dopaminergic mechanisms appear to be important mediators of the phenomenon of cocaine-induced behavioral sensitization, the precise role of the CRF in cocaine-related phenomena remains to be delineated and will be briefly discussed below.

Cocaine-induced behavioral sensitization helps to elucidate the possible role of conditioning phenomena in increased responsivity to the same stimulation over time. Conditioning appears to be involved, as the behavioral sensitization is environmental context-dependent. That is, animals pretreated and tested in the same environment show increased responsivity to cocaine (Figure 1) while those pretreated in a different environment from which they are tested show no greater cocaine-induced hyperactivity than saline-injected controls (Post *et al.*, 1981; Weiss *et al.*, 1988a; Post, Weiss and Pert, 1987). This environmental context-dependent effect shows stimulus generalization as the greater the similarity between pretreatment and test environment, the

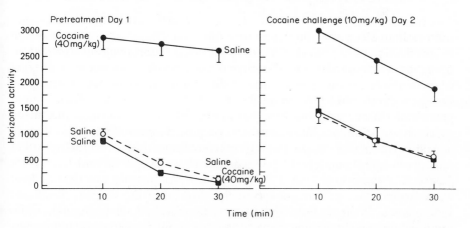

Figure 1. Influence of environmental context on cocaine-induced behavioral sensitization. Only rats previously treated with cocaine (40 mg/kg) in the test cage (filled circles) show increased response to cocaine (10 mg/kg) the next day. Animals receiving cocaine (40 mg/kg) in the home cage (filled squares) were no more responsive the next day than saline controls

greater the degree of sensitization. Moreover, if the initial degree of cocaine-induced behavior is blocked with neuroleptics or nonspecifically with high doses of benzodiazepines, the sensitization effect does not occur (Weiss *et al.*, 1988a). Following repeated cocaine pretreatment, animals also show an increased reactivity to a saline challenge administered i.p. or to amphetamine or saline administered into the nucleus accumbens. Dopamine appears to be important, since selective dopaminergic lesions of the nucleus accumbens or the amygdala are capable of blocking the induction of cocaine-induced behavioral sensitization (Weiss, Pert and Post, unpublished data, 1888). Since lesions of the nucelus accumbens also block the self-administration of cocaine (Pettit *et al.*, 1984), we suggest that the nucleus accumbens lesions may interfere with sensitization by similarly blocking the rewarding effects of the prior cocaine administration. Lesions of the amygdala may affect the ability of the rats to associate the environmental context with the prior cocaine experience (Murray and Mishkin, 1985).

The conditioned component of cocaine-induced behavioral sensitization is of interest in its own right, but also provides an important emerging concept for several phenomena that might be relevant to the understanding of affective illness. To the extent that cocaine provides a relevant model of a stressor, the data suggest the possibility that the increased behavioral responsibility to repetition of the same stimulus may be, in part, due to conditioned behavioral and biochemical effects (Post, Rubinow and Ballenger, 1984b).

ELECTRICAL AND PHARMACOLOGICAL KINDLING

As originally described by Goddard, McIntyre and Leech (1969), repeated subthreshold electrical stimulation on a once-daily basis eventually results in the production of full-blown seizures to previously subconvulsant stimulation. If kindled seizures are repeated enough times, a phase of spontaneity emerges where animals demonstrate seizures in the absence of exogenous electrophysiological stimulation (Pinel and Rovner, 1978a, b; Racine, 1978). Similar phenomena occur with the local anesthetic lidocaine as well as the mixed psychomotor stimulant-local anesthetic cocaine. Repeated administration of lidocaine (65 mg/kg) in an initially subconvulsant dose, eventually evokes seizures in approximately 40% of animals (Post, Kopanda and Lee, 1975; Post *et al.*, 1984; Post, 1981). If these seizure inductions are repeated for weeks to months, we have observed that several of the animals developed spontaneous seizures (Post and Contel, unpublished observations). Lidocaine-induced seizures show many behavioral similarities to those induced by electrical stimulation of the amygdala, and show similar electrophysiological spiking in the amygdala. Moreover, lidocaine-induced kindling shows cross-sensitization to electrical kindling of the amygdala (Post *et al.*, 1984). Animals also show pharmacological kindling to cocaine, although the cocaine-induced seizures are poorly tolerated and most of the animals die after the first or second cocaine-induced seizure episode (Weiss *et al.*, 1988b). Thus, spontaneity has not yet been observed with cocaine seizure.

Three phases of kindling may, therefore, be described:

(1) The initial development phase where the processes resulting in the culmination of seizure occur;
(2) completed kindled phase where repeated seizures are reliably induced;
(3) the spontaneous phase where seizures occur in the absence of exogenous stimulation (pharmacological or electrical).

As we will describe below, there is a differential pharmacology in these three stages of kindling. We have postulated that similar stages of evolution occur in some subictal phenomena, such as the 'kindling' of cocaine-induced panic attacks (Post *et al.*, 1986, 1987c).

A variant on pharmacological kindling is observed with intrathecal [intra-cerebroventricular (i.c.v.)] administration of CRF. Following a single CRF administration i.c.v., typical limbic-like seizures develop with a considerable delay (usually 4–8 h following injection) (Weiss *et al.*, 1986). These seizures are also associated with afterdischarges in the amygdala and Ehlers *et al.* (1983) have postulated that the delay in the appearance of seizures is related to a kindling-like phenomenon over time following the single dose. Repeated daily administration of CRF i.c.v. results in the appearance of tolerance to the convulsive and aggression-inducing effects (Weiss *et al.*, 1986). Thus, it remains to be delineated whether the CRF effect is mediated through a kindling-like process or some other mechanism which also requires a several hour delay before the onset of seizures. Nonetheless, the data are of considerable interest in relationship to the possibility that an endogenous occurring stress-related peptide may be capable not only of inducing a variety of behavioral effects that are relevant to depression (i.e., changes in motor activity, appetite, interest in sex, and changes in aggression), but also of inducing limbic seizures at high enough doses. We have not been able to ascertain which areas of brain are critical to the CRF seizure using either CRF intracerebral application to areas including the amygdala, hippocampus, septum, hypothalamus, periaqueductal gray, or endopyriform cortex, or by lesioning areas including the amygdala, hippocampus, olfactory bulb, or endopyriform cortex in attempts to block the effects of i.c.v. CRF (Weiss, Pert and Post, unpublished 1989).

In contrast to CRF, repeated application of enkephalin into regionally selective areas of the amygdala does result in a bona fide pharmacologic kindling-like effect, where initial injections are unsuccessful but later ones produce afterdischarges and seizure behaviors (Cain and Corcoran, 1984).

It is of interest that handling stress may re-trigger these seizures once they have been pharmacologically kindled.

It is also of interest that the local anesthetics lidocaine, procaine, and cocaine all appear to release CRF in hypothalamic mince preparations (Calogero et al., 1987, 1988), and the effect of lidocaine can be blocked with the anticonvulsant carbamazepine (Calogero et al., 1987). Chronic oral administration of carbamazepine blocks the development of lidocaine- and cocaine-induced pharmacological kindled seizures, although the role of CRF in this effect remains to be determined (Weiss, Pert and Post, unpublished 1989). Moreover, once these seizures are fully developed, carbamazepine is not able to block completed lidocaine seizures or high-dose cocaine seizures. Conversely, we have found that carbamazepine is ineffective in the initial development phases of electrically kindled seizures, although it is highly effective as an anticonvulsant in blocking completed electrically kindled seizures (Weiss and Post, 1987).

Thus, there is a double dissociation with carbamazepine in which it blocks the development but not the completed phase of pharmacological kindling with local anesthetics, but the converse is true for electrical kindling of the amygdala. This dissociation appears to be a general principle in the pharmacological interventions in kindling which appear to differ as a function of stage of kindling. Perhaps this is most strikingly demonstrated in the work of Pinel and colleagues (1983). They observed that diazepam was highly effective in the initial development and completed phases of electrical kindling, while it was ineffective on the spontaneous seizures. In contrast, phenytoin, which is largely ineffective in the initial stages, was highly effective in preventing spontaneous seizures (Figure 2).

RELATIONSHIP TO AFFECTIVE ILLNESS

We are now in a position to consider how the principles elucidated in behavioral sensitization to psychomotor stimulants and electrical and pharmacological kindling may guide us in thinking about the course of manic-depressive illness. The course of affective illness tends to be one associated with recurrences and these may increase in severity and/or rapidity. The median course of 82 bipolar affectively ill patients admitted to the NIMH is illustrated in Figure 3. Longer intervals without illness occur between the initial episodes compared with those after many recurrences. This decrease in the duration of the well interval has been observed in multiple studies in more than 4000 patients since the time of Kraepelin. Figure 4 illustrates a patient with such a course of illness. This 47-year-old bipolar patient experienced depressions initially at menarche and post-partum with a subsequent mania and depression occurring after the deaths of relatives or pets, or other psychosocial stressors. However, with further progression of the illness,

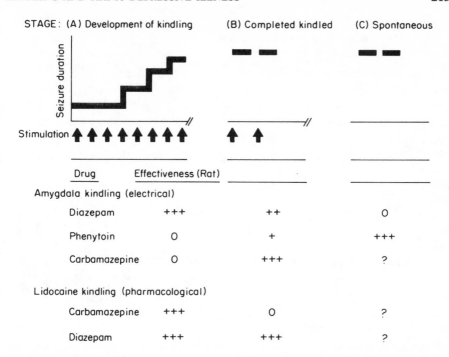

STAGE: (A) Development of kindling   (B) Completed kindled   (C) Spontaneous

Drug	Effectiveness (Rat)		
Amygdala kindling (electrical)			
Diazepam	+++	++	O
Phenytoin	O	+	+++
Carbamazepine	O	+++	?
Lidocaine kindling (pharmacological)			
Carbamazepine	+++	O	?
Diazepam	+++	+++	?

Figure 2. Anticonvulsants are effective in some stages of amygdala kindling but not others. Moreover, the same anticonvulsant, carbamazepine, is differentially effective in different stages of amygdala kindling compared with lidocaine kindling, a double dissociation

episodes appeared to emerge spontaneously and rhythmically, independent of clear psychosocial precipitants. To the extent that initial episodes of illness are triggered by exogenous stresses or even endogenous pharmacological pertubations, the kindling and sensitization models suggest a series of processes that could account for the eventual emergence of full-blown episodes to stimuli that were previously subthreshold, as well as the increase of severity of these episodes upon recurrence or rechallenge.

In behavioral sensitization to the psychomotor stimulants, alterations in responsivity are associated with not only increases in magnitude of response, but also in the rapidity of onset of the response. In this regard, it is of interest that patients with greater numbers of prior episodes had steeper and more rapid onsets of individual affective episodes than those with fewer numbers of previous episodes (Post et al., 1981). The possibility that an episode of the opposite valence (mania or depression) could emerge from similar inducing properties is also of interest in relationship to the phenomenon of Siegel's conditioned compensatory responses, as discussed elsewhere (Post, Rubinow and Ballenger, 1984). This mechanism could give potential

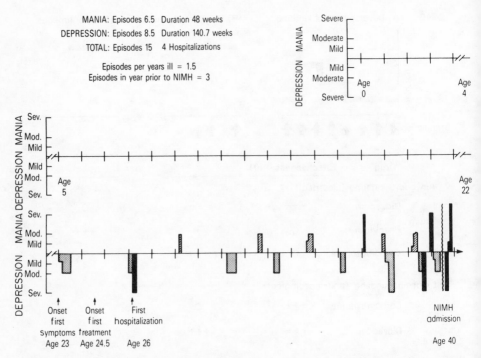

Figure 3. Note decreasing duration of well intervals between episodes (faster cycling) severity of illness in this group of treatment-refractory patients studied in a tertiary referral center

explanation for the emergence of moods of the opposite phase that occur in response to the same stressful stimuli, in this fashion providing a neurobiological bridge for a concept that has its many psychodynamic hypothetical mechanisms as well.

As the neural substrates involved in the emergence of affective episodes are repeatedly engaged with the occurrence of successive episodes, the theory would postulate that they would not only be increasingly vulnerable to reactivation, but also be triggered by repetition of lesser inducing stimuli. That is, as illustrated in Figure 5, the occurrence of a full-blown stressful experience triggered by a loss may not be required for subsequent activation of episodes. Imagining the possible occurrence of an undesirable event, under laws of secondary and tertiary conditioning, might be sufficient to induce an episode. With sufficient repetitions, like the phenomenon of spontaneity in kindling, episodes may then begin to emerge in an autonomous or rapid-cycling fashion independent of external events.

Since the pharmacology of kindled seizures differs as a function of stage of development, we can ask whether a similar phenomenon may not also be occurring in the psychopharmacology of the affective disorders as a function

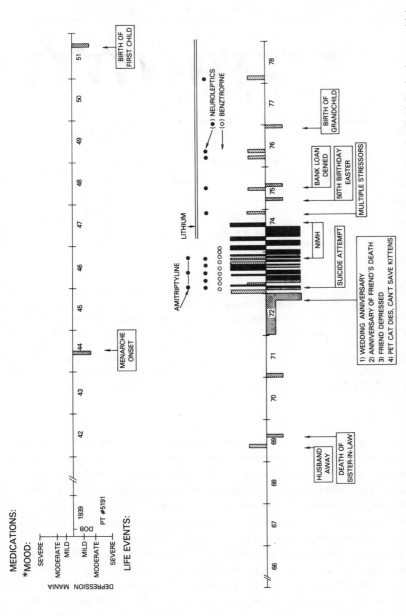

Figure 4. This patient demonstrates several patterns of illness evolution not uncharacteristic of bipolar disorder. Initial episodes are widely spaced, but with recurrence become more closely clustered with shorter well intervals. Tricyclic treatment may have been associated with the induction of rapid and continuous cycling, a pattern observed in 34 per cent and 16 per cent, respectively, of our tricyclic-treated patients. Initial episodes were associated with apparent endocrine and psychosocial precipitants, while this was not always the case with later episodes, especially those in 1973 during the pattern of rapid cycling, and many episodes thereafter. Does this correspond to the stage of spontaneity in the kindling analogy (see Figure 5)? At NIMH, many episodes appeared to be triggered by second-order stimuli or more 'symbolic' events. Lithium treatment made a substantial input on the course of illness, but breakthrough episodes still occurred with or without apparent stressors

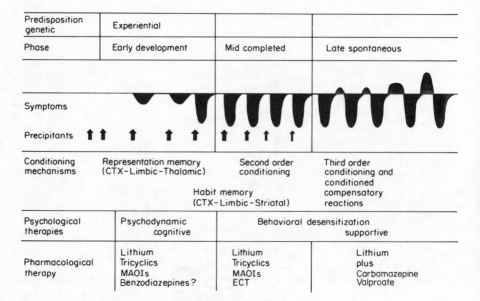

Predisposition genetic	Experiential		
Phase	Early development	Mid completed	Late spontaneous
Symptoms			
Precipitants			
Conditioning mechanisms	Representation memory (CTX-Limbic-Thalamic)	Second order conditioning	Third order conditioning and conditioned compensatory reactions
		Habit memory (CTX-Limbic-Striatal)	
Psychological therapies	Psychodynamic cognitive	Behavioral desensitization supportive	
Pharmacological therapy	Lithium Tricyclics MAOIs Benzodiazepines?	Lithium Tricyclics MAOIs ECT	Lithium plus Carbamazepine Valproate

Figure 5. Schematic for the evolution of affective illness emphasizes that increases in frequency and severity of episodes may occur initially in response to psychosocial precipitants, but, with sufficient repetition, episodes may occur spontaneously (i.e. without clearcut environmental precipitants). As discussed by Mishkin and associates, this progression may be paralleled by differences in anatomical substrates subserving representational versus habit memory. In this latter instance, with sufficient repetitions, memory may be encoded in the habit system and require differential psychotherapeutic as well as pharmacotherapeutic interventions

of stages of their development. As schematized in Figure 6, we would wonder whether psychotherapy and benzodiazepines may not be effective in the initial phases of stress-related dysphorias, while tricyclic and monoamine oxidase inhibitor (MAOI) antidepressants are usually required for the more major depressive episodes that show more endogenous characteristics. With psychotic components of depression, adjunctive treatment with neuroleptics or ECT may also be required. However, in the later, rapid-cycling or spontaneous phases of the illness, tricyclics or MAOIs may, in some instances, accelerate rapid cycling and thus be relatively contraindicated. Similarly, there is a wealth of evidence suggesting that rapid-cycling manic-depressive patients show lesser degrees of responsivity to lithium carbonate than those in the earlier phases of the illness. Several studies (Post *et al.*, 1987b; Joffe, 1988; Kishimoto and Okuma, 1985) have suggested that rapid cycling may be a positive predictor of acute or long-term response to carbamazepine.

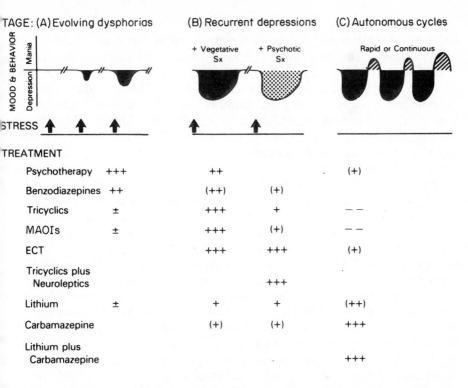

STAGE:	(A) Evolving dysphorias	(B) Recurrent depressions		(C) Autonomous cycles
TREATMENT				
Psychotherapy	+++	++		(+)
Benzodiazepines	++	(++)	(+)	
Tricyclics	±	+++	+	– –
MAOIs	±	+++	(+)	– –
ECT		+++	+++	(+)
Tricyclics plus Neuroleptics			+++	
Lithium	±	+	+	(++)
Carbamazepine		(+)	(+)	+++
Lithium plus Carbamazepine				+++

Figure 6. MAOIs (monoamine oxidase inhibitors), ECT (electroconvulsive therapy). Just as different stages of kindling are differentially responsive to pharmacological interventions (Figure 2), we postulate a differential effectiveness of therapeutic agents as a function of the longitudiinal course of affective illness (see Post *et al.* (1986a) for details). This schema remains to be directly tested. While there is clear evidence for lesser effectiveness of lithium in rapid- compared with nonrapid-cycling patients, it is not clear whether this is a subgroup effect or a change with progression of the illness. Moreover, recent data suggest that carbamazepine may also be effective early in the illness and not just in rapid cyclers

Thus, while the responsivity to carbamazepine in early phases of the illness may also occur (but remains to be adequately delineated, see Placidi *et al.*, 1984; Lerer *et al.*, 1987; Bellaire, Demish and Stoll, 1988; Okuma *et al.*, 1988), it would appear that carbamazepine and other adjunctive anticonvulsants may be of particular use in the later, more rapid-cycling phases of the illness that tend to be refractory to lithium carbonate. Obviously, this schema remains to be more directly examined from the clinical and pharmacological perspectives, but it is presented with the idea that in addition to a variety of other variables which may affect pharmacoresponsivity (such as genetic predisposition, severity of illness, subtype, and atypicality) that course of illness variables may also be relevant.

In a similar fashion we would also wonder whether psychotherapeutic interventions might not also be differentially appropriate as a function of stage of illness. The differential pharmacotherapy of kindling as a function of stage clearly implies that different neurophysiological or anatomical substrates are engaged in different stages of the illness. Similar evidence occurs for different types of learning and memory where different substrates have been postulated for long- and short-term memory. In addition, Mishkin and Appenzeller (1987) have recently elucidated two different memory systems, one involving representational memory, thought to involve a limbic–thalamic–frontal cortical circuit and another involving habit memory, thought to involve a limbic-striatal circuit. Habit memory appears to be engaged by paradigms which, among other things, involve many repetitions of the learning process. When this happens, even lesions of the amygdala and hippocampus which severely disrupt representational memory, leave habit memory unimpaired. Perhaps in an analogous fashion, with sufficient repetition of affective episodes, the recurrence develops sufficient automaticity such that cognitive or representational maneuvers are without effect (Figure 5). That is, they are based highly on 'harder-wired' circuits related to probable outcomes. In this fashion, one might consider that psychodynamic psychotherapies might have the greatest impact with patients in early phases of their illness when early developmental issues, stress and losses, are critically involved. With some repetition of episodes, a role for cognitive techniques might come into play as adequate management of stressors may help avoid episode induction. Finally, in the later phases of the illness, one might conceive of more behavioral and deconditioning techniques where attempts are made to 'disconnect' and desensitize previously facilitated circuits between triggering events and biochemical and affective reactions that might occur on an almost automatic basis. These types of interventions may be helpful for the patient who indicates that he has 'insight' but is still unable to ward off the almost automatic triggering of anxiety and dysphoria that some events bring on.

CONTINGENT INEFFICACY AND CONTINGENT TOLERANCE

The kindling model also has led to the elucidation of the concept of contingent inefficacy and tolerance to the anticonvulsant effects of clinically used drugs such as carbamazepine. Previously, the behavioral sensitization and kindling models have helped to explain possible differential pharmaco-responsivity as a function of when the intervention is applied. In the current analysis, we are emphasizing that it is the temporal contingencies of drug in relationship to treated episodes that may be critical to drug responsivity or lack thereof. As previously indicated, carbamazepine treatment prior to each kindling stimulation is not sufficient to block the development of amygdala kindling. We have, however, observed that this treatment renders the drug subsequently ineffective in the completed stage of kindling when, in contrast, drug-naïve animals or animals that have been treated with carbamazepine after each kindled stimulation are highly responsive to the anticonvulsant effects of carbamazepine (Figure 7). These data indicate that treatment with a drug during a phase when it is ineffective may affect its later utility, in this case rendering a potentially useful drug ineffective, i.e. contingent inefficacy.

Drug-responsive, fully kindled animals repeatedly pretreated with carbamazepine will develop tolerance to the anticonvulsant effects of the drug (contingent tolerance). This contingent tolerance can be reversed by a period of treatment with the drug after each kindled stimulation or by a period of kindling the animals without drug. In contrast, merely waiting for as long as 3 weeks or treating with carbamazepine alone (in the absence of seizures) is insufficient to reverse the contingent tolerance.

These preclinical data may have relevance for treatment of a variety of neuropsychiatric syndromes. Tolerance develops to the antinociceptive effects of carbamazepine in trigeminal neuralgia (Fromm et al., 1981). Perhaps a period of experiencing episodes of trigeminal neuralgia in the absence of drug would be sufficient to reinstitute efficacy, similar to that observed in the kindling paradigm. These data may also have more direct implications for drug refractoriness in epileptic patients as well as for the recently observed phenomena that ineffectiveness of seizure control in the first several years of treatment (Reynolds, 1987) is a very accurate predictor of subsequent poor prognosis. Perhaps once anticonvulsant inefficacy is established clinically, like that in the experimental situation, it prejudices against subsequent responsivity. Similarly, in patients who may have become tolerant, perhaps appropriate 'reversal' procedures may be required; i.e. a period of time off medications when seizures are experienced.

Finally, we wonder whether a similar process might not be occurring in some patients with manic-depressive illness. We have followed 24 patients for an average of four years during carbamazepine maintenance. Patients were treated either with carbamazepine alone (a minority) or in combination with lithium carbonate (which had previously been inadequately effective when used alone). Half this population showed stable and long-lasting clinical improvement to the addition of carbamazepine. However, the other half showed a pattern of reemergence of episodes in the first or second year of treatment. Such a patient is illustrated in Figure 8.

In instances where carbamazepine was initially effective, we would again question whether or not temporary withdrawal of medication that had become ineffective in preventing the reemergence of episodes might not renew its effectiveness. Clearly, such a mechanism deserves further clinical and preclinical exploration, along with strategies that might retard the development of conditioned tolerance. We have preliminarily observed that con-

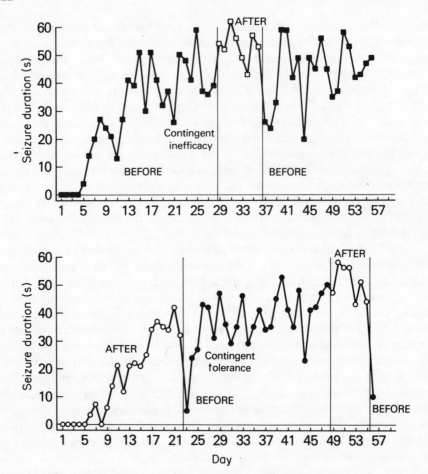

Figure 7. The group mean seizure duration is illustrated for the animals given once-daily electrical stimulation of the amygdala for 1 s and once-daily carbamazepine, either before or after kindling. Top panel: the carba-before group did not respond to treatment at a time when the carba-after group was responsive (contingent inefficacy: for comparison see bottom panel days 23–25). Carbamazepine treatment after kindled seizures in this group (days 29–36) reslted in only a modest reinstatement of anticonvulsant efficacy ($P < 0.12$ for seizure stage; $P < 0.05$ for afterdischarge duration; data not shown). Bottom panel: the carba-after group showed a good anticonvulsant response to treatment before kindled seizures (days 23–25) ($P < 0.01$) but became tolerant to this effect. A subsequent 7-day carba-after treatment (days 49–55) reinstated anticonvulsant efficacy ($P < 0.05$). A period of time off medications is also effective if animals are kindled, but not if they are left unstimulated; i.e. tolerant animals must experience a seizure in the absence of drug pretreatment for renewal of efficacy

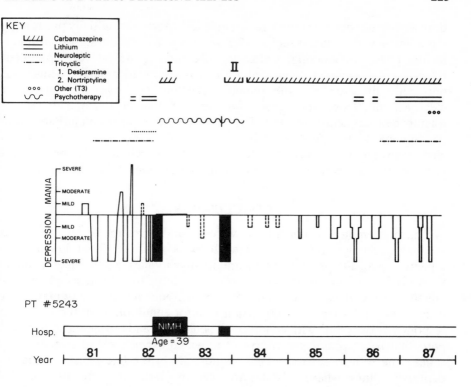

Figure 8. This patient showed good acute response to carbamazepine (I and II), but after initial partially successful prophylaxis with carbamazepine, developed a pattern of progressive loss of efficacy. In contrast to the severe depression requiring hospitalization at the end of 1983 while on no medications, carbamazepine prophylaxis was initially associated with only brief mild to moderate depressions. These progressed in severity and duration in spite of continued medication with carbamazepine and the addition of supplemental lithium, tricyclics, and even neuroleptics for the episodes in 1987. This pattern is consistent with the development of tolerance, and to the extent this is the case, the patient may benefit from a period of time off carbamazepine in order to reinstitute efficacy

ditioned tolerance does not show cross-tolerance to drugs of a different class. For example, animals showing conditioned tolerance to the anticonvulsant effects of carbamazepine on amygdala-kindled seizures still respond to the benzodiazepine diazepam, even though this agent itself can become less effective through conditioned tolerance development. Further rotating pretreatment drugs or increasing doses does not appear to delay the development of tolerance. Thus, other alterations need to be investigated.

We emphasize the contingent nature of the tolerance and inefficacy phenomena. Animals treated with equal doses of carbamazepine given immediately *after*, rather than *before*, seizures do not become tolerant to the drug and do not develop contingent inefficacy. Moreover, initially pretreating the animals with carbamazepine *after* seizure induction during the developmental phases of kindling, yields no difference in the rate of subsequent tolerance development compared with vehicle-treated animals. Thus, it is only when the drug is in the animal at the time of the seizure episode or electrical stimulation (i.e. during kindling development) that inefficacy or tolerance subsequently develop. The molecular mechanisms underlying these phenomena deserve further study as they imply a progressive 'learning' to circumvent the anticonvulsant effects of a drug, which may also be relevant to or dependent upon the mechanisms that are responsible for kindling itself.

CONCLUSIONS

We have attempted to illustrate how consideration of the sensitization and kindling preclinical phenomena may help us to think about longitudinal aspects of manic-depressive illness and its psychopharmacotherapeutic interventions. These models provide conceptual bridges for considering how progression of the illness in terms of severity or frequency of cycling may occur over time. They suggest an important role for conditioning in the increased responsivity over time with conditioned behavioral and biochemical reactions potentially occurring in the course of repeated experiences of affective episodes. The transition to apparent spontaneity in the late phases of manic-depressive illness where episodes are occurring autonomously also provides a bridge between early psychodynamic and later neurobiological explanations of the illness. Rather than these two types of processes being mutually exclusive, the foregoing analysis suggests the possibility that within individual patients, there may be a gradual emergence of episodes and evolution from the precipitated to the spontaneous variety. Clearly, this is postulated by the model and early evidence suggests that psychosocial precipitants may be more evident with episodes early in the course than later in the course (Ambelas, 1979).

The kindling and sensitization models further raise the possibility that psychopharmacological interventions would have a dual positive effect in adequate prophylaxis. Not only would they prevent potentially catastrophic episodes of depression and mania from occurring, but they might also prevent whatever sensitization and kindling-like process were occurring with the repetition of these episodes. Thus, it would be postulated that adequate prevention of these episodes in itself, to the extent it impacted on underlying processes akin to sensitization and kindling, may ultimately leave the patient less vulnerable than another patient who had experienced repeated episodes.

The conditioned component of the behavioral sensitization to cocaine also provides an interesting model for neuroleptic nonresponsiveness once initial 'episodes' of cocaine-induced behavior are induced. That is, if neuroleptics are given prior to the initial cocaine, they are able to block the development of behavioral sensitization, but once cocaine-induced behaviors occur, even highly sedating doses of neuroleptics are unable to block the resulting behavioral sensitization (Weiss *et al.*, 1988a; Tadokoro and Kuribara, 1986; Beninger and Hahn, 1983; Beninger and Herz, 1986). This phenomenon may have a variety of clinical equivalents in various psychotic syndromes. Wyatt *et al.* (1988) recently reviewed the data which support the notion that late or delayed treatment with neuroleptics, after psychotic symptoms have been expressed for a considerable period of time, may be less effective than early intervention. Again, this is an area for further clinical study, but the foregoing analysis provides a preclinical model for further systematic testing. It is of interest that in the behavioral sensitization model, two agents are able to block both the development and expression of cocaine-induced sensitization; e.g. diazepam and clonidine. These drugs are of interest in that both clonazepam and clonidine have been reported to be antimanic agents. It is also of interest that carbamazepine is unable to block either the development or the expression of cocaine-induced behavioral sensitization, in contrast to its effects on some stages of kindling development.

In a parallel fashion to the phenomena just described for behavioral sensitization, where neuroleptic intervention varies in effectiveness as a function of when it is applied in the sequence of evolution of the phenomenon, a similar process has been explicated for kindled seizures. As illustrated in Figure 5, it now appears to be a general principle that different phases of the development of kindling are differentially pharmacologically responsive. We have raised the possibility that not only is the psychopharmacotherapy of recurrent affective disorders also differentially effective as a function of stage of development of the illness, but that such a concept also be relevant for development of different types of therapies which might be targeted to stage of development of the illness.

Lastly, we have introduced the concept of conditioned inefficacy and tolerance to the anticonvulsant effects of carbamazepine. In parallel with the role of conditioning in the development of behavioral sensitization to the psychomotor stimulant cocaine, we have elucidated a conditioned component to the opposite phenomenon of tolerance to the effectiveness of an anticonvulsant drug. In this instance, the contingencies and relationships of drug to episode being treated appear to determine its effectiveness. Once inefficacy or tolerance has developed to the anticonvulsant effects of carbamazepine it persists for extended periods of time and can only be reversed by a period of kindling with the drug administered *after* stimulation or with kindling alone. It is possible that parallel maneuvers in epilepsy, trigeminal neuralgia, or affective illness may be effective in reinstituting efficacy when contingent inefficacy or tolerance has developed in these clinical siituations as well.

Thus, we have attempted to illustrate the interplay between the preclinical models of sensitization and kindling and various clinical phenomena in the longitudinal course of manic-depressive illness. It is obvious that these models have the most direct clinical relevance for cocaine-induced behavioral syndromes in man (cocaine sensitization and the kindling of panic attacks) (Post et al., 1986, 1987c) and for epileptic phenomena in man (kindling), but we have attempted to illustrate how they may also be relevant for various aspects of the course of manic-depressive illness, which does not involve a convulsive process. In this fashion, we are using seizures as an easily measurable endpoint and model system, not with the literal idea that affective illness is a seizure phenomenon.

Nonetheless, studies of amygdala kindling and considerations of limbic system excitability and modulation of emotion and affect were, in fact, instrumental in our initiation of studies of the efficacy of carbamazepine in the treatment of manic-depressive illness (Post et al., 1978; Ballenger and Post, 1978; Post et al., 1985). It is noteworthy, however, that little evidence exists to date that suggests that the psychotropic effects of carbamazepine in manic-depressive illness are based on its ability to stabilize limbic system substrates (Post and Uhde, 1986). In fact, there is no evidence of a relationship of EEG or clinically assessed psychosensory abnormalities (Silberman et al., 1985) to be associated with degree of psychotropic response to carbamazepine. In addition, there is no evidence for 'hot spots' on PET scans in this disorder (Post et al., 1987a) as there is for stimulant-induced syndromes (Baxter et al., 1988). In contrast, relative hypometabolism in temporal lobes and other areas of the brain has been observed during depressive illness. Thus, while the ability of carbamazepine to stabilize limbic system excitability has been postulated as a potential mechanism of its action, it is noteworthy that carbamazepine also exerts anticonvulsant effects on a variety of nonlimbic seizures (Post et al., 1985) and affects a panoply of neurotransmitter systems which have been implicated in either its anticonvulsant or psychotropic effects (Post, 1987, 1988b). Several systems have been closely linked to the anticonvulsant effects of carbamazepine on amygdala-kindled seizures. These include peripheral-type benzodiazepine receptors and the necessary (but not sufficient) condition of unblocked $alpha_2$-noradrenergic receptors. A variety of data also strongly implicate type–2 sodium channels in the anticonvulsant effects of carbamazepine. However, while the anticonvulsant effects of carbamazepine on amygdala kindling are observable following a single dose, the psychotropic effects of carbamazepine in mania and depression appear to require considerable time to emerge (Post et al., 1987b; Post, 1988b). These data suggest that elucidating mechanisms requiring a time lag and chronic carbamazepine administration in order to be observed, may be more closely associated with its psychotropic properties. In this regard, we have recently established that chronic carbamazepine (but not acute, or repeated acute intermittent treatment), is required in order to block the development of lidocaine- and cocaine-kindled seizures (Weiss *et al.*, 1988b). As such, this seizure model might be of use to help elucidate mechanisms that are more closely related to carbamazepine's psychotropic as opposed to anticonvulsant effects.

The kindling story provides a menu for a series of clinical and preclinical studies to be conducted in regard to the longitudinal course of affective syndromes and the mechanism of action of carbamazepine. The sensitization and kindling models may also provide a conceptual bridge between earlier psychoanalytic and psychodynamic formulations of psychiatry and/or current concepts involving conditioning, endogenous, and autonomous processes. Classical neurotransmitters such as the catecholamines, and neuropeptides, such as corticotropin-releasing factor and endogenous opiates, deserve further study as mediators of potential clinical analogues of sensitization and kindling in man.

REFERENCES

Ambelas, A. (1979). Psychologically stressful events in the precipitation of manic episodes. *Psychoneuroendocrinology*, **9**, 233.

Antelman, S. M. and Chioco, L. A. (1984). Stress: its effect on interactions among biogenic amines and role in the induction and treatment of disease. In: *Handbook of Psychopharmacology*, Vol. 18 (eds L. S. Iverson, S. D. Iverson and S. H. Snyder), pp. 279–341.

Ballenger, J. C. and Post, R. M. (1978). Therapeutic effects of carbamazepine in affective illness: a preliminary report. *Commun. Psychopharmacol.*, **2**, 159–175.

Baxter Jr L. R., Schwartz, J. M., Phelps, M. E., Mazziotta, J. C. Barrio, J., Rawson, R. A., Engel, J., Guze, B. H., Selin, C. and Sumida, R. (1988). Localization of neurochemical effects of cocaine and other stimulants in the human brain. *J. Clin. Psychiat.*, **49**, 23–26.

Bellaire, W., Demish, K. and Stoll, K.-D. (1988). Carbamazepine versus lithium in prophylaxis of recurrent affective disorders (poster). *16th Collegium Internationale Neuropsychopharmacolgicum (C.I.N.P.) Congress*, Munich, 15–19 August 1988.

Beninger, R. J. and Hahn, B. L. (1983). Pimozide blocks establishment but not expression of amphetamine-produced environment-specific conditioning. *Science*, **220**, 1304–1306.

Beninger, R. J. and Herz, R. S. (1986). Pimozide blocks establishment but not expression of cocaine-produced environment-specific conditioning. *Life Sci.*, **38**, 1425.

Cain, D. P. and Corcoran, M. E. (1984). Intracerebral beta-endorphin, met-enkephalin and morphine: kindling of seizures and handling-induced potentiation of epileptiform effects. *Life Sci.*, **34**, 2535.

Calogero, A. E., Kling, M. A., Gallucci, W. T., Saoutis, C., Post, R. M., Chrousos, G. P. and Gold, P. W. (1987). 'Local anaesthetics procaine and lidocaine stimulate corticotropin releasing hormone secretion *in vitro*: clinical implications. Abstract, Society for Neuroscience, New Orleans, 16–20 November 1987, p. 1163.

Calogero, A. E., Kling, M. A., Bernardini, R., Gallucci, W. T., Post, R. M., Chrousos, G. P. and Gold, P. W. (1988). Cocaine stimulates rat hypothalamic corticotropin releasing hormone secretion *in vitro*. *Clin. Res.*, **36**, 361.

Ehlers, C. L., Henriksen, S. J., Wang, M., Rivier, J., Vale, W. and Bloom, F. E. (1983). Corticotropin releasing factor produces increases in brain excitability and convulsive seizures in rats. *Brain Res.*, **278**, 332.

Fromm, G. H., Chatthe, A. S., Terrance, C. F. and Glass, J. D. (1981). Role of inhibitory mechanisms in trigeminal neuralgia. *Neurology*, **3**, 683–687.

Goddard, G. V., McIntyre, D. C. and Leech, C. K. (1969). A permanent change in brain function resulting from daily electrical stimulation. *Exp. Neurol.*, **25**, 295–330.

Joffe, R. T. (1988). Lithium and carbamazepine in manic-depressive illness: a clinical evaluation. *Pharmacopsychiatry* (in press).

Kelly, P. H. and Iversen, S. D. (1975). Selective 6-OHDA-induced destruction of mesolimbic dopamine neurons: abolition of psychostimulant-induced locomotor activity in rats. *Eur. J. Pharmacol.*, **40**, 45–56.

Kishimoto, A. and Okuma, T. (1985). Antimanic and prophylactic effects of carbamazepine in affective disorders. Abstract, *IVth World Congress of Biological Psychiatry*, Philadelphia, 8–13 September 1985, p. 363.

Lerer, B., Moore, N., Meyendorff, E., Cho, S. R. and Gershon, S. (1987). Carbamazepine versus lithium in mania: a double-blind study. *J. Clin. Psychiat.*, **48**, 89–93.

Manschreck, T. C., Allen, D. F. and Neville, M. (1987). Freebase psychosis: cases from a Bahamian epidemic of cocaine abuse. *Compr. Psychiat.*, **28**, 555–564.

Mishkin, M. and Appenzeller, T. (1987). The anatomy of memory. *Sci. Am.*, **256**, 80–89.

Murray, E. A. and Mishkin, M. (1985). Amygdalectomy impairs crossmodal association in monkeys. *Science*, **228**, 604–606.

Okuma, T., Yamashita, I., Takahashi, R., Itoh, H., Kuribara, M., Otsuki, S., Watanabe, S., Sarai, K., Hazama, H. and Inanaga, K. (1988). Double-blind controlled studies on the therapeutic efficacy of carbamazepine in affective and schizophrenic patients. *Psychopharmacology*, **96**, 102, Abstract TH18.05.

Pettit, H. O., Ettenberg, A., Bloom, F. E. and Koob, G. F. (1984). Destruction of dopamine in the nucleus accumbens selectively attenuates cocaine but not heroin self-administration in rats. *Psychopharmacology*, **84**, 167–173.

Pinel, J. P. (1983). Effects of diazepam and diphenylhydantoin on elicited and spontaneous seizures in kindled rats: a double dissociation. *Pharmacol. Biochem. Behav.*, **18**, 61.

Pinel, J. P. J. and Rovner, L. I. (1978a). Electrode placement and kindling-induced experimental epilepsy. *Exp. Neurol.*, **58**, 335–346.

Pinel, J. P. J. and Rovner, L. I. (1978b). Experimental epileptogenesis: kindling-induced epilepsy in rats. *Exp. Neurol.*, **58**, 190–202.

Placidi, G. F., Lenzi, A., Rampello, E., Andreani, M. F., Cassano, G. B. and Grossi, E. (1984). Long-term double-blind prospective study on carbamazepine versus lithium in bipolar and schizoaffective disorders: preliminary results. In: *Anticonvulsants in Affective Disorders* (eds H. M. Emrich, T. Okuma, and A. A. Muller), pp. 188–197. Excerpta Medica, Amsterdam.

Post, R. M. (1975). Cocaine psychoses: a continuum model. *Am. J. Psychiat.*, **132**, 225–231.

Post, R. M. (1976). Clinical aspects of cocaine: assessment of acute and chronic effects in animals and man. In: *Cocaine: Chemical, Biological, Clinical, Social, and Treatment Aspects* (ed. S. J. Mule), pp. 203–215. CRC Press, Cleveland.

Post, R. M. (1981). Lidocaine kindled limbic seizures: behavioral implications. In: *Kindling 2* (ed. J. A. Wada), pp. 149–160. Raven, New York.

Post, R. M. (1987). Mechanisms of action of carbamazepine and related anticonvulsants in effective illness. In: *Psychopharmacology: A Generation of Progress* (eds H. Meltzer and W. E. Bunney Jr), pp. 567–576. Raven, New York.

Post, R. M. (1988a). Non-homologous animal models of affective illness: clinical relevance of sensitization and kindling. In: *Animal Models of Depression* (eds G. Koob and C. Ehlers). University of Chicago Press, Chicago (in press).

Post, R. M. (1988b). Time course of clinical effects of carbamazepine: implications for mechanisms of action. *J. Clin. Psychiat.*, **49**, 35–46.

Post, R. M. and Uhde, T. W. (1985). Are the psychotropic effects of carbamazepine in manic-depressive illness mediated through the limbic system? *Psychiatr. J. Univ. Ottawa*, **10**, 205–219.

Post, R. M. and Uhde, T. W. (1986). Carbamazepine in the treatment of affective illness. In: *The Limbic System: Functional Organization and Clinical Disorders* (eds B. K. Doane and K. E. Livingston), pp. 229–249. Raven, New York.

Post, R. M., Kopanda, R. T. and Lee, A. (1975). Progressive behavioral changes during chronic lidocaine administration: relationship to kindling. *Life Sci.*, **17**, 943–950.

Post, R. M., Rubinow, D. R. and Ballenger, J. C. (1984). Conditioning, sensitization, and kindling: implications for the course of affective illness. In: *Neurobiology of Mood Disorders* (eds R. M. Post and J. C. Ballenger), pp. 432–466. Williams & Wilkins, Baltimore.

Post, R. M., Weiss, S. R. B. and Pert, A. (1987). The role of context in conditioning and behavioral sensitization to cocaine. *Psychopharmacol. Bull.*, **23**, 425–429.

Post, R. M., Ballenger, J. C., Rey, A. C. and Bunney Jr, W. E. (1981). Slow and rapid onset of manic episodes: implications for underlying biology. *Psychiat. Res.*, **4**, 229–237.

Post, R. M., Kennedy, C., Shinohara, M., Squillace, K., Miyaoka, M., Suda, S., Ingvar, D. H. and Sokoloff, L. (1984). Metabolic and behavioral consequences of lidocaine-kindled seizures. *Brain Res.*, **324**, 295–304.

Post, R. M., Uhde, T. W., Joffe, R. T. and Bierer, L. (1986). Psychiatric manifestations and implications of seizure disorders. In: *Medical Mimics of Psychiatric Disorders* (eds I. Extein and M. Gold), pp. 33–91. APA Press, Washington, DC.

Post, R. M., DeLisi, L. E., Holcomb, H. H., Uhde, T. W., Cohen, R. and Buchsbaum, M. S. (1987a). Glucose utilization in the temporal cortex of affectively ill patients: positron emission tomography. *Biol. Psychiat.*, **22**, 46–54.

Post, R. M., Uhde, T. W., Roy-Byrne, P. P. and Joffe, R. T. (1987b). Correlates of antimanic response to carbamazepine. *Psychiat. Res.*, **21**, 71–83.

Post, R. M., Weiss, S. R. B., Pert, A. and Uhde, T. W. (1987c). Chronic cocaine administration: sensitization and kindling effects. In: *Cocaine: Clinical and Biobehavioral Aspects* (eds S. Fisher, A. Raskin and E. R. Uhlenhuth), pp. 109–173, Oxford University Press, New York.

Racine, R. (1978). Kindling: the first decade. *Neurosurgery*, **3**, 234–252.

Reynolds, E. H. (1987). Early treatment and prognosis of epilepsy. *Epilepsia*, **28**, 97–106.

Rivier, C. and Vale, W. (1987). Cocaine stimulates adrenocorticotropin (ACTH) secretion through a corticotropin-releasing factor (CRF)-mediated mechanism. *Brain Res.*, **422**, 403–406.

Sherer, M. A., Kumor, K. M., Cone, E. J. and Jaffe, J. H. (1988). Suspiciousness induced by four-hour intravenous infusions of cocaine. Preliminary findings. *Arch. Gen. Psychiat.*, **45**, 673–677.

Silberman, E. K., Post, R. M., Nurnberger, J., Theodore, W. and Boulenger, J.-P.

(1985). Transient sensory, cognitive, and affective phenomena in affective illness: a comparison with complex partial epilepsy. *Br. J. Psychiat.*, **146**, 81–89.

Tadokoro, S. and Kuribara, H. (1986). Reverse tolerance to the ambulation-increasing effect of methamphetamine in mice as an animal model of amphetamine-psychosis. *Psychopharmacol. Bull.*, **22**, 757.

Washton, A. M. and Gold, M. S. (1894). Chronic cocaine abuse: evidence for adverse effects on health and functioning. *Psychiatr. Ann.*, **14**, 733–743.

Weiss, S. R. B. and Post, R. M. (1987). Carbamazepine and carbamazepine–10,11-epoxide inhibit amygdala kindled seizures in the rat but do not block their development. *Clin. Neuropharmacol.*, **10**, 272–279.

Weiss, S. R. B., Pert, A. and Post, R. M. (1989). Studies on the localization of the effects of CRF on seizures and aggressive behavior. Unpublished manuscript.

Weiss, S. R. B., Post, R. M., Gold, P. W., Chrousos, G., Sullivan, T. L., Walker, D. and Pert, A. (1986). CRF-induced seizures and behavior: interaction with amygdala kindling. *Brain Res.*, **372**, 345–351.

Weiss, S. R. B., Post, R. M., Pert, A., Woodward, R. and Murman, D. (1988a). Role of conditioning in cocaine-induced behavioral sensitization: differential effect of haloperidol. *Neuropharmacology* (submitted for publication).

Weiss, S. R. B., Szele, F., Nierenberg, J. and Post, R. M. (1988b). Carbamazepine inhibits local anesthetic kindled seizures by cocaine and lidocaine. *Brain Research* (submitted for publication).

Wyatt, R. J., Alexander, R. C., Egan, M. S., and Kirsch, D. G. (1988). Schizophrenia: just the facts. What do we know, how well do we know it. *Schizophrenia Res.*, **1**, 3–18.

The Clinical Relevance of Kindling
Edited by T. G. Bolwig and M. R. Trimble
© 1989 John Wiley & Sons Ltd

15

Addictive behavior and kindling: relationship to alcohol withdrawal and cocaine

JAMES C. BALLENGER and ROBERT M. POST[1]
Department of Psychiatry and Behavioral Sciences, Medical University of South Carolina, USA and [1]Biological Psychiatry Branch, National Institute of Mental Health, Bethesda, Maryland, USA

INTRODUCTION

Most of the theories and research potentially linking kindling and drugs of abuse have been with alcohol, cocaine, and, to a lesser extent, amphetamines. The kindling model has been utilized in the attempt to understand potential brain mechanisms for progressive aspects of the syndromes of abuse of these three drugs. In this chapter we will review first the animal and human experiments linking kindling and alcohol abuse, primarily in the alcohol withdrawal syndrome. We will then review evidence potentially linking kindling-like changes with cocaine and other stimulant drugs.

PART I: KINDLING AND ALCOHOL WITHDRAWAL PHENOMENA

In 1978 we hypothesized that a kindling model appeared to be consistent with multiple aspects of the etiology, presentation, and progression of the alcohol withdrawal syndrome (Ballenger and Post, 1978). We hypothesized that the limbic system hyperirritability which accompanies each alcohol withdrawal over time serves to kindle increasingly widespread central nervous system structures. Available evidence suggested that these 'kindling-like' changes might constitute the underlying pathophysiology of alcohol withdrawal symptoms both in terms of the physiological symptoms of tremor, seizures, or delirium and the observed personality changes between episodes

231

of withdrawal in alcoholics. This analogy between kindling and its various characteristics and stages and the stages of alcohol withdrawal and chronic alcoholism is schematized in Figure 1.

The data available then and subsequently from both the literature and our own studies seem consistent with such a model. If kindling-like changes are occurring after repeated episodes of alcohol withdrawal, we reasoned that certain predictions would be true. These predictions follow, and the data supporting or failing to support each of these predictions are summarized in the following section.

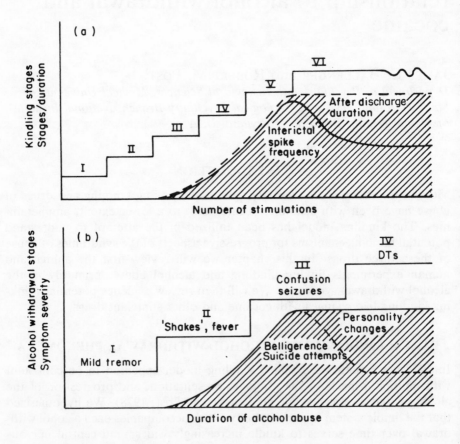

Figure 1. Kindling model for symptomatology of chronic alcoholism (a) electrical kindling; (b) chronic alcoholism. [Reproduced with permission from Ballenger and Post (1978)]

Predictions based on the kindling model of alcohol withdrawal

(1) The kindling stimulus (presumably withdrawal from alcohol) would occur many times separated in time, and the symptoms of withdrawal should be related to the recurrence of this kindling stimulus.
(2) Withdrawal symptoms should become progressively more severe with repeated episodes of withdrawal.
(3) The withdrawal syndrome should be organized into stages analogous to kindling stages and the progression of severity of the withdrawal syndrome should be cumulative, and in general unidirectional as in the kindling paradigm.
(4) Symptoms should be understandable as secondary to subcortical kindling-like changes in neuronal excitablity and potentially involve seizures.
(5) Over time if a kindling process is occurring, there should be evidence of an altered central nervous system between episodes of withdrawal. These might involve sequential changes in personality or emotional difficulties, progress over time, and be apparent during the interval between alcohol withdrawals.
(6) There should be a predictable interaction between alcohol withdrawal and its symptoms and the medications and procedures known to influence the kindling process.

Evidence Supportive of Predictions:

Alcohol withdrawal as the kindling stimulus

Alcohol is a powerful central nervous system (CNS) depressant, and when alcohol levels fall in the brain, hyperirritability of the CNS occurs (Kalant, LeBlanc and Gibbins, 1971; McQuarrie and Fingl, 1958; Mendelson, 1972). This has been demonstrated by multiple methods including exaggeration of evoked responses during withdrawal (Begleiter, Gross and Porjesz, 1973; Macdonell, Fessock and Brown, 1971; Victor and Brausch, 1967), lowering of the electroshock startle threshold (Edmonds and Bellin, 1976), and threshold for either spontaneous seizures (Kalant, 1961; Mendelson, 1972) or seizures induced by various stimuli, handling (Goldstein, 1973), chemical (Hunt, 1973), auditory (Freund and Walker, 1971) or electroconvulsive (McQuarrie and Fingl, 1958). Convulsive withdrawal effects are observed even after brief ethanol exposure (Pinel, 1980).

Although most studies in man of the cortical EEG during alcohol withdrawal show only minor abnormalities, these abnormalities are thought to reflect more widespread abnormalities subcortically (Begleiter and Platz, 1972). This assumption is supported by animal studies in which clear abnormalities are observed in subcortical limbic structures during alcohol withdrawal. This has been demonstrated in the cat (Guerrero-Figueroa et al., 1970; Perrin, Kalant and Livingstone, 1975), mouse (Walker and Zornetzer, 1974), and rat (Hunter et al., 1973). In these animals during withdrawal, epileptiform spikes are observed which increase in both severity and frequency until they are organized into bursts of spikes, and ultimately sustained seizure discharges occur. As withdrawal proceeds, sustained epileptic discharges are observed in increasingly widespread anatomical areas and spread from limbic areas (hippocampus and amygdala) to thalamus, septal nucleus and frontal cortex. These spikes are observed either just before, or concurrently with the behavioral signs of withdrawal.

It was the similarity of these EEG abnormalities in the limbic areas to those seen during electrical kindling that led us to hypothesize that this hyperirritability and actual epileptic spiking during alcohol withdrawal could serve as a kindling stimulus in alcoholics. Also these EEG abnormalities and behavioral symptoms of withdrawal were observed to be cumulative and to become progressively more severe with repeated episodes of withdrawal (Baker and Cannon, 1979; Branchey, Rauscher and Kissin, 1971; Hunter et al., 1973; Poldrugo and Snead, 1984; Clemmesen and Hemmingsen, 1984; Walker and Zornetzer, 1974).

In alcoholics, withdrawal from alcohol occurs both in major bouts of prolonged withdrawal but also on an approximately 24-h basis as the alcoholic sleeps. Again the similarity to the optimal interval (approximately every 24 h) for kindling in animals was striking. This led to the dual predictions that years of alcohol abuse (and daily withdrawals), as well as episodes of major withdrawal, would correlate with the severity of alcohol withdrawal symptomatology. We will present data supportive of both predictions.

Consistent with the kindling model, individuals who drink heavily but only sporadically in binges do not appear to reliably develop severe alcohol withdrawal syndromes (Feuerlein, 1967). Although it is unclear and certainly complex what factors are involved in the development of withdrawal symptoms in man, available evidence suggests that heavy and regular, if not daily, use appears to be necessary for the development of the full-blown alcohol withdrawal syndrome (Mello and Mendelson, 1976).

Progression of the severity of the alcohol withdrawal syndrome over time

The preponderance of evidence suggests that the withdrawal syndrome is cumulative and requires many years of alcohol abuse for significant withdrawal syndromes to emerge (Gross et al., 1972; Johnson, 1961; Lundqvist, 1961; Mendelson, Stein and McGuire, 1966; Nielsen, 1965; Segal et al., 1970; Wolfe and Victor, 1971). The most severe components of the syndrome, including hallucinations and delirium tremens (DTs) (Victor and Adams, 1953), seizures (Brown et al., 1988; Gross et al., 1972), clouding of consciousness (Gross et al., 1972) and alcoholic psychosis (Singer and Wong, 1973) generally only occur after years of alcohol abuse. There is a striking concurrence in the large questionnaire studies from multiple countries documenting that the physical symptoms of withdrawal generally only occur after a decade of heavy alcohol abuse (Horn and Wanberg, 1969; Jellinek, 1952; Park, 1973; Trice and Wahl, 1958). However, certain data are inconsistent with this hypothesis including recent data that seizures are primarily related to levels of recent alcohol use (Ng et al., 1988) and that DTs are not correlated with duration of abuse (Feuerlein, 1974; Whitwell, 1975), but with pattern of drinking (Mello, 1973), or an interaction of duration and pattern (Mello and Mendelson, 1976). In animals, it is relatively noncontroversial that the withdrawal syndrome is related to duration of exposure and dose (Ellis and Pick, 1970; Freund, 1969; Goldstein, 1972a, b; Walker and Zornetzer, 1974).

Most pertinent to the model we have proposed are the studies indicating that alcohol withdrawal is more severe in animals previously addicted to alcohol (Branchey, Rauscher and Kissin, 1971; Goldstein, 1974; Hunter et al., 1973; Clemmesen and Hemmingsen, 1984; Poldrugo and Snead, 1984; Walker and Zornetzer, 1974). Consistent with the kindling model, the behavioral symptoms and the EEG abnormalities in mice (Walker and Zornetzer, 1974) and rats (Branchey, Rauscher and Kissin, 1971; Goldstein, 1974; Hunter et al., 1973) become progressively more severe with repeated episodes of withdrawal. In the studies of Branchey, Rauscher and Kissin (1971) and Goldstein (1974), the cumulative changes appear to be dependent on an optimal interval between episodes of withdrawal, reminiscent of the kindling paradigm. Also, some investigators feel that with readdiction, a shorter period of ethanol intake is required to produce the same symptomatology (Baker and Cannon, 1979; Branchey, Rauscher and Kissin, 1971; Ellis and Pick, 1970; Kalant et al., 1971, 1978; LeBlanc et al., 1969). In chronic alcoholics who are experimentally administered alcohol, they develop withdrawal symptoms after less alcohol exposure than do abstinent morphine addicts (Isbell et al., 1955) or normals (Gross, Lewis and Hastey, 1974; Mello, 1973; Mendelson and La Dou, 1964).

In 1978 we presented evidence from 200 consecutive admissions to a Navy alcohol rehabilitation unit documenting a progression of the severity of the alcohol withdrawal syndrome over years of alcohol abuse (Ballenger and Post, 1978). The subjects met DSM-II criteria for diagnosis of habitual excessive drinking or alcohol addiction and Research Diagnostic Criteria (RDC) for alcoholism. They had been drinking more than 7 ounces of absolute alcohol daily, e.g. greater than 10 beers or approximately 1 pint of whiskey, for at least 6 months preceding admission and had sufficient data present in their records to retrospectively assess the intensity of their current and past withdrawal symptomatology. Since many of the alcoholics were hospitalized early in their illness, we defined the onset of alcohol abuse as the beginning of heavy drinking, i.e. daily drinking greater than 7 ounces of absolute alcohol or when classic symptoms of alcoholism appeared, e.g. loss of control, blackouts, loss of job, divorce, or arrest secondary to drinking. Records were reviewed for age, years of drinking, years of alcohol abuse, and withdrawal symptoms both by history and during the index hospitalization. Data on withdrawal symptoms were available from both the physicians' and social workers' histories and two self-report inventories of alcohol use and withdrawal symptoms. It was assumed that the number of years of alcohol abuse could be reliably approximated by the alcoholics as had been done in multiple previous studies (Jellinek, 1952; Mello and Mendelson, 1976; Mendelson and LaDou, 1964; Park, 1973). Withdrawal symptoms were globally rated on a scale of 5 stages: Stage 0—no withdrawal symptoms; Stage 1—mild tremulousness; Stage 2—gross tremors ('shakes'), autonomic hyperactivity (fever, diaphoresis); Stage 3—seizures, confusion, or isolated hallucinations; Stage 4—delirium tremens (DTs). Diagnosis of DTs was made when delirium, increased autonomic activity, tremors and visual hallucinations were all present during alcohol withdrawal. In this retrospective review we only identified four cases of DTs; however, we also reviewed records of all patients on other medical services in the same hospital during the same years and located an additional 15 patients with the discharge diagnosis of DTs. Our results are reported on these 19 patients with DTs.

As is seen in Table 1, 91% of the alcoholics who had been drinking less than 3 years prior to their index admission were observed to have no withdrawal symptoms and none of the patients experienced more than a mild tremor (Stage 1). However, after 3 to 5 years of alcohol abuse, 36% of patients were observed to have symptoms of mild tremor (Stage 1) and 22% had histories of Stage 2 or greater symptomatology. After 10 or more years of abuse, two-thirds of patients had withdrawal symptoms which were rated Stage 2 or worse. The most serious withdrawal reactions (seizures and DTs —

Table 1. Duration of alcohol and withdrawal symptomatology (index admission)

Years of alcohol abuse		Severity of withdrawal				
		0	1	2	3	4
		None	Mild tremor	'Shakes' automatic hyperactivity	Seizures confusion	DTs
½–3	(n 95)	87 (91%)	8 (9%)	0	0	0
3–5	(n 36)	15 (42%)	13 (36%)	8 (22%)	0	0
5–10	(n 48)	15 (31%)	12 (25%)	17 (35%)	3 (6%)	1 (3%)
10–15	(n 15)	3 (20%)	2 (14%)	6 (40%)	3 (20%)	1 (6%)
15–20	(n 4)	1 (25%)	0	1 (25%)	0	2 (50%)
> 20	(n 2)	0	1 (50%)	1 (50%)	0	0

Stages 3 and 4) were not observed until after 6 years of alcohol abuse and 60% occurred after 10 years or greater. The finding that more serious withdrawal symptomatology was associated with longer duration of alcohol abuse was significant by both Chi square analysis ($\chi^2 < 160.89$, $P < 0.001$) and Kendall's tau (tau $= 0.55$, $P < 0.001$).

In the 19 cases of DTs, the onset of DTs occurred in 80% of the patients only after 10 years with almost half of the patients reporting the first episode after 15 or more years of alcohol abuse.

Although this research was based on a retrospective review of charts and the assumption that years of alcohol abuse correlated with episodes of withdrawal, these data are certainly consistent with the prediction that the alcohol withdrawal syndrome progresses over time in the direction of increasing severity.

The kindling withdrawal syndrome should progress in a stepwise unidirectional manner

Consistent with this prediction, the alcohol withdrawal syndrome has been generally seen to be organized into serially progressive stages in which one stage is incorporated into the next in a unidirectional manner similar to the kindling model. In both circumstances once a level of severity is obtained, subsequent episodes of withdrawal (or kindling), usually, although not invariably, again reach that level of severity (Mello and Mendelson, 1976).

In multiple species there is a similar sequence of severity of withdrawal which begins with tremor which worsens as the withdrawal syndrome progresses, followed by autonomic hyperactivity, then seizures, hallucinations and in humans, in its most extreme form to DTs. Alcohol withdrawal symptomatology has been observed in monkeys (Ellis and Pick, 1970), mice (Walker and Zornetzer, 1974), dogs (Essig and Lam, 1971), rats (Hunter *et al.*, 1973), and in humans (Gross *et al.*, 1971; Isbell *et al.*, 1975; Victor and Adams, 1953). Analogous to the kindling stages, the alcohol withdrawal syndrome appears to be organized in stages such that there is an 'all or none' quality in some of the alcohol symptoms, clusters or stages. For instance, although as many as a third of cases of DTs began with withdrawal seizures, once DTs begin, invariably the seizures remit and do not recur (Victor, 1973; Victor and Brausch, 1967; Wolfe and Victor, 1971). Similar to the reorganization of the behavioral and EEG responses in the kindling process which occurs just prior to the onset of seizures (Pinel and Van Oot, 1975), Whitwell (1975) has described the appearance of a lucid period just prior to the onset of alcoholic delirium. Also at the onset of DTs there is evidence of a change in the evoked potentials (Victor and Brausch, 1967).

Symptoms should be understandable as secondary to a subcortical 'kindling-like process

EEG changes in subcortical areas should be similar in alcohol withdrawal and kindling. When they have been directly measured during alcohol withdrawal with depth electrodes in the rat (Hunter *et al.*, 1973) and mouse (Walker and Zornetzer, 1974), a consistent progression of EEG abnormalities is observed which is strikingly similar to the EEG changes observed in the kindling process. There is a progression from high amplitude slow waves to isolated, and then grouped epileptiform spikes, culminating in sustained epileptic discharges. Concomitantly, the animals display behavioral changes of increasingly severe hyperactivity, tremor, tail arching, dorsiflexion of the spine, and ultimately convulsions. Therefore both the behavioral and EEG findings of these animals withdrawing from alcohol are similar to those in animals which are being electrically kindled.

Again, seizures are involved in both processes. The generalized seizures which are a central feature of severe alcohol withdrawal are perhaps the most obvious similarity between the kindling model and alcohol withdrawal. Seizures occur in both situations only after repeated exposure to the kindling stimuli, i.e. electrical stimulation in the kindling paradigm and theoretically, multiple episodes of CNS hyperirritability accompanying alcohol withdrawal.

We have recently reported (Brown *et al.*, 1988) that the number of detoxifications alcoholics had previously undergone correlated with the predisposition to withdrawal seizures. We retrospectively studied 74 male alcoholics with alcohol withdrawal seizures documented in our VA Hospital over the 14 years from 1972–1985. We contrasted them to a comparison group of male alcoholics admitted to the same alcohol detoxification unit over the same period of time, but who had no history of alcohol withdrawal seizures. Records were carefully examined to obtain data for demographics, alcohol use, detoxification history, clinical variables, and laboratory data. A significantly higher ($P < 0.05$) percentage (48%) of the alcoholics with withdrawal seizures had undergone five or more detoxifications, compared to only 12% of the comparison group (see Figure 2). Age of the first detoxification was 11.6 years earlier (mean age 36.5 years) in the withdrawal seizures group than controls ($P < 0.001$), but detoxification history, not age, accounted for the observed differences in withdrawal seizure susceptibility. Other indices of alcohol use did not differ between the groups, e.g. alcohol use in the month prior to admission, years of significant use, or age when first beginnning to drink (see Table 2). Obviously the observations that withdrawal seizures were not related to number of years of previous abuse is inconsistent with the data presented above, although the correlation with number of previous detoxifications is consistent with the proposed model. Also, 72% of the patients who had seizures during the index hospitalization had previously

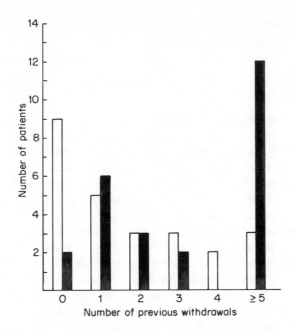

Figure 2. Number of previous withdrawals (detoxifications) in the seizure (■) and control (□) groups. [Reproduced with permission from Brown *et al.* (1988)]

Table 2. Alcohol use history of alcholics with and without alcohol withdrawal seizures

Variable	Withdrawal seizures (*n* = 25)	Control (*n* = 25)	Significance
Reported alcohol use (oz/day) during month prior to admission (mean ± SD)	35.4±15.4 (25)*	41.3±34.6 (25)	NS
< 20 oz	12% (3)	16% (4)	
20–40 oz	60% (15)	60% (4)	NS
> 40 oz	28% (7)	(24%)	
Years of significant use			
0–9	16% (4)	17% (4)	
10–20	52% (13)	46% (11)	NS
> 21	32% (8)	37% (9)	
Age started drinking (mean ± SD)	16.6±3.0 (17)	16.4±3.5 (18)	NS

* Numbers in parentheses are the number of patients who had data available for analysis of this variable.

experienced withdrawal seizures. This is consistent with a stage-like, unidirectional quality of the progressive changes.

There should be evidence of residual changes between 'kindling stimulations' i.e. alcohol withdrawals

Perhaps most important in the kindling process are the observed changes in behavioral patterns as kindling progresses, e.g. aggressivity (Adamec, 1975; Pinel *et al.*, 1977) and multiple other behaviors (Post, Rubinow and Ballenger, 1984). We have hypothesized that the personality changes which are observed in chronic alcoholics would be the analogous behavioral changes and that they should therefore be sequential, of a more or less continuous nature, and not be confined to withdrawal periods.

There are multiple reports of severe psychiatric difficulties which occur not only during intoxication (Mendelson, 1964) but that various symptoms, particularly psychological ones (Feuerlein, 1974; Segal *et al.*, 1970) beginning in the withdrawal period continue on into the abstinence period in alcoholics. Also large scale questionnaire studies report that psychological symptoms occur outside the withdrawal period. Beginning with Jellinek's studies (1946, 1952), multiple investigators (Glatt, 1961; Park, 1973; Trice and Wahl, 1958) have identified a strikingly similar serial progression of behavioral abnormalities associated with chronic alcoholism in thousands of alcoholics from multiple countries. They report a sequence of symptoms which begins after 5–10 years of alcohol abuse which includes major psychological problems of grandiosity, aggressive behavior, persistent remorse, and unreasonable resentments (Jellinek, 1952). As alcohol abuse continues, some of these early behavioral difficulties recede in importance, but new difficulties appear, e.g. alcoholic jealousy, decreased sexual drive, deterioration in ethics, decreases in the ability to think clearly, and late in the course, alcoholic psychoses. Glatt (1961) has reported that asocial or antisocial behavior and suicide attempts which often appear after 5–10 years of alcohol abuse tend to disappear only after prolonged sobriety (greater than 6 months). Others have reported an increase in 'emotionality' and anxiety with chronic alcohol abuse (McNamee, Mello and Mendelson, 1968; Tamerin and Mendelson, 1969). There is general agreement that the end stage alcoholic after 15–20 years of alcohol abuse generally no longer has difficulty with the aggressive and destructive behavior which appeared earlier in the course, but has often developed a striking syndrome of religiosity, indefinable fears, compulsive behaviors, psychomotor inhibition, loss of craving for alcohol, and severe physical symptoms (Gross *et al.*, 1976; Jellinek, 1952).

The closest analogy to the kindling model in humans is probably the complex partial seizure syndrome, which may represent an 'experiment in nature' of the kindling model in humans. The direct effects of chronic epileptic spiking and seizure discharges in limbic and related cortical areas in man are obviously unknown, but all types of psychiatric difficulties have been reported (Flor-Henry, 1969; Gibbs, 1951; Hill, 1953), and an interictal behavioral disorder has been described which is similar in many respects to the syndrome of chronic alcoholism mentioned above. Many of the features, religiosity (Bear and Fedio, 1977; Dewhurst and Beard, 1970), decreased sexual interest (Blumer, 1970), obsessionalism, guilt, humorless over-generalized serious concern (Bear and Fedio, 1977; Geschwind, 1973) and emotionality overlap directly with the behavioral and personality features reported with chronic alcohol abuse. Other personality features associated with the complex partial seizure syndrome such as denial, dependency (Blumer, 1974), an increase in philosophical concerns, sadness (Dewhurst and Beard, 1970), paranoid ideation (Flor-Henry, 1969), and difficulty with aggression (Bear and Fedio, 1977; Serafetinides, 1965) are obviously features commonly associated with chronic alcoholism.

Interaction of alcohol withdrawal and medications and procedures which affect kindling

Those medications which promote or retard kindling should have similar effects on the alcohol withdrawal syndrome if our hypothesis is correct. A direct interaction between kindling and alcohol withdrawal has been demonstrated in that previous withdrawal does facilitate electrical kindling (Carrington, Ellinwood and Kirshnan, 1984; Hoffer et al., 1980). Also previous kindling of the amygdala results in a marked increase in severity of subsequent alcohol withdrawal reactions (Carrington and Ellinwood, 1981; Pinel, 1980; Pinel and Van Oot, 1975, 1978). Severity of the withdrawal syndrome is greatly increased not only with the full kindling procedure but also with stimulation below the after-discharge threshold so that there are no observable EEG or behavioral effects from the stimulation. Thus the presence of convulsive phenomena or even recordable after-discharges is not a prerequisite for kindling (Racine, 1972). According to the proposed model, cumulative physiologic changes would occur in the alcoholic with each withdrawal, even if no overt symptoms were observed.

There are also pharmacological data which indirectly connect kindling and alcohol withdrawal. The benzodiazepines and especially diazepam have antikindling effects (Babington and Wedeking, 1973; Racine, 1975; Wise and Chinerman, 1974) and can be quite effective in reducing the full range of alcohol withdrawal symptoms including DTs and alcohol seizures (Thompson, Johnson and Maddrey, 1975).

The anticonvulsive carbamazepine (Tegretol) has been shown to have inhibitory effects on the development of kindling in cats and primates (Wada and Osawa, 1976; Post et al., 1986b) and against established kindling in multiple species, including rats (Weiss and Post, 1987; Albright and Burnham, 1980; Schmutz, Chapter 4). In Europe, carbamazepine has been demonstrated to be effective in treating alcohol withdrawal (Agricola, Mazzanino and Urani, 1982; Bjorkovist et al., 1976; Poutanen, 1979; Ritola and Malinon, 1981). Open trials have demonstrated its effectiveness in the alcohol withdrawal syndrome and even possibly its superiority in ameliorating certain aspects of the alcohol withdrawal syndrome (Brune and Busch, 1971; Poutanen, 1979). In four double-blind controlled trials, carbamazepine (CBZ) was superior to placebo (Bjorkovist et al., 1976), and equal in efficacy to tiapride (Agricola, 1982), clomethiazole (Ritola and Malinen, 1981) and barbital (Flygerring, 1984). These trials suggest the CBZ may result in more rapid decreases in symptoms, perhaps especially psychiatric symptoms (Agricola et al., 1982). We and others (Ballenger and Post, 1978; Brown et al., 1988; Butler and Messiha, 1986; Pinel, 1980) have suggested that treatment of alcohol withdrawal with anticonvulsants with antikindling properties may be superior to the benzodiazepines in potentially reducing or preventing long-term neurological, psychiatric, or behavioral complications of alcoholism if in fact kindling is involved in some way with the progressive aspects of alcoholism.

We have performed a double-bind comparison of carbamazepine and oxazepam, a commonly used benzodiazepine in hospitalized withdrawing alcoholics (Malcolm et al., 1989). To our knowledge this is the first study to compare CBZ in a double-blind trial with a standard benzodiazepine utilized in the treatment of alcohol withdrawal. We screened 512 consecutive daytime admissions to our VA alcohol detoxification unit for subjects for this study. Patients had to be male, meet DSM-III-R criteria for alcohol dependence, and have a score of 20 or more on the Clinical Institute Withdrawal Assessment for Alcohol (CIWA-A). On this scale, a score of 20 or more indicates significant withdrawal symptomatology requiring treatment (Shaw et al., 1981). Further exclusion criteria included daily use of CNS active drugs including drugs of abuse, or other significant psychiatric or medical difficulties. Out of the potential 512 subjects, 83% failed to meet study criteria, primarily because of low CIWA-A scores (40%). Eighty-six subjects met initial study criteria and participated in the study although five subjects were dropped between days 2–3 because of abnormalities in their initial laboratory assessments. Patients were followed with the CIWA-A scale which rates patients along 15 clinical dimensions. It was administered twice daily, 1 h after the administration of medication. Patients were also followed with various physiological measures including pulse, blood pressure, and tremor. Patients were examined neurologically utilizing deep tendon reflexes and a standardized rating of ataxia twice daily. Patients also rated themselves on 11 self-report measures including sleepiness, anxiety, alcohol craving, energy, anger, craving for sweets, hunger, shakiness, nausea, need for alcohol, and quality of the previous night's sleep. The patients completed these scales once a day in the afternoon. They also completed the Hopkins symptom checklist (SCL-90) (Derogatis, 1977). The Beck Depression Inventory (Beck *et al.*, 1961), and the State-Trait Inventory (Speilberger, 1977) were utilized to assess depression and anxiety and the Wechsler Memory Scale to evaluate memory. These psychometric measures were evaluated at baseline and on days 3 and 7 of treatment.

Study subjects were blindly assigned to either 200 mg of CBZ or 30 mg of oxazepam (OX) every 6 h for 7 days with matching placebo for both medications (double-dummy design). All patients, research staff and ward clinical personnel were blinded to the study drugs.

The initial demographics for both groups were well matched. Mean CBZ level on day 3 (9.8 ± 2.9 µg/ml) was significantly higher than day 7 (8.7 ± 2.5 µg/ml) although this was not considered to be clinically significant. Both CBZ and OX treatment resulted in significant improvement in withdrawal symptomatology ($P < 0.0001$) as measured by the CIWA-A (see Figure 3). However, there were no significant differences between CBZ and OX on this scale. There were similar significant declines ($P < 0.01$) in tremor, systolic blood pressure, gait and self-reported shakiness, nervousness, and craving for alcohol. These did not differ between the drug groups. There were also no significant differences in side effects of the two medications.

These results document that CBZ is as effective as OX, a traditional benzodiazepine, in the treatment of acute alcohol withdrawal. Although this

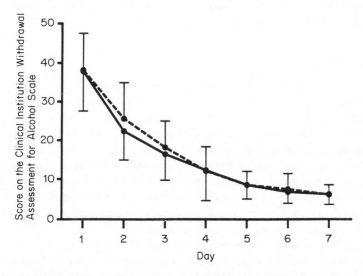

Figure 3. CIWA-A scores plotted for carbamazepine (solid line, $n = 39$) and oxazepam (broken line, $n = 42$) groups over seven days. [Reproduced with permission from Malcolm *et al.* (1989)]

is consistent with the alcohol kindling model we have proposed, its effectiveness in the syndrome obviously may not relate to its anti-kindling properties but to other unknown properties. The proposed kindling model would suggest that carbamazepine might have potentially greater efficacy against behavioral symptoms than do the benzodiazepines since it has more powerful effects against established kindled foci (Post et al., 1986b; Weiss and Post, 1987). However, benzodiazepines do have less potent antikindling effects and this would minimize potential differences. In this study we did observe evidence that some of the psychopathological aspects of the withdrawal syndrome did, in fact, respond better to CBZ than OX. CBZ was superior in reducing global symptoms of psychopathology, and analysis of the subscales of the SCL-90 also demonstrated that CBZ was significantly greater in reducing obsessive-compulsive scores and anxiety scores compared to OX. In addition there were greater improvements on the SCL-90 factors of somatization, depression, hostility, paranoid ideation, and psychoticism which approached significance. Actually the SCL-90 scores for total psychopathology increased on OX over the 7-day trial while they significantly decreased on CBZ. On the other hand, OX reduced phobic anxiety scores more than CBZ, although this difference failed to reach significance. These observations are similar to the reports from Europe suggesting that CBZ has perhaps more extensive and certainly more rapidly appearing effects against psychopathology. It is also of interest that in one study (Carlsson and Pettersson, 1972) CBZ reduced dysphoric symptoms in abstinent chronic alcoholics, suggesting CBZ might have positive effects against symptoms of alcoholism beyond the withdrawal period.

Discussion

If this model is correct and repeated episodes of withdrawal over years of alcohol abuse do lead to a 'kindled state', treatment of episodes of withdrawal in alcoholism could involve different strategies aimed at retarding the establishment of or expression of kindling-like changes. Potentially, treatment of each episode of withdrawal with antikindling agents (benzodiazepines or anticonvulsants) could modify future withdrawal reactions or other symptoms of alcoholism, e.g. the psychiatric and behavioral problems. Also, treatment with antikindling agents of alcohol-kindling-related psychiatric problems, e.g. depression, anxiety, and aggressiveness, could potentially modify the progressive course of these common problems.

Similarly it appears that this model may offer some potential understanding of the addictive process in alcoholism. Certainly previous alcohol addiction leads to greater subsequent alcohol consumption in animals (Deutsch and Koopmans, 1973; Hunter et al., 1973), and rats which have been physically addicted to alcohol subsequently become addicted again more rapidly and with less exposure (Branchey, Rauscher and Kissin, 1971; Kalant, LeBlanc and Gibbins, 1971; Walker and Zornetzer, 1974). Also alcoholics demonstrate an increased susceptibility to relapse for at least the first 6 months of abstinence (Davies, Shepherd and Myers, 1956; Jellinek, 1952; Kissin and Charnoff, 1967). These and other data suggest that the addictive process involves long-lasting physiological changes. Although kindling-like processes could be involved in such long-lasting physiologic changes, there is no evidence currently available to support that hypothesis.

PART II: COCAINE-INDUCED SENSITIZATION AND KINDLING

Cocaine is both a psychomotor stimulant and a local anesthetic. This combination of properties accounts for its broad and unique spectrum of behavioral toxicities. On the one hand, cocaine is a powerful blocker of catecholamine and indoleamine reuptake. It is thought that its ability to enhance catecholamines, particularly dopamine, accounts for its stimulant effects. If lesions of dopaminergic systems are made in the nucleus accumbens, animals show decreases in cocaine- and amphetamine-induced hyperactivity (Kelly and Iverson, 1975). Moreover, recent evidence indicates that these lesions decrease cocaine-induced self-administration in animals (Pettit et al., 1984; Roberts et al., 1980). While cocaine is a less potent releaser of dopamine and norepinephrine than is amphetamine, its effects on reuptake lead to increases in synaptic dopamine. Dose-related increases in dopamine have recently been documented in striatum and in nucleus accumbens with in vivo dialysis (Glue et al., 1988). Interestingly, significant dose-related increases were not observed in prefrontal cortex in the rat. Nonetheless, it is into this area in the rat that intracerebral administration of cocaine appears rewarding (Goeders and Smith, 1986) in contrast to amphetamine, where both intravenous self-administration and intracerebral administration appear to depend on a nucleus accumbens substrate (Hernandez, Lee and Hoebel, 1987).

Thus, the ability of the psychomotor stimulants to produce alertness, arousal, motor activation, and euphoria is thought to be related to catecholaminergic systems. Experienced users have a great deal of difficulty distinguishing amphetamine and cocaine (Fischman et al., 1976). They are also unable to discriminate a wide variety of psychomotor stimulants with direct or indirect sympathomimetic effects (Martin et al., 1971). Behavioral toxicities that emerge from repeated psychomotor stimulant administration can be modeled in the animal laboratory. Behavioral sensitization appears characteristic of psychomotor stimulants and dopamine agonists and involves increased behavioral activation upon repeated administration of the same dose. Since amphetamine and cocaine can both produce behavioral sensitization and, in some instances, cross-sensitization to each other (Post and Contel, 1983), it appears that this component of cocaine's long-term effects is dependent on its stimulant (dopaminergic) properties rather than on its local-anesthetic effects.

In contrast, a true kindling phenomenon appears to be attributable to cocaine's properties as a local anesthetic. Repeated administration of high but subconvulsant doses of cocaine will eventually lead to the development of limbic-type seizures (Post et al., 1987). Weiss et al. (1987) have demonstrated that this phenomenon is dose-related, with rare seizures being produced by 40 mg/kg i.p., but more ready seizure induction being more rapidly achieved with 50 and 65 mg/kg. With the latter dose, approximately 50% of the animals may seize on the first day and all succumb within the first week of cocaine administration, usually after the first or second cocaine-induced seizure. It is likely that this effect is attributable to a kindling phenomenon based on observations with the purely local anesthetic lidocaine (Post, Kopanda and Lee, 1975; Post et al., 1984).

Using a dose of lidocaine (either 60 or 65 mg/kg i.p., once daily), most of the animals do not seize during the first or second day of administration. However, after several weeks, approximately 40% of the animals develop seizures. These seizures bear many similarities to those observed with amygdala kindling. They are associated with after-discharges in the amygdala and are behaviorally similar, involving tonic–clonic movements of head, trunk, and forepaws with rearing and falling. Moreover, there is cross-sensitization in both directions between lidocaine kindling and amygdala kindling. Lidocaine-kindled animals demonstrate amgydala-kindled seizures at twice the rate of controls (Post et al., 1984). Amygdala-kindled animals show a much higher incidence of lidocaine-induced seizures on challenge after the completion of kindling compared with implanted, sham-stimulated controls (Post et al., 1981). Lidocaine-kindled animals show prominent increases in glucose utilization in amygdala and hippocampus or perirhinal areas (Post et al., 1984).

Lidocaine is the local anesthetic with equal potency to cocaine on a mg/kg basis, but it does not share cocaine's psychomotor-stimulant properties, as it lacks the ability to affect firing of catecholamine and indoleamine neurons (Pitts and Marwah, 1988). While procaine is also classified as a purely local anesthetic, it has been demonstrated to induce a pharmacological kindling-like pattern of seizure induction, and has minimal effects on firing of catecholaminergic and indoleaminergic neurons in the locus coeruleus, substantia nigra, and raphe nucleus (Pitts and Marwah, 1986, 1988). However, it does appear to have a slightly different profile compared with lidocaine, as it will be self-administered by animals (Woolverton and Balster, 1979) and it has been included in some preparations as a potential mood-elevating compound. Moreover, experienced volunteers appear able to discriminate cocaine from lidocaine but this is less readily achieved with procaine (Fischman, Schuster and Hatano, 1983).

Thus, it is important to distinguish between the psychomotor stimulant and local-anesthetic properties of cocaine in assessing its addicting and kindling properties, as well as in distinguishing its behavioral and physiological toxicities. It would appear that the properties of cocaine most directly attributable to its euphorogenic effects, and thus most closely related to its addiction potential, in fact demonstrate tolerance rather than sensitization. Fishman (1984) reported that a second i.v. administration of cocaine shortly after the first was associated with attenuation of psychological and physiological effects, suggesting the development of tolerance if not tachyphylaxis, at least given this temporal patterning of administration. These data are also convergent with those of Kumor et al. (1988) and Sherer et al. (1988), who demonstrated an inability to maintain peak euphoric effects of cocaine in spite of continuous intravenous infusions to maintain blood levels. Instead of the euphoria, increases in dysphoria and in paranoia (suspiciousness) were observed with maintenance of this infusion. These data are convergent with those in the animal literature suggesting that, on repeated administration of the stimulant amphetamine or cocaine, different components of its effects can show tolerance, no change over time, or sensitization (Robinson and Becker, 1986). Differences appear to depend on the endpoint measured as well as on the temporal characteristics of the drug administration (Post, 1980). Thus, the behavioral and convulsive toxicological effects of cocaine, rather than its euphorogenic effects, are the ones that demonstrate sensitization and kindling.

We would, again, like to draw a careful distinction between behavioral sensitization, with its typical endpoint in animal studies of motor activity or stereotypy, and those of the pharmacological kindling effects, where seizures are the endpoint. Pharmacological intervention in these two effects also differ considerably. For example, there is preliminary evidence that lithium can impair the development of some aspects of behavioral sensitization while it is without effect on kindling (at least of the electrical variety elicited from amygdala or hippocampus) (Post, Weiss and Pert, 1984). Conversely, carbamazepine is a potent anticonvulsant in many types of kindled seizures, but is without effect in blocking the major components of behavioral sensitization (Post, Rubinow and Ballenger, 1984; Weiss et al., 1988, unpublished observations).

Important disjunctions occur in the efficacy of carbamazepine as an anticonvulsant on different stages of kindled seizures, and this varies according to the type of kindling. For example, carbamazepine will not block the development of amygdala-kindled seizures in the rat, while it is the most potent drug in inhibiting completed seizures kindled from the amygdala (Post et al., 1986b; Weiss and Post, 1987). The opposite is true for the effects of carbamazepine on local-anesthetic-induced kindled seizures. In this instance, chronic oral treatment with carbamezpine is highly effective in blocking the development of lidocaine- and cocaine-induced kindled seizures, but it is not effective on completed lidocaine-kindled seizures or on high-dose cocaine seizures (Weiss *et al.*, 1988b).

In contrast to lidocaine-kindled seizures, which are generally well tolerated by animals, even after extended periods of repeated seizure induction (weeks to months), seizures induced by cocaine are associated with a high incidence of mortality (Weiss *et al.*, 1988b). The cocaine seizure appears highly similar to that observed with lidocaine in terms of its behavioral characteristics, but during or at the end of a seizure episode, animals cease breathing and succumb in this immediate postictal period. Carbamazepine not only blocks cocaine-kindled seizure development, but also the associated lethality. Again, it should be reemphasized that acute administration of carbamazepine is not only not effective in blocking a high-dose cocaine seizure, but in some instances may actually increase lethality (Weiss *et al.*, 1988b). Thus, carbamazepine cannot be used acutely in the treatment of cocaine seizures. Chronic carbamazepine administration is also without effect on acute high-dose cocaine seizures on day 1, although with repeated administration it does appear to block seizure development and the associated lethality (Weiss *et al.*, 1988b).

Just as there are temporal dissociations in the ability of pharmacological interventions to be effective in different phases of kindling, a similar phenomenon occurs in cocaine-induced behavioral sensitization. Pretreatment with neuroleptics appears to block the development of behavioral sensitization, but once it is manifest, even high doses of neuroleptics are without effect (Weiss *et al.*, 1988a). Thus, it appears that it is not prior experience with cocaine alone that is responsible for cocaine-induced behavioral sensitization, but experience with cocaine in the same environmental context that leads to greater degrees of reactivity upon rechallenge. Therefore, it is to be expected that if animals' hyperactivity on day 1 is inhibited by neuroleptics or diazepam, they show lesser degrees of behavioral sensitization upon rechallenge on day 2 (Weiss *et al.*, 1988a). However, once cocaine-induced hyperactivity is experienced on day 1, neuroleptics given prior to the day 2 challenge are ineffective in blocking the expression of cocaine-induced behavioral sensitization (Weiss *et al.*, 1988a). These findings are parallel to those reported by Tadokoro and Kuribara (1986) as well as Beninger and Hahn (1983) and Beninger and Herz (1986) using other psychomotor stimulants and neuroleptics. Thus, to the extent that this conditioned component of behavioral sensitization is relevant to some elements of psychosis evolution in man, one would predict that aspects of behavioral sensitization that show a prominent conditioned component may not respond adequately to neuroleptics. Clearly, the predictions derived from this model require direct clinical testing in order to assess their relevance in man.

Post and associates (1986a, 1987) have postulated that the local anaesthetic component of cocaine may be associated with kindling-like effects not only for seizures themselves but also for subictal phenomena. In particular, they postulated that the high incidence of panic attacks reported in cocaine users requesting assistance (50% of the first 500 callers to the Cocaine Hotline reported panic attacks) may be attributable to cocaine's local-anesthetic properties. This is based on reports of 'doom anxiety' associated with administration of local anesthetics for cardiac arrhythmias and a high incidence of dysphoria associated with intravenous procaine administration in subjects with borderline personality disorder or affective illness, and a lower incidence in controls (Kellner et al., 1987). Moreover, the evolution of panic anxiety phenomena appears to very closely parallel the stages of kindling (Post et al., 1986a, 1987). In 1986 Post and colleagues reported a case of apparent cocaine-induced panic attacks that progressed in stages paralleling the evolution of kindling; i.e. development, completed, spontaneous (Post et al., 1986a).

Given the foregoing analyses, it is apparent that the rewarding aspects of cocaine self-administration that appear to be most closely associated with the addictive process, are not the components that show true kindling-like evolution. In fact, it appears that the behavioral and convulsive toxicities are more likely to emerge as a secondary consequence of cocaine addiction because of patterns of repeated intermittent and compulsive use that drive the user to higher and more frequent doses of cocaine. These, in turn, become sufficient to allow for the emergence of the local-anesthetic effects of cocaine due to the high doses employed. Thus, it appears that it is the components of cocaine's catecholaminergic potentiation (most closely associated with behavioral sensitization) that appear more integrally related to the addictive process. Considerable evidence implicates dopaminergic effects in nucleus accumbens and related areas of brain, not only with the reward properties of cocaine, but also with those of opiates and direct electrical brain stimulation reward, leading to the formulation that dopamine may play a key role in the addictive process (Koob, Le and Creese, 1987; Scheel-Krüger et al., 1977; Wise, 1981, 1984).

The prominent conditioned components of behavioral sensitization to cocaine that have been uncovered in animal models (Weiss et al., 1988b) are of great interest to the increasing reports of the very powerful conditioned cueing effects that can occur with cocaine use in man. Gawin and Kleber (1987) and Gawin and Ellinwood (1988) have reported anecdotes of users 'automatically' driving their cars off exits where they had previously habitually driven to purchase cocaine, even after many months of abstinence. Childress et al. (1988) have systematically demonstrated the powerful effects of cocaine cues in the laboratory; showing addicts pictures of cocaine paraphernalia induces intense craving, again even after many months of abstinence. Repeated attempts to decondition and desensitize this craving have been partially successful, but even when they are capable of reducing the craving, conditioned hypothermic effects may still be observed.

This suggests that the physiological consequences of the cocaine experience in man, like behavioral sensitization in animals, may persist on a conditioned basis for extraordinarily long periods of time and be extremely refractory to attempts at therapeutic intervention. Perhaps the use of combined approaches, including pharmacotherapy with such agents as desipramine or the first dopamine agonist bromocriptine, in conjunction with behavioral techniques, will reduce this long-lasting residual and apparent vulnerability to release and addiction.

CONCLUSIONS

Thus, it would appear necessary to distinguish behavioral endpoints that seem to show kindling-like progression with repeated episodes of intoxication or withdrawal, from those that are associated with a true pharmacological kindling of seizures. Clearly, in the alcohol withdrawal syndromes, behavioral toxicities may gradually emerge prior to (or exlcusive of) the occurrence of seizures. A panoply of symptoms appears to increase in severity, eventually climaxing in the appearance of DTs, whether or not seizures eventually become manifest. The case is even more complicated with cocaine as a potential pharmacological kindling agent. In this instance, it would appear that some of the behavioral syndromes are directly analogous to the kindling-like process, perhaps attributable to local-anesthetic properties of the drug. In contrast, other behaviors may show a sensitization-like pattern but occur through completely independent mechanisms more closely related to those of other psychomotor stimulants and linked to dopaminergic mechanisms. The ability of cocaine to produce both sensitization and kindling may account for a panoply of psychological and physiological side effects.

Based on well-tested preclinical models, as well as a growing clinical experience that is convergent with this formulation, it appears that kindling-like phenomena are important to understanding a range of toxicities that emerge with repeated episodes of alcohol withdrawal or cocaine intoxication. The lay public, as well as clinical and basic scientists, should be educated to these additional covert dangers of alcohol and cocaine use which are not readily apparent on initial experiences with these agents. It is only after repeated experiences that the phenomena of sensitization and kindling appear to be engaged.

Thus, not only do these models emphasize the potential for progressive evolution of symptomatology over time, but also that pharmacological interventions may differ as a function of stage of evolution. In some phases, drugs that are initially successful in preventing the development of sensitization and kindling may not be effective in blocking the expression of sensitization or late phases of kindled seizures (Post *et al.*, 1986b). Further basic studies of the preclinical models of pharmacological kindling with alcohol withdrawal and cocaine may help delineate the factors that are critical for kindling evolution, its prevention, and reversal.

REFERENCES

Adamec, R. (1975). Behavioral and epileptic determinants of predatory attack behavior in the cat. *Can. J. Neurol. Sci.*, **2**, 457–466.

Agricola, R., Mazzanino, M. and Urani, R. (1982). Treatment of acute alcohol withdrawal with carbamazepine: A double-blind comparison with tiapride. *J. Int. Med. Res.*, **10**, 160–165.

Albright, P. S. and Bruni, J. (1980). Development of a new pharmacological seizure model: effects of anticonvulsants on cortical and amygdala-kindled seizures in the rat. *Epilepsia*, **21**, 681–689.

Albright, P. S. and Burnham, W. M. (1980). Development of a new pharmacological seizure model: effects of anticonvulsants on cortical- and amygdala-kindled seizures in the rat. *Epilepsia*, **21**, 681–689.

Babington, R. and Wedeking, P. (1973). The pharmacology of seizures induced by sensitization with low intensity brain stimulation. *Pharmacol. Biochem. Behav.*, **1**, 461–467.

Baker, T. B. and Cannon, D. S. (1979). Potentiation of ethanol withdrawal by prior dependence. *Psychopharmacology*, **60**, 105–110.

Ballenger, J. C. and Post, R. M. (1978). Kindling as a model for alcohol withdrawal syndromes. *Br. J. Psychiat.*, **133**, 1–14.

Bear, D. and Fedio, P. (1977). Quantitative analysis of interictal behavior in temporal lobe epilepsy. *Arch. Neurol.*, **34**, 454–467.

Beck, A. T., Ward, C. H., Mendelson, M., Mock, J. E. and Enbaugh, J. K. (1961). An inventory for measuring depression. *Arch. Gen. Psychiat.*, **4**, 561–571.

Begleiter, H. and Platz, A. (1972). The effects of alcohol on the central nervous system in humans. In: *The Biology of Alcoholism: Physiology and Behavior*. Vol. II (eds B. Kissin and H. Beglieter). Plenum Press, New York.

Begleiter, H., Gross, M. M. and Porjesz, B. (1973). Recovery function and clinical symptomatology in acute alcoholization and withdrawal. In: *Alcohol Intoxication and Withdrawal: Experimental Studies* (ed. M. M. Gross). Plenum Press, New York.

Beninger, R. J. and Hahn, B. L. (1983). Pimozide blocks establishment but not expression of amphetamine-produced environment-specific conditioning. *Science*, **220**, 1304–1306.

Beninger, R. J. and Herz, R. S. (1986). Pimozide blocks establishment but not expression of cocaine-produced environment-specific conditioning. *Life Sci.*, **38**, 1425.

Bjorkqvist, S. G., Isohanni, M., Makela, R. and Malinen, L. (1976). Ambulant treatment of alcohol withdrawal symptoms with carbamazpine: a formal multicentre double-blind comparison with placebo. *Acta Psychiatr. Scand.*, **53**, 333–342.

Blumer, D. (1970). Changes in sexual behavior related to temporal lobe disorder in man. *J. Sex Res.*, **6**, 173–180.

Blumer, D. (1974). Organic personality disorder. In: *Personality Disorders: Diagnosis and Management* (ed. J. Lion). Williams and Wilkins, Baltimore.

Branchey, M., Rauscher, G. and Kissin, B. (1971). Modifications in the response to alcohol following the establishment of physical dependence. *Psychopharmacologia*, **22**, 314–322.

Brown, M. E., Anton, R. F., Malcolm, R. and Ballenger, J. C. (1988). Alcohol detoxification and withdrawal seizures: clinical support for a kindling hypothesis. *Biol. Psychiat.*, **23**, 507–514.

Brune, F. and Busch, H. (1971). Anticonvulsive-sedative treatment of delirium alcoholism. *Q. J. Stud. Alcohol.*, **32**, 334–342.

Butler, D. and Messiha, F. (1986). Alcohol withdrawal and carbamazepine. *Alcohol*, **3**, 113–129.

Carlsson, C. and Pettersson, L. (1972). Dysphoric symptoms in chronic alcoholics and the effects of carbamazepine (Tegretol). *Int. J. Clin. Pharmacol.*, **5**, 403–405.

Carrington, C. and Ellinwood, E. H. (1981). Effects of alcohol withdrawal on kindling. Alcoholism — The Search for the Sources Symposium. NC Alcoholism Research Authority, Raleigh, NC, January 1981. *Alc. Clin. Exp. Res.*, **5**, 348.

Carrington, C. D., Ellinwood, E. H. and Krishnan, R. R. (1984). Effects of single and repeated alcohol withdrawal on kindling. *Biol. Psychiat.*, **19**(4), 525–537.

Childress, A., Ehrman, R., McLellan, A. T. and O'Brien, C. P. (1988). Conditioned craving and arousal in cocaine addiction: a preliminary report. *Natl. Inst. Drug Abuse Res. Monog. Ser.*, **81**, 74–80.

Clemmesen, L. and Hemmingsen, R. (1984). Physical dependence on ethanol during multiple intoxication and withdrawal episodes in the rat: evidence of potentiation. *Acta Pharmacol. Toxicol.*, **55**, 345–350.

Davies, D. L., Shepherd, M. and Myers, E. (1956). The two year prognosis of fifty alcohol addicts after treatment in hospitals. *Q. J. Stud. Alcohol.*, **17**, 485–502.

Derogatis, L. R. (1977). *SCL–90. Administration, Scoring, and Procedure Manual—I*. John Hopkins University School of Medicine, Baltimore.

Deutsch, J. A. and Koopmans, H. S. (1973). Preference enhancement for alcohol by passive exposure. *Science*, **179**, 1242–1243.

Dewhurst, K. and Beard, A. W. (1970). Sudden religious conversions in temporal lobe epilepsy. *Br. J. Psychiat.*, **117**, 497–507.

Edmonds, H. L. and Bellin, S. I. (1976). Quantification of alcohol intoxication and withdrawal in the rat. *Neuroscience Abstracts, 6th Annual Meeting of the Society for Neuroscience*, 7–11 November 1976, II, Abstract #1250.

Ellis, F. W. and Pick, J. . (1970). Experimentally induced ethanol dependence in rhesus monkeys. *J. Pharmacol. Exp. Ther.*, **175**, 88–93.

Essig, C. F. and Lam, R. C. (1971). The alcohol abstinence syndrome in dogs and its treatment with pentobarbital. In: *Recent Advances in Studies of Alcoholism: An Interdisciplinary Symposium* (eds N. K. Mello and J. Mendelson), Washington, DC, 1970. US Government Printing Office, Washington, DC, NIH Publication Number (HSM)71–9045.

Feuerlein, W. (1967). Klinisch-statistische Untersuchengen Uber die Entstehungsbedengungen und die Prognose des Alkoholdelirs. *Nervenarzt*, **38**, 206–212.

Feuerlein, W. (1974). The acute alcohol withdrawal syndrome: findings and problems. *Br. J. Addict.*, **69**, 141–148.

Fischman, M. W. (1984). The behavioral pharmacology of cocaine in humans. *Natl. Inst. Drug Abuse Res. Monogr. Ser.*, **50**, 72–91.

Fischman, M. W., Schuster, C. R. and Hatano, Y. (1983). A comparison of the subjective and cardiovascular effects of cocaine and lidocaine in humans. *Pharmacol. Biochem. Behav.*, **18**, 123–127.

Fischman, M. W., Schuster, C. R., Resnikov, L., Shick, J. F. F., Krasnegor, N. A.,

Fennell, W. and Freedman, D. X. (1976). Cardiovascular and subjective effects of intravenous cocaine administration in humans. *Arch. Gen. Psychiat.*, **33**, 983–989.

Flor-Henry, P. (1969). Schizophrenic-like reactions and affective psychoses associated with temporal lobe epilepsy: etiological factors. *Am. J. Psychiat.*, **126**, 400–403.

Flygerring, J., Hansen, J., Holst, B., Peterson, E. and Sorensen, A. (1984). *Acta Psychiatr. Scand.*, **69**, 398–408.

Freund, G. (1969). Alcohol withdrawal syndrome in mice. *Arch. Neurol.*, **21**, 315–320.

Freund, G. and Walker, D. W. Sound-induced seizures during ethanol withdrawal in mice. *Psychopharmacologia*, **22**, 24–49.

Gawin, F. H. and Ellinwood, E. H. (1988). Cocaine and other stimulants. *N. Engl. J. Med.*, **38**, 1173–1182.

Gawin, F. H. and Kleber, H. (1987). Issues in cocaine abuse treatment research. In: *Cocaine: Clinical and Biobehavioral Aspects* (eds S. Fisher, A. Raskin and E. H. Uhlenhuth), pp. 174–192. Oxford University Press, New York.

Geschwind, N. (1973). Effects of temporal lobe surgery on behavior. *N. Engl. J. Med.*, **286**, 480–481.

Gibbs, F. A. (1951). Ictal and nonictal psychiatric disorders in temporal lobe epilepsy. *N. Nerv. Ment. Dis.*, **113**, 522–528.

Glatt, M. M. (1961). Drinking habits of English (middle class) alcoholics. *Acta Psychiatr. Scand.*, **37**, 88–113.

Glue, P., Mele, A., Chiueh, C. C., Nutt, D. J. and Pert, A. (1988). Microdialysis and tissue level studies of presynaptic dopamine function in chronically cocaine-treated rats. *Abstracts, Society for Neuroscience 18th Annual Meeting*, Toronto, 1988, p. 740, Abst. #294.3.

Goeders, N. E. and Smith, J. E. (1986). Reinforcing properties of cocaine in the medial prefrontal cortex: primary action on presynaptic dopaminergic terminals. *Pharmacol. Biochem. Behav.*, **25**, 191–199.

Goldstein, D. B. (1972a). Relationship of alcohol dose to intensity of withdrawal signs in mice. *J. Pharmacol. Exp. Ther.*, **180**, 203–215.

Goldstein, D. B. (1972b). An animal model for testing effects on drugs and alcohol withdrawal reactions. *J. Pharmacol. Exp. Ther.*, **183**, 14–22.

Goldstein, D. B. (1973). Relationship of alcohol dose to intensity of withdrawal signs in mice. *J. Pharmacol. Exp. Ther.*, **12**, 1097–1102.

Goldstein, D. B. (1974). Rates of onset and decay of alcohol physical dependence in mice. *J. Pharmacol. Exp. Ther.*, **190**, 377–383.

Gross, M. M., Lewis, E. and Hastey, J. (1974). Acute alcohol withdrawal syndrome. In: *The Biology of Alcoholism: Clinical Pathology*, Vol. III (eds B. Kissin and H. Begleiter). Plenum Press, New York.

Gross, M. M., Rosenblatt, S. M., Malinowski, B., Broman, M. and Lewis, E. (1971). A factor analytic study of the clinical phenomena in the acute alcohol withdrawal syndromes. In: *Selected Papers given at the 16th International Institute on the Prevention and Treatment of Alcoholism*, Vol. II. Press of Addiction Research Foundation, Toronto.

Gross, M. M., Rosenblatt, S. M., Lewis, E. Chartoff, S. and Malenowski, B. (1972). Acute alcoholic psychoses and related syndromes: psychosocial and clinical characteristics and their implications. *Br. J. Addict.*, **67**, 15–31.

Gross, M. M., Kierszenbaum, H. S., Lewis, E. and Lee, Y. (1976). Desire to drink: relationship to age, blood alcohol concentration, and severity of withdrawal syndrome on admission for detoxification. *Ann. N.Y. Acad. Sci.*, **273**, 360–363.

Guerrero-Figueroa, R., Rye, M. M., Gallant, D. M. and Bishop, M. (1970). Electrographic and behavioral effects of diazepam during alcohol withdrawal stage in cats. *Neuropharmacology*, **9**, 143–150.

Hernandez, L., Lee, F. and Hoebel, B. G. (1987). Simultaneous microdialysis and amphetamine infusion in the nucleus accumbens and striatum of freely moving rats: increase in extracellular dopamine and serotonin. *Brain Res. Bull.*, **19**, 623–628.

Hill, D. (1953). Psychiatric disorders of epilepsy. *Med. Res.*, **20**, 473–475.

Hoffer, B. J., Taylor, D., Baker, R., Deitrich, R., Seiger, A. and Olson, L. (1980). Ethanol withdrawal seizures in hippocampus transplanted to the anterior chamber of the eye. *Life Sci.*, **26**, 239–244.

Horn, J. and Wanberg, K. (1969). Symptom patterns related to excessive use of alcohol. *Q. J. Stud. Alcohol.*, **30**, 35–58.

Hunt, W. A. (1973). Changes in the neuro-excitability of alcohol-dependent rats undergoing withdrawal as measured by the pentylenetetrazole seizure threshold. *Neuropharmacology*, **12**, 1097–1102.

Hunter, B. E., Boast, C. A., Walker, D. W. and Zornetzer, S. F. (1973). Alcohol withdrawal syndrome in rats: neural and behavioral correlates. *Pharmacol. Biochem. Behav.*, **11**, 719–725.

Isbell, H., Fraser, H. F., Wikler, A., Belleville, R. and Eisenman, A. (1955). An experimental study of the etiology of 'rum fits' and delirium tremens. *Q. J. Stud. Alcohol.*, **16**, 1–33.

Jellinek, E. M. (1946). Phases in the drinking histories of alcoholics. *Q. J. Stud. Alcohol.*, **7**, 1–88.

Jellinek, E. M. (1952). Phases of alcohol addiction. *Q. J. Stud. Alcohol.*, **13**, 673–684.

Johnson, R. M. (1961). The alcohol withdrawal syndrome. *Q. J. Stud. Alcohol.*, Suppl. **1**, 66–76.

Kalant, H. The pharmacology of alcohol intoxication. *Q. J. Stud. Alcohol.*, Suppl. **1**, 1–23.

Kalant, H., Leblanc, A. and Gibbins, R. (1971). Tolerance to, and dependence on, ethanol. In: *Biological Basis of Alcoholism* (eds Y. Israel and J. Mardones). Wiley, New York.

Kalant, H., LeBlanc, A. E., Gibbins, R. S. and Wilson, A. (1978). Accelerated development of tolerance during repeated cycles of ethanol exposure. *Psychopharmacologia*, **60**, 69–65.

Kellner, C. H., Post, R. M., Putnam, F., Cowdry, R., Gardner, D., Kling, M. A., Minichiello, M. A., Trettau, J. R. and Coppola, R. (1987). Intravenous procaine as a probe of limbic system activity in psychiatric patients and normal controls. *Biol. Psychiat.*, **22**, 1107–1126.

Kelly, P. H. and Iversen, S. D. (1975). Selective 6-OHDA induced destruction of mesolimbic dopamine neurons: abolition of psychostimulant induced locomotor activity in rats. *Eur. J. Pharmacol.*, **40**, 45–56.

Kissin, B. and Charnoff, S. M. (1967). Clinical evaluations of tranquilizers and antidepressants in the long term treatment of chronic alcoholism. In: *Alcoholism: Behavioral Research, Therapeutic Approaches* (ed. R. Fox). Springer, New York.

Koob, G. F., Le, H. T. and Creese, I. (1987). The D1 dopamine receptor antagonist SCH 23390 increases cocaine self-administration in the rat. *Neurosci. Lett.*, **79**, 315–320.

Kumor, K., Sherer, M., Thompson, L., Cone, E., Mahaffey, J. and Jaffe, J. H. (1988). Lack of cardiovascular tolerance during intravenous cocaine infusions in human volunteers. *Life Sci.*, **42**, 2063–2071.

LeBlanc, A. F., Kalant, H., Gibbius, R. J. and Berman, N. P. (1969). Acquisition and loss of tolerance to ethanol by the rat. *J. Pharmacol. Exp. Ther.*, **168**, 244–250.

Lundqvist, G. (1961). Delirium tremens: a comparative study of pathogenesis, course, and prognosis with delirium tremens. *Acta Psychiatr. Scand.*, **36**, 443–446.

Macdonnell, M. F., Fessock, L. and Brown, S. H. (1971). Ethanol and the neural substrate for affective defense in the cat. *Q. J. Stud. Alcohol.*, **32**, 406–419.

Malcolm, R., Ballenger, J. C., Sturgis, E. F. and Anton, R. (1989). A double-blind controlled trial comparing carbamazepine to oxazepam in the treatment of alcohol withdrawal. *Am. J. Psychiat.* (in press).

Martin, W. R., Sloan, J. W., Sapira, J. D. and Jasinski, D. R. (1971). Physiological subjective, and behavioral effects of amphetamine, methamphetamine, ephedrine, phenmetrazine, and methylphenidate in man. *Clin. Pharmacol. Ther.*, **12**, 245–258.

McNamee, H. Mello, N. and Mendelson, J. (1968). Experimental analysis of drinking patterns of alcoholics: concurrent psychiatric observations. *Am. J. Psychiat.*, **124**, 1063–1069.

McQuarrie, D. and Fingl, E. (1958). Effect of single doses and chronic administration of ethanol on experimental seizures in mice. *J. Pharmacol. Exp. Ther.*, **124**, 264–271.

Mello, N. K. (1973). A review of methods to induce alcohol addiction in animals. *Pharmacol. Biochem. Behav.*, **1**, 89–101.

Mello, N. K. and Mendelson, J. H. (1976). The development of alcohol dependence: a clinical study. *McLean Hosp. J.*, **1**, 64–84.

Mendelson, J. H. (ed.) (1964). Experimentally-induced chronic intoxication and withdrawal in alcoholics. *Q. J. Stud. Alcohol.*, *Suppl.* **2**.

Mendelson, J. H. (1972). Biochemical mechanisms of alcohol addiction. In: *The Biology of Alcoholism: Biochemistry*, Vol. 1 (eds B. Kissin and H. Begleiter). Plenum Press, New York.

Mendelson, J. H. and La Dou, J. (1964). Experimentally induced chronic intoxication and withdrawal in alcoholics: psychophysiological findings. *Q. J. Stud. Alcohol.*, *Suppl.* **2**, 14–39.

Mendelson, J. H., Stein, S. and McGuire, M. T. (1966). Comparative psychophysiological studies of alcoholic and non-alcoholic subjects undergoing experimentally induced ethanol intoxication. *Psychosom. Med.*, **28**, 1–12.

Ng, S. K. C., Hauser, W. A., Brust, J. C. M. and Susser, M. (1988). Alcohol consumption and withdrawal in new-onset seizures. *New Engl. J. Med.*, **319** (11), 666–673.

Nielsen, J. (1965). Delirium tremens in Copenhagen: part of a cross-national investigation of delirium tremens in the Nordic countries sponsored by the Nordic Committee for alcohol research. *Acta Psychiatr. Scand.*, **187**, 1–92.

Park, P. (1973). Developmental ordering of experiences in alcoholism. *Q. J. Stud. Alcohol*, **34**, 473–488.

Perrin, R. K., Kalant, H. and Livingston, K. E. (1975). Electroencephalographic signs of ethanol tolerance and dependence in the cat. *Electroencephalog. Clin. Neurophysiol.*, **39**, 157–162.

Pettit, H. O., Ettinberg, A., Bloom, F. E. and Koob, G. F. (1984). Destruction of dopamine in the nucleus accumbens selectively attenuates cocaine but not heroin self-administration in rats. *Psychopharmacology*, **84**, 167–173.

Pinel, J. P. J. (1980). Alcohol withdrawal seizures: implications of kindling. *Pharmacol. Biochem. Behav.*, **13**(1), 225–231.

Pinel, J. P. J. and Van Oot, P. H. (1975). Generality of the kindling phenomen: some clinical implications. *Can. J. Neurol. Sci.*, **2**, 467–475.

Pinel, J. P. J. and Van Oot, P. H. (1978). Increased susceptibility to the epileptic effects of alcohol withdrawal following periodic electroconvulsive shocks. *Biol. Psychiat.*, **13**, 353–368.

Pinel, J. P. J., Treit, D. and Rovener, L. I. (1977). Temporal lobe aggression in rats. *Science*, **197**, 1088–1089.

Pitts, D. K. and Marwah, J. (1986). Electrophysiological effects of cocaine on central monoaminergic neurons. *Eur. J. Pharmacol.*, **131**, 95–98.

Pitts, D. K. and Marwah, J. (1988). Cocaine and central monoaminergic neurotransmission: a review of electrophysiological studies and comparison to amphetamine and antidepressants. *Life Sci.*, **42**, 949–968.

Poldrugo, F. and Snead, O. C. (1984). Electroencephalographic and behavioral correlates in rats during repeated ethanol withdrawal syndromes. *Psychopharmacology*, **83**, 140–146.

Post, R. M. (1980). Intermittent versus continuous stimulation: effect of time interval on the development of sensitization or tolerance. *Life Sci.*, **26**, 1275–1282.

Post, R. M. and Contel, N. R. (1983). Human and animal studies of cocaine: implications for development of behavioral pathology. In: *Stimulants: Neurochemical, Behavioral, and Clinical Perspective* (ed. I. Creese), pp. 169–203. New York, Raven Press.

Post, R. M., Kopanda, R. T. and Lee, A. (1975). Progressive behavioral changes during chronic lidocaine administration: relationship to kindling. *Life Sci.*, **17**, 943–950.

Post, R. M. Rubinow, D. R. and Ballenger, J. C. (1984). Conditioning, sensitization, and kindling: implications for the course of affective illness. In: *Neurobiology of Mood Disorders* (eds R. M. Post and J. C. Ballenger), pp. 432–466. Williams and Wilkins, Baltimore.

Post, R. M., Weiss, S. R. B. and Pert, A. (1984). Differential effects of carbamazepine and lithium on sensitization and kindling. *Prog. Neuropsychopharmacol. Biol. Psychiat.*, **8**, 425–434.

Post, R. M., Squillace, K. M., Pert, A. and Sass, W. (1981). Effect of amygdala kindling on spontaneous and cocaine-induced motor activity and lidocaine seizures. *Psychopharmacology*, **72**, 189–196.

Post, R. M., Kennedy, C., Shinohara, M., Squillace, K., Miyaoka, M., Suda, S., Ingvar, D. H. and Sokoloff, L. (1984). Metabolic and behavioral consequences of lidocaine-kindled seizures. *Brain Res.*, **324**, 295–304.

Post, R. M., Uhde, T. W., Joffe, R. T. and Bierer, L. (1986a). Psychiatric manifestations and implications of seizure disorders. In: *Medical Mimics of Psychiatric Disorders* (eds I. Extein and M. Gold), pp. 35–91. American Psychiatric Association Press, Washington, DC.

Post, R. M., Weiss, S. R. B., Szele, F. and Woodward, R. (1986b). Differential anticonvulsant effects of carbamazepine as a function of stage and type of kindling. *Abstracts, Society for Neuroscience, 16th Annual Meeting*, Washington, DC, p. 1375, #374.1.

Post, R. M., Weiss, S. R. B., Pert, A. and Uhde, T. W. (1987). Chronic cocaine administration: sensitization and kindling effects. In: *Cocaine: Clinical and Biobehavioral Aspects* (eds A. Raskin and S. Fisher), pp. 109–173. Oxford University Press, New York.

Poutanen, P. (1979). Experience with carbamazepine in the treatment of withdrawal symptoms in alcohol abusers. *Br. J. Addict.*, **74**, 201–204.

Racine, R. J. (1972). Modification of seizure activity by electrical stimulation: II. Motor seizures. *Electroencephalogr. Clin. Neurophysiol.*, **32**, 281–294.

Racine, R. J., Livingston, K. and Joaquin, A. (1975). Effects of procaine hydrochloride, diazepam, and diphenylhydantoin on seizure development in cortical and subcortical structures in rats. *Electroencephalogr. Clin. Neurophysiol.*, **38**, 355–365.

Racine, R. J., Livingston, K. and Joaquin, A. (1975). Effects of procaine hydrochloride, diazepam, and diphenylhydantoin on seizure development in cortical and subcortical structures in rats. *Electroencephalogr. Clin. Neurophysiol.*, **38**, 355–365.

Ritola, E. and Malinen, L. (1981). A double-blind comparison of carbamazepine and clomethiazole in the treatment of alcohol withdrawal syndrome. *Acta Psychiat. Scand.*, **64**, 254–259.

Roberts, D. C. S., Koob, G. F., Klonoff, P. and Fibiger, H. C. (1980). Extinction and recovery of cocaine self-administration following 6-hydroxydopamine lesions of the nucelus accumbens. *Pharmacol. Biochem. Behav.*, **12**, 781–787.

Robinson, T. E., Becker, J. B. (1986). Enduring changes in brain and behavior produced by chronic amphetamine administration: a review and evaluation of animal models of amphetamine psychosis. *Brain Res. Rev.*, **1**, 157–198.

Scheel-Krüger, J., Braestrup, C., Nielson, M., Golembrowska, K. and Mogilnicka, F. (1977). Cocaine: discussion on the role of dopamine in the biochemical mechanism of action. In: *Advances in Behavioral Biology*, Vol. 21. *Cocaine and Other Stimulants* (eds E. H. Ellinwood and M. M. Kilbey), pp. 373–408. Plenum Press, New York.

Segal, B. M., Kushnarev, V. M., Urakov, I. G. and Misionzhnik, E. U. (1970). Alcoholism and disruptions of activity of deep cerebral structures. *Q. J. Stud. Alcohol.*, **31**, 587–601.

Serafetinides, E. A. (1965). Aggressiveness in temporal lobe epileptics and its relation to cerebral dysfunction and environmental factors. *Epilepsia*, **6**, 33–42.

Shaw, J. M., Kolesar, G. S., Sellers, E. M., Kaplan, H. L. and Sandor, P. (1981). Development of optimal treatment tactics for alcohol withdrawal. I. Assessment and effectiveness of support care. *J. Clin. Psychopharmacol.*, **1**, 382–387.

Sherer, M. A., Kumor, K. M., Cone, E. J. and Jaffe, J. H. (1988). Suspiciousness induced by four-hour intravenous infusions of cocaine. Preliminary findings. *Arch. Gen. Psychiat.*, **45**, 673–677.

Singer, K. and Wong, M. (1973). Alcoholic psychoses and alcoholism in the Chinese. *Q. J. Stud. Alcohol.*, **34**, 878–886.

Spielberger, C. D. (1977). *Self Evaluation Questionnaire*. Consulting Psychologists Press, Palo Alto, CA.

Tadokoro, S. and Kuribara, H. (1986). Reverse tolerance to the ambulation-increasing effect of methamphetamine in mice as an animal model of amphetamine psychosis. *Psychopharmacol. Bull.*, **22**, 757–762.

Tamerin, J. S. and Mendelson, J. H. (1969). The psychodynamics of chronic inebriation: observations of alcoholics during the process of drinking in an experimental group setting. *Am. J. Psychiat.*, **125**, 886–899.

Thompson, W. L., Johnson, A. D. and Maddrey, W. L. (1975). Diazepam and paraldehyde for treatment of severe delirium tremens: a controlled trail. *Ann. Intern. Med.*, **82**, 175–180.

Trice, H. and Wahl, R. (1958). A rank order analysis of symptoms of alcoholism. *Q. J. Stud. Alcohol.*, **19**, 636–648.

Victor, M. (1973). Withdrawal, neurological syndromes, and EEG. *Ann. N.Y. Acad. Sci.*, **215**, 210–213.

Victor, M. and Adams, R. D. (1953). The effect of alcohol on the nervous system. *Proc. A. Res. Nerv. Ment. Dis.*, **32**, 526–573.

Victor, M. and Brausch, J. (1967). The role of abstinence in the genesis of alcoholic epilepsy. *Epilepsia*, **8**, 1–20.

Wada, J. and Osawa, T. (1976). Spontaneous recurrent seizure state induced by daily electric amygdaloid stimulation in Senegalese baboons (Papio papio). *Neurology*, **26**, 273–286.

Walker, D. W. and Zornetzer, S. F. (1974). Alcohol withdrawal in mice: electroencephalographic and behavioral correlates. *Electroencephalogr. Clin. Neurophysiol.*, **36**, 233–243.

Weiss, S. R. B. and Post, R. M. (1987). Carbamazepine and carbamazepine–10,11-epoxide inhibit amygdala-kindled seizures in the rat but do not block their development. *Clin. Neuropharmacol.*, **10**, 272–279.

Weiss, S. R. B., Costello, M., Woodward, R., Nutt, D. J. and Post, R. M. (1987). Chronic carbamazepine inhibits the development of cocaine-kindled seizures. *Abstract, Society of Neuroscience 17th Annual Meeting*, New Orleans, November 1987, p. 950. Abstract 262.20.

Weiss, S. R. B., Post, R. M., Pert, A., Woodward, R. and Murman, D. (1988a). Role of conditioning in cocaine-induced behavioral sensitization: differential effect of haloperidol. *Neuropsychopharmacology* (in press).

Weiss, S. R. B., Post, R. M., Szele, F., Woodward, R. and Nierenberg, J. (1988b). Chronic carbamazepine inhibits the development of local-anesthestic seizures kindled by cocaine and lidocaine. *Brain Res.* (in press).

Whitwell, F. D. (1975). A study into the etiology of delirium tremens. *Br. J. Addict.*, **70**, 156–161.

Wise, R. A. (1981). Brain dopamine and reward. In: *Theory in Psychopharmacology*, Vol. 1 (ed. S. J. Cooper), pp. 103–122. Academic Press, London.

Wise, R. A. (1984). Neural mechanisms of the reinforcing action of cocaine. *Natl. Inst. Drug Abuse Monogr. Ser.*, **50**, 15–33.

Wise, R. and Chinerman, J. (1974). Effects of diazepam and phenobarbitol on electrically induced amigdoloid seizures and seizure development. *Exp. Neurol.*, **45**, 355–363.

Wolfe, S. M. and Victor, M. (1971). The alcohol withdrawal syndrome. In: *Recent Advances in Studies of Alcoholism: An Interdisciplinary Symposium* (eds M. K. Mello and J. Mendelson). Washington, DC, 25–27 June, 1970. US Government Printing Office, Washington, DC, NIH Publication Number (HSM)71–9045.

Woolverton, W. L. and Balster, R. L. (1979). Reinforcing properties of some local anesthetics in rhesus monkeys. *Pharmacol. Biochem. Behav.*, **11**, 669–672.

The Clinical Relevance of Kindling
Edited by T. G. Bolwig and M. R. Trimble
© 1989 John Wiley & Sons Ltd

Discussion — Session 5

ECT AND KINDLING

J. Majkowski   Electroconvulsive therapy and kindling do not have anything to do with one another. There are completely different paradigms which are required for kindling. We are dealing practically, with ECT in human beings, with neurochemical changes. In kindling, we are starting with electrical phenomena. That is a very important difference.

M. Fink   I agree with you, and I thank you for agreeing with me in that the two phenomena are distinct.

T. G. Bolwig   Another difference between ECT and kindling lies in the permanency of the kindling phenomenon and the very transient effects that ECT has. Clinically, we know that patients will very often relapse after a few months, so that we have to give them a new series of ECT or drugs. We also know that all changes — electrophysiological or neurochemical — are fully reversible, even after enormous amounts of ECT or electroconvulsive shock in animals.

R. Racine   I have nothing to say about the therapeutic use of ECT. It may be quite effective, and the benefits may outweigh the risks; but at the same time I think it is very clear that any treatment that produces a forebrain discharge will leave a lasting effect in brain function. We have looked at ECS treatment in rats, using a probe stimulation like a kindling stimulation. If the ECS is repeated and spaced once a week, you see that there is in fact a lasting change in brain function. The animal responds as if he has been partially kindled, and it takes far fewer stimulations then to subsequently kindle that animal. The other point I would like to make is that I think it is a mistake to compare the treatments that you might expect would produce a spontaneous seizure with kindling, which in most experiments have not gone to the stages of producing spontaneous seizures. If you take a kindled

259

animal to its typical endpoint (that is, the typical criterion that's used) that animal will never have shown a spontaneous seizure, and he never will! If you give an animal repeated ECS, you may never see a spontaneous seizure. That does not mean the brain has not been changed. That does not mean that the tissue has not been made, at least to some extent, epileptogenic.

M. Fink There is, in the whole world literature, one case of human brain kindling. The patient developed phantom pain after a hand injury. She underwent coagulation of part of the left nucleus ventralis posterior medialis of the thalamus, and had daily electrical stimulation of the thalamus. In the third week of stimulation, she perceived spontaneous mild movements of the right half of her face. I think that this single case exemplifies what Dr Racine is saying. I do not think that we can accept as psychiatrists that experiments in which an electrode is put into a rat's brain has anything to do with man. That is: once you have put an electrode in a rat's brain, you have produced clear and present damage. There is no question that it is easy for any pathologist to tell you whether the brain presented to him has had electrodes put in or not — any time after the electrodes have been put in. I do not see those experiments have anything to do with electroconvulsive therapy. The issue has been to ask, if we produce seizures in patients, externally, or produce seizures in animals externally, without a probe, what is the evidence of cellular change? Can you separate those animals who have had exposure to repeated seizures from those animals who have not been exposed to seizures — control animals? The answer is that the pathologist cannot do that. You cannot see any permanent change.

M. R. Trimble Professor Post, could you just distinguish clearly between sensitization and kindling.

R. Post Sensitization is the behavioral endpoint of increased motor activity, for example running behavior in the rat, and you can get that with amphetamine, or a dopamine agonist. That is just increased responsivity to the same dose over time. Motor activity has nothing to do with seizures. In fact, the biochemistry of sensitization in some cases is quite opposite to the biochemistry of kindling. Stresses will increase sensitization, stresses may actually, by increasing noradrenergic count, decrease kindling. So sensitization is the *behavioural* component. Since cocaine is a dirty drug, it sensitizes as well as kindles, and the kindling is the seizure endpoint that we have all been talking about.

R. Adamec Do panic attacks in cocaine use persist after periods of abstinence? Is this a lasting change following their induction, or is it dependent on continued cocaine use?

R. Post Some patients continued to have spontaneous panic attacks.

R. Adamec I was curious to why you emphasized panic attacks.

J. C. Ballenger The reason is because the pure local anaesthetics can give you anxiety without the catecholamine stimulation. That is a thing called 'doom' anxiety in patients who get lidocaine for their cardiac problems. When we gave procaine to our patients, we got mixed effects. Some patients got euphoric, some got extremely dysphoric. So we think the local anaesthetics alone are capable of tapping into something in the temporal lobes, which can bring on panic. It is clear that with chronic use of amphetamine or cocaine, patients get more and more dysphoric. The euphoria is very difficult to maintain or sustain, and patients get increasingly dysphoric and paranoid. I think that the panic is probably more related to local anaesthetic than cocaine *per se*.

M. Fink Do you see the development eventually of spontaneous seizures with cocaine?

J. Ballenger Not spontaneous seizures. We have seen spontaneous seizures with lidocaine kindling, because the animals survived lidocaine kindling long enough. We have never seen spontaneous cocaine seizures, because the animals all die before that.

M. Fink What would be the effect in a lidocaine produced seizure if you interrupt the process by giving the animal ECS. Does that change the seizure threshold so spontaneity does not occur?

J. Ballenger We have not done that with lidocaine, but we have clearly done that with regular amygdalar kindling. ECS in the rat blocks the development of amygdala kindling, and it also blocks completely kindled seizures.

W. Rutz In Sweden, the psychiatrists are very concerned about alcoholism. Our drinking pattern is very special: we drink a lot once or twice a week. May this be the cause of our heavy alcoholism in Sweden; is a more steady state of drinking better?

R. Post Actually, binge drinking is less associated with withdrawal reactions than steady drinking. What leads to withdrawal reactions, particularly withdrawal reactions that get worse over time, is somewhat controversial. It often has to do with daily drinking of a heavy nature, in animals and in man; but it is harder in man to know what the adequate stimulus has to be.

The Clinical Relevance of Kindling
Edited by T. G. Bolwig and M. R. Trimble
© 1989 John Wiley & Sons Ltd

16

Kindling and panic disorder

RABEN ROSENBERG
*Department of Psychiatry, Rigshospitalet, University of Copenhagen,
DK-2100 Copenhagen, Denmark*

INTRODUCTION

Kindling, first described by Goddard, McIntyre and Leech (1969), refers to the progressive after-discharges following repeated stimulation of a given brain site with an initially subthreshold current (Post and Ballenger, 1981). Kindling-like phenomena have been suggested as models of various kinds of psychopathology, including temporal lobe epilepsy, alcohol withdrawal syndromes, tardive dyskinesia and rapid cycling affective disorders (Post and Ballenger, 1981). In its most general sense, kindling refers to neural processes which mediate lasting changes in brain function in response to repeated, temporally spaced application of neurobehaviorally active agents (Adamec and Stark-Adamec, 1983).

Fear and autonomic nervous system hyperactivity are often experienced by patients with partial seizures (McLachlan and Blume, 1980, Weilberg, Bear and Sachs, 1987), and affective dimensions are added to perceptual and mnemonic phenomena in limbic activation by brain stimulation endowing an experiential immediacy (Gloor *et al.*, 1982). In 1962 Roth and Harper described phenomenological similarities, for instance depersonalization and sudden paroxysms of fear, but also clear differences between a phobic-depersonalization syndrome and temporal lobe epilepsy. The relation of anxiety to epilepsy has been obscured by the ambiguity of the clinical meaning of anxiety and the absence of a reliable and valid classification of anxiety disorders.

With the appearance of the third edition of Diagnostic and Statistical Manual of Mental Disorders (DSM-III) (American Psychiatric Association, 1987), some of these limitations were circumvented as a descriptive-operational approach to classification was provided. Issues such as empirical testing of reliability and evaluation of validity have had high priority developing the DSM-III. A new terminology was introduced. Within a surprisingly short period of time, the DSM-III and DSM-III-R, a revised edition, have been accepted worldwide as a fruitful classification system to psychiatry research.

A new diagnostic entity, panic disorder, is delineated in DSM-III. The main feature of this disorder is recurrent panic attacks, i.e. acute paroxysms of anxiety (Table 1). Previously, panic attacks, phenomenological similar to the anxiety attacks of neurosis anxiosa [ICD8 (World Health Organization, 1967)], had been conceptualized in psychoanalytical or behavioral terms (Klein, 1981). Recent epidemiological, genetic, clinical, therapeutic and neurobiologic studies have changed the scene, and leading theories now relate panic disorder to neurobiological abnormalities (Klein, 1981; Sheehan 1982). From case histories demonstrating concomitant panic attacks and seizure disorders (Weilberg, Bear and Sachs, 1987, Wall, Tuchman and Mielke, 1985) common pathophysiological mechanisms have been suggested involving temporolimbic systems.

Table 1. Panic disorder, diagnostic criteria according to DSM-III-R*

A. At least once unexpected panic attacks
B. Either four attacks/four weeks or one attack followed by persistent fear during one month of having another attack
C. At least four of the following symptoms during at least one of the attacks:
    (1) dyspnoea
    (2) dizziness
    (3) palpitations
    (4) trembling
    (5) sweating
    (6) choking
    (7) nausea
    (8) depersonalization or derealization
    (9) paresthesias
    (10) flushes
    (11) chest pain
    (12) fear of dying
    (13) fear of going crazy
D. Development of symptoms:
    suddenly with maximum intensity within 10 min during at least some of the attacks
E. No organic factor

---

* Abridged by the author.

It is tempting to hypothesize that kindling-like phenomena might underly the evolution of panic disorder. The relevance and evidence of this hypothesis is the topic for this chapter.

PANIC DISORDER

Natural history

Panic disorder is characterized by recurrent spontaneous attacks ('coming out of the blue'). Situational attacks, precipitated by phobic stimuli such as supermarkets, buses, crowds or canteens eventually follow. The disorder may progress from uncomplicated panic disorder to panic disorder with agoraphobia (DSM-III-R), defined as the presence of mild to moderate and or severe phobic avoidance behavior.

Comorbidity between major depression and panic disorder have often been reported (Breier, Charney and Heninger, 1985). According to the demoralization hypothesis major depression is a secondary phenomenon to the anxiety disorder due to the increasing distress and social disability imposed by recurrent panic attacks and agoraphobia. The relation between major depression and panic disorder is, however, subject to uncertainty as major depressive episodes may precede the panic attacks. Hence, panic disorder and major depression have been conceived as sharing a common diathesis (Breier, Charney and Heninger, 1985).

Untreated panic disorder follows a chronic course (Breier, Charney and Heninger, 1986), but periods with mild or few symptoms may alternate with periods dominated by panic attacks, eventually precipitated by various life events (Roy-Burne, Garaci and Uhde, 1986).

Evidence has been provided that childhood anxiety, particularly over-anxious disorder (Aronson and Logue, 1987) and separation anxiety disorder (Gittelman and Klein, 1984) are associated with later development of panic disorder and agoraphobia.

Epidemiology and genetics

Several epidemiological surveys have been conducted in the USA applying the DSM-III. Prevalences of panic disorder of about 0.6–1.0% and of agoraphobia of 2.7–6.8% have been reported (Regier et al., 1988, Weissman, 1988). The rates are two- to fourfold higher in women than men.

Panic disorder is familial (Weissman, 1988). Thus, Crowe et al. (1983) reported a morbidity risk of 17.3% for panic disorder in first degree relatives, but only 1.8% for control relatives. A twin study applying DSM-III criteria brings support to a genetic disposition to panic disorder (Torgersen, 1983). Furthermore, a linkage between panic disorder and a chromosomal marker locus (alpha-haptoglobin) has been indicated (Crowe et al., 1987).

Biology of panic disorder

Evidence of a biologic dysfunction underlying panic disorder has recently been obtained. The most consistent finding has been the precipitation of panic attacks by lactate infusions in a majority of panic disorder patients (Liebowitz et al., 1984). Interestingly, this phenomenon is blocked by pretreatment with some antidepressant drugs (Gorman et al., 1987), which also are clinically efficacious in panic disorder. Carbon-dioxide inhalation may also provoke panic attacks (Fyer et al., 1987).

A series of clinical studies of noradrenergic and serotonergic cerebral functions have been performed by Charney, Heninger and coworkers, indicating a locus coeruleus mediated dysregulation of noradrenergic activity in panic disorder (Charney and Heninger, 1986; Charney et al., 1987).

Treatment

An important early finding was the efficacy of antidepressant drugs on panic attacks (Klein, 1964). Reviewing the literature, Liebowitz et al. (1988) found 'dramatic efficacy for all tested tricyclics in disorders involving panic attacks'. Recently, the benzodiazepine alprazolam has been found efficacious against panic attacks and phobic avoidance behavior (Ballenger et al., 1988), but at higher dosages than normally recommended for anxiety disorders.

Behavior therapy involving exposure-in vivo techniques has been found effective against phobic avoidance behavior (Jansson, Jerremalm and Oest, 1986). It is under debate whether panic attacks can also be treated effectively by behavior therapy (Marks, 1986, Klein, Ross and Cohen, 1987).

NEUROBIOLOGICAL MODELS OF ANXIETY

The presence of basic strategies of defensive behavior in animals (withdrawal, immobility, aggressive behavior and deflections of attacks) and emotional behaviour is reliant on innate biological mechanisms. The neurobiological bases of such innate anxiety mechanisms in human are but vaguely understood. It is widely accepted that limbic areas including the amygdala are main brain areas for emotional behaviors. According to Gray (1982), benzodiazepines reduce anxiety by impairing the function of the septo-hippocampal system. LeDoux (1987), reviewing the literature, considers the amygdala as a critical brain area for the processing of emotions.

Noradrenergic neurones in the locus coeruleus play an activating role for alarm with increased motor and autonomic activity, and stimulation in monkeys of the locus coeruleus produces fear-like behavior (Redmond, 1987). Panic disorder has been conceived as involving a locus coeruleus dysfunction. Clonidine and yohimbine, a presynaptic alpha-1-adrenoceptor agonist and antagonist, respectively, reduces vs augments anxiety level in humans, including panic attacks (Charney and Heninger, 1986; Charney *et al*, 1987). Tricyclic antidepressants and monoamine oxidase inhibitors (MAOI), all effective drugs in the treatment of panic disorder, slow the firing rate of the locus coeruleus (Redmond, 1987).

Serotonin-selective antidepressants [clomipramine (Johnston, Troyer and Whitsett, 1988), fluvoxamine (Den Boer and Westenberg, 1988)] have been found efficacious in treating panic attacks. Hence, a serotonergic disturbance is indicated too, probably involving the raphe nuclei system, but also several other brain areas as both brain stem nuclei (the locus coeruleus and the raphe nuclei) have abundant efferent neurons to the limbic system, including the amygdala (Ottersen, 1981).

As most benzodiazepines (at ordinary therapeutic dosages) have been conceived as relatively poor antipanic agents, the supramolecular GABA/benzodiazepine receptor complex (Insel *et al.*, 1984) has not had a prominent role in panic disorder theories. However, the benzodiazepines receptors are widely distributed in the CNS, including the locus coeruleus and the raphe nuclei, and some benzodiazepines *do* have strong antipanic efficacy [alprazolam and probably also clonazepam (Fountaine and Chouinard, 1984)].

In summary, genetic, clinical, therapeutic and biological studies have provided evidence for the validity of panic disorder as a classificatory entity, and for a dysfunction of catecholaminergic systems in the CNS as the underlying neurobiological disturbance.

PANIC DISORDER AND THE KINDLING PARADIGM

To elucidate whether panic disorder might be conceived within the frame of reference of the kindling paradigm, the following main variables (according to Ballenger and Post, 1981) are to be considered:

(1) application of repetitive subthreshold stimuli;
(2) at certain intervals;
(3) the sudden appearance of the kindling phenomenon;
(4) the stable duration of the phenomenon.

Repetitive subthreshold stimuli

An important function of innate anxiety mechanisms is a behavioral change to novel, threatening and nonreward stimuli including inhibition of all ongoing behavior, increased attention to the environment and increased readiness for rapid and vigorous action (Gray, 1982). In the awake monkey locus coeruleus activity associates with vigilance and arousal, and to fear-eliciting stimuli (Redmond, 1987).

Genetic influences may determine how active the locus coeruleus (or other relevant structure such as the raphe nuclei) is in each individual. If disposed to panic disorder a conditioned emotional response (CER) to fairly harmless (novel and mild threatening stimuli) may take place early in life according to classical Pavlovian conditioning. Secondarily, phobic avoidance behavior develops due to the reinforcement of avoidance behavior by drive (= anxiety) reduction (Thorpe and Burns, 1983). Phenomenologically, the CER is experienced as egodysthymic apprehension, not linked to specific environmental stimuli, but to any stimuli of novel, threatening or nonreward quality. According to this two-factor learning theory the escape behavior protects the CER from extinction due to unfavorable interstimulus intervals for environmental CER triggering stimuli.

The easily elicited alarm and anxiety reactions and the avoidance behavior brings about an overanxious (Aronson and Logue, 1987) and behaviorally restricted child. Separation anxiety (Gittelman and Klein, 1984) or school phobia eventually develop.

At certain intervals

Now and then — inevitably — the child is exposed to threatening or nonrewarding stimuli [including 'life events' (Roy-Burne, Geraci and Uhde, 1986)] of more pronounced intensity, from which escape is not possible. Hence, at certain intervals innate anxiety mechanisms are activated at much higher levels than usual, precipitating subpanic attacks. Due to the long time periods between these exposures, no significant habituation of the subpanic attacks takes place. In terms of theories involving brain stem nuclei as part of alarm and anxiety systems, perturbations recurrently spread from the brain stem via efferent neurons to limbic areas including the amygdala, i.e. to regions susceptible to kindling-like phenomena (Adamec and Stark-Adamec, 1983).

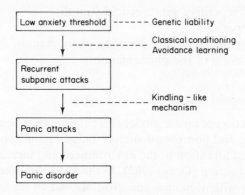

Figure 1. Panic disorder as a kindling-like phenomenon

Appearance of the kindling phenomenon

It is hypothesized that the first major panic attack (i.e. fulfilling the DSM-III criteria) arises as a kindling phenomenon. In congruence with this view, the first attack appears suddenly and spontaneously, i.e. by subtle changes of environmental stimuli out of proportion to the intensity of the panic attack. As panic disorder typically debuts at the age of 20–30 (Breier, Charney and Heninger, 1985), the kindling phenomenon seems to depend on a fairly large period of recurrent subthreshold stimulation. In this respect panic disorder is similar to other conditions conceived within the kindling paradigm, i.e. manic-depressive psychosis (Post and Ballenger, 1981) and tardive dyskinesia (Post and Ballenger, 1981, Glenthøj, Hemmingsen and Bolwig, 1988).

During a panic attack extreme fear as well as depersonalization may be experienced in agreement with a temporolimbic involvement. Interestingly, positron emission tomography (PET) in patients vulnerable to lacate-induced panic has revealed several abnormalities in the resting, nonpanic state: an abnormal hemispheric asymmetry of parahippocampal blood flow, blood volume, and oxygen metabolism; and an abnormal susceptibility to episodic hyperventilation (Reiman et al., 1986). Recently, Reiman et al. (1988) found an increased cerebral blood flow in a bilateral region corresponding to the temporopolar cortex *during* lactate-induced panic.

The mechanisms of the antipanic efficacy of tricyclic antidepressants are not known. With respect to the kindling hypothesis, the reduction of locus coeruleus activity by these drugs and the down regulation of beta-adrenergic receptors which are abundant in the hippocampus (Palacios and Kuhar, 1982), attract considerable interest. Other antipanic drugs such as alprazolam or clonazepam are anticonvulsant and probably exert their therapeutic action via temporolimbic structures.

Against a theory involving locus coeruleus mediated kindling of limbic areas in panic disorder, are some experimental findings that grafted nor-adrenergic neurons suppress seizure development in kindling-induced epilepsy (Barry et al., 1987). However, panic disorder patients do seldom have seizures, and although some phenomenological similarities are found (Roth and Harper, 1962) between panic disorder and temporal lobe epilepsy, and common pathophysiological mechanisms have been suggested, no firm evidence is available that these disorders do have identical pathogenical mechanisms.

Stable duration of kindling phenomenon

Panic disorder follows a chronic course. Although periods relatively free of panic attacks do sometimes appear (Breier, Charney and Heninger, 1985, 1986), panic attacks might be precipitated by chemical means in predisposed individuals. Thus, many (but not all) panic disorder patients are susceptible to lactate- or CO_2-induced panic attacks (Liebowitz *et al.*, 1984; Fyer *et al.*, 1987). Various life events (Roy-Burne, Geraci and Uhde, 1986) may also initiate periods with disabling panic attacks in certain individuals, indicating a long-lasting vulnerability to panic attacks.

Improvement by drug treatment (tricyclic or benzodiazepine antidepressants) (Liebowitz *et al.*, 1988; Ballenger *et al.*, 1988), or by behavior therapy (Marks, 1986) is far from satisfactory for many patients, and relapse rates are high after discontinuation of drug treatment (Ballenger *et al.*, 1988).

A robust finding has been an association between the duration of the disorder and avoidance behavior (Breier, Charney and Heninger, 1985, Ballenger *et al.*, 1988). Agoraphobic behavior is often conceptualized as a secondary phenomenon to the panic attacks, developed in accordance with learning theory principles.

Although behavior therapy significantly improves avoidance behavior (Jansson, Jerremalm and Oest, 1986; Marks, 1986), firm evidence is lacking that panic attacks diminish in intensity or frequency as they have only seldom been specified as an outcome variable in behavioral studies. According to Klein, Ross and Cohen (1987), drug treatment is required to abolish panic attacks. Furthermore, learning theory predicts that spontaneous panic attacks should be extinguished as they are reinforced by exposition to phobic stimuli (Klein, 1981). A kindling-like phenomenon may explain the limited applicability of learning theory to account for the development of uncomplicated panic disorder as well as the sparse success of behavior therapy for panic attacks. The fact that many patients with panic disorder and agoraphobia still do have an unsatisfactory improvement in spite of drug or behavioral treatment may indicate a long-lasting neurobiological dysfunction in panic disorder.

CONCLUSION

Although speculative, the kindling hypothesis of panic disorder does have some degree of validity from available empirical evidence. Several critical variables of the kindling paradigm can be subjected to empirical testing. The clinical course (natural history) and outcome by various treatment modalities should be investigated considering a variety of different variables, including panic attacks, phobic avoidance behavior and depression. A high-risk design may yield important information about a basic pattern of learning processes in children disposed to panic disorder as well as the relation between anxiety disorders in children and panic disorder in adults. In terms of a locus coeruleus mediated development of panic disorder by a kindling mechanism, it is predicted that drugs such as tricyclic antidepressants and certain benzodiazepines, which diminish the firing rate of the locus, may suppress the development of panic disorder in predisposed individuals.

The different clinical features of panic and seizure disorders do of course question the relevance of applying the concept of kindling, suggested for the development of seizures, to the development of panic disorder. A kindling-like phenomenon may be a more proper term for a clinical spectacle involving recurrency and development of a symptom or a syndrome of increasing severity and disability. The attempts to account for different clinical syndromes such as temporal lobe epilepsy, alcohol withdrawal syndromes, tardive dyskinesia, rapid cycling affective disorders and finally panic disorder by a kindling-like phenomenon certainly demonstrate some heuristic value of this concept in biological psychiatry. However, a claim for construct validity definitely awaits future animal and clinical studies.

REFERENCES

Adamec, R. E. and Stark-Adamec, C. (1983). Limbic kindling and animal behavior — implications for human psychopathology associated with complex partial seizures. *Biol. Psychiat.*, **18**, 269–293.

American Psychiatric Association (1980). *Diagnostic and Statistical Manual of Mental Disorders*, Third Edition, APA, Washington, DC (Third Edition, Revised, 1987).

Aronson, T. A. and Logue, C. M. (1987). On the longitudinal course of panic disorder: development history and predictors of phobic complications. *Compr. Psychiat.*, **28**, 344–355.

Ballenger, J. C., Burrows, G. D., DuPont Jr, R. L., Lessser, I. M., Noyes Jr, R., Pecknold, J. C., Rifkin, A. and Swinson, R. P. (1988). Alprazolam in panic disorder and agoraphobia: results from a multicenter trial. I. Efficacy in short-term treatment. *Arch. Gen. Psychiat.*, **45**, 413–422.

Barry, D. I., Kikvadze, I., Brundin, P., Bolwig, T. G., Bjorklund, A. and Lindvall, O. (1987). Grafted noradrenergic neurons suppress seizure development in kindling-induced epilepsy. *Proc. Natl. Acad. Sci.*, **84**, 8712–8715.

Breier, A., Charney, D. S. and Heninger, G. R. (1985). The diagnostic validity of anxiety disorders and their relationship to depressive illness. *Am. J. Psychiat.*, **142**, 787–797.

Breier, A., Charney, D. S. and Heninger, G. R. (1986). Agoraphobia with panic attacks: development, diagnostic stability, and course of illness. *Arch. Gen. Psychiat.*, **43**, 1029–1036.

Charney, D. S. and Heninger, G. R. (1986). Abnormal regulation of noradrenergic function in panic disorders. *Arch. Gen. Psychiat.*, **43**, 1042–1058.

Charney, D. S., Woods, S. W., Goodman, W. K. and Heninger, G. R. (1987). Neurobiological mechanisms of panic anxiety: biochemical and behavioral correlates of yohimbine-induced panic attacks. *Am. J. Psychiat.*, **144**, 1030–1036.

Crowe, R. R., Noyes, R., Pauls, D. L. and Slymen, D. (1983). A family study of panic disorder. *Arch. Gen. Psychiat.*, **40**, 1065–1069.

Crowe, R. R., Noyes, Jr, R., Wilson, A. F., Elston, R. C. and Ward, L. J. (1987). A linkage study of panic disorder. *Arch. Gen. Psychiat.*, **44**, 933–937.

Den Boer, J. A. and Westenberg, H. G. M. (1988). Effect of a serotonin and noradrenaline uptake inhibitor in panic disorder: a double-blind comparative study with fluvoxamine and maprotiline. *Int. Clin. Psychopharmacol.*, **3**, 59–74.

Fountaine, R. and Chouinard, G. (1984). Antipanic effect of clonazepam. *Am. J. Psychiat.*, **141**, 149–149.

Fyer, M. R., Uy, J., Martinez, J., Goetz, R., Klein, D. F., Fyer, A., Liebowitz, M. R. and Gorman, J. (1987). CO_2 challenge of patients with panic disorder. *Am. J. Psychiat.*, **144**, 1080–1082.

Gittelman, R. and Klein, D. F. (1984). Relationship between separation anxiety and panic and agoraphobic disorders. *Psychopathology*, **17** (Suppl. 1), 56–65.

Glenthøj, B., Hemmingsen, R. and Bolwig, T. G. (1988). Kindling: a model for the development of tardive dyskinesia? *Behav. Neurol.*, **1**, 29–40.

Gloor, P., Olivier, A., Quesney, L. F., Andermann, F. and Horowitz, S. (1982). The role of the limbic system in experiential phenomena of temporal lobe epilepsy. *Ann. Neurol.*, **12**, 129–144.

Goddard, G. V., McIntyre, D. C. and Leech, C. K. (1969). A permanent change in brain function resulting from daily electrical stimulation. *Exp. Neurol.*, **25**, 295–330.

Gorman, J. M., Liebowitz, M. R., Dillon, D., Fyer, A. J., Cohen, B. S. and Klein, D. F. (1987). Antipanic drug effects during lactate infusion on lactate-refractory panic patients. *Psychiat. Res.*, **21**, 205–212.

Gray, J. A. (1982). *The Neuropsychology of Anxiety: An Enquiry into the Function of the Septo-hippocampal System*. Oxford University Press, Oxford.

Insel, T. R., Ninan, P. T., Aloi, J., Jimerson, D. C., Skolnick, P. and Paul, S. M. (1984). A benzodiazepine receptor-mediated model of anxiety. *Arch. Gen. Psychiat.*, **41**, 741–750.

Jansson, L., Jerremalm, A. and Oest, L. G. (1986). Follow-up of agoraphobic patients treated with exposure *in vivo* or applied relaxation. *Br. J. Psychiat.*, **149**, 486–490.

Johnston, D. G., Troyer, I. E. and Whitsett, S. F. (1988). Clomipramine treatment of agoraphobic women. *Arch. Gen. Psychiat.*, **45**, 353–462.

Klein, D. F. (1964). Delineation of two drug-responsive anxiety syndromes. *Psychopharmacologia*, **5**, 397–408.

Klein, D. F. (1981). Anxiety reconceptualized. In: *Anxiety: New Research and Changing Concepts* (eds D. F. Klein and J. Rabkin), pp. 235–263. Raven Press, New York.

Klein, D. F., Ross, D. C. and Cohen, P. (1987). Panic and avoidance in agoraphobia. *Arch. Gen. Psychiat.*, **44**, 377–389.

LeDoux, J. E. (1987). Emotion. In: *Handbook of Physiology, Section 1: The Nervous System* (eds V. B. Mountcastle, F. Plum and S. R. Geiger), pp. 419–459. American Physiological Society, Bethesda, Maryland.

Liebowitz, M. R., Fyer, A. J., Gorman, J. M., Dillon, D. Appleby, I. L., Levy, G., Anderson, S., Levitt, M., Palij, M., Davies, S. O. and Klein, D. F. (1984). Lactate provocation of panic attacks. *Arch. Gen. Psychiat.*, **41**, 764–770.

Liebowitz, M. R., Fyer, A. J., Gorman, J. M., Campeas, R. B., Sandberg, D. P., Hollander, E., Papp, L. A. and Klein, D. F. (1988). Tricyclic therapy of the DSM-III anxiety disorders: a review with implications for further research. *J. Psychiatr. Res.*, **22** (Suppl. 1), 7–32.

Marks, I. M. (1986). Genetics of fear and anxiety disorders. *Br. J. Psychiat.*, **149**, 406–418.

McLachlan, R. S. and Blume, W. T. (1980). Isolated fear in complex partial status epilepticus. *Ann. Neurol.*, **8**, 639–641.

Ottersen, O. P. (1981). The afferent connection of the amygdala of the rat as studied with retrograde transport of horseradish peroxidase. In: *The Amygdaloid Complex* (ed. Y. Ben-Ari), pp. 91–104. Elsevier, Amsterdam.

Palacios, J. M. and Kuhar, M. J. (1982). Beta adrenergic receptor localization in rat brain by light microscopic autoradiography. *Neurochem. Int.*, **4**, 473–490.

Post, R. M. and Ballenger, J. C. (1981). Kindling models for the progressive development of psychopathology: sensitization to electrical, pharmacological, and psychological stimuli. In: *Handbook of Biological Psychiatry*, Vol. IV (eds H. W. Van Praag, M. H. Lader, O. J. Rafaelsen and E. J. Sachar, pp. 609–651.

Redmond, D. E. (1987). Studies of the nucleus locus coeruleus in monkeys and hypothesis for neuropsychopharmacology. In: *Psychopharmacology: The Third Generation of Progress* (ed. H. Y. Meltzer), pp. 967–975. Raven Press, New York.

Regier, D. A., Boyd, J. H., Burke Jr, J. D., Rae, D. S., Myers, J. K., Kramer, M., Robins, L. N., George, L. K., Karno, M. and Locke, B. Z. (1988). One-month prevalence of mental disorders in the United States. *Arch. Gen. Psychiat.*, **45**, 977–986.

Reiman, E. M., Raichle, M. E., Robins, E., Butler, F. K., Herscovitch, P., Fox, P. and Perlmutter, J. (1986). The application of positron emission tomography to the study of panic disorder. *Am. J. Psychiat.*, **143**, 469–477.

Reiman, E. M., Raichle, M. E., Robins, E., Fusselman, M., Mintun, M., Fox, P. and Price, J. (1988). Neuroanatomical correlates of lactate-induced panic and anticipatory fear. *Psychopharmacologia*, **96** (Suppl), 36 ((Abstr.).

Roth, M. and Harper, M. (1962). Temporal lobe epilepsy and the phobic anxiety-depersonalization syndrome: Part II: practical and theoretical considerations. *Compr. Psychiat.*, **3**, 215–226.

Roy-Burne, P., Geraci, M. and Uhde, T. W. (1986). Life events and the onset of panic disorder. *Am. J. Psychiat.*, **143**, 1424–1431.

Sheehan, D. V. (1982). Panic attacks and phobias. *New Engl. J. Med.*, **307**, 156–158.

Thorpe, G. L. and Burns, L. E. (1983). *The Agoraphobic Syndrome*. Wiley, New York.

Torgersen, S. (1983), Genetic factors in anxiety disorders. *Arch. Gen. Psychiat.*, **40**, 1085–1089.

Wall, M., Tuchman, M. and Mielke, D. (1985). Panic attacks and temporal lobe seizures associated with a right temporal lobe arteriovenous malformation: case report. *J. Clin. Psychiat.*, **46**, 143–145.

Weilberg, J. B., Bear, D. M. and Sachs, G. (1987). Three patients with concomitant panic attacks and seizure disorder: possible clues to the neurology of anxiety. *Am. J. Psychiat.*, **144**, 1053–1056.

Weissman, M. M. The epidemiology of anxiety disorders: rates, risks and familial patterns. *J. Psychiatr. Res.*, **22** (Suppl. 1), 99–114.

World Health Organization (1967). *Manual of the International Statistical Classification of Diseases, Injuries and Causes of Death* (ICD–8), WHO, Geneva.

with corticosterone transport of horseradish peroxidase. In: *The Amygdaloid Complex* (ed. Y. Ben-Ari), pp. 91–104. Elsevier, Amsterdam.

Wamsley, J. M., and Kuhar, M. J. (1982). Benzodiazepine receptor localization in rat brain by light microscopic autoradiography. *Neuropeptides* No. 4, 47–59.

Weill, W. M., Bernstein, C. (1984). Kindling model for the progressive development of psychopathology: sensitization to electrical, pharmacological, and psychological stimuli. In: *Handbook of Biological Psychiatry*, Vol. IV (eds H. W. Van Praag, M. H. Lader, O. J. Rafaelsen and E. J. Sachar, pp. 499–531.

Weiskrantz, L. E. (1956). Studies of the amygdala focus functions in monkeys and hypothesis for psychopharmacology. In: *Psychopharmacology: The Third Generation of Progress* (ed. H. Y. Meltzer), pp. 959–975. Raven Press, New York.

Regier, D.A., Boyd, J. H., Burke, J. D., Rae, D. S., Myers, J. K., Kramer, M., Robins, L. N., George, L. K., Karno, M. and Locke, B. Z. (1988). One-month prevalence of mental disorders in the United States. *Arch. Gen. Psychiat.* 45, 977–986.

Reiman, E. M., Raichle, M. E., Robins, E. R., Mintun, M. A., Fox, P. T. and Fusselman, D. (1989). The application of positron emission tomography to the study of panic disorder. *Am. J. Psychiat.* 145, 469–477.

Reznik, R. M., Reiman, M. E., Fyer, A., Gorman, J. M., Mintun, M. A., Fox, P. T. and Price, J. (1986). Neuroanatomical correlates of anticipated panic and anticipatory fear. *Psychopharmacologia* 96 (Suppl.) 87 (Abstr.)

Reiss, M. and Harris, M. (1985). Temporal lobe epilepsy and the phobic anxiety-depersonalization syndrome. Part II: clinical and theoretical considerations. *Compr. Psychiat.* 1, 215–226.

Rosenbaum, H., Gersten, M. and Hirshfeld, D. W. (1986). Life events and the onset of panic disorder. *Am. J. Psychiat.* 143, 1424–1448.

Shehan, D. V. (1982). Panic attacks and phobias. *New Engl. J. Med.* 307, 156–158.

Thorpe, G. L. and Burns, L. E. (1983). *The Agoraphobic Syndrome.* Wiley, New York.

Tyrer, S. (1984). Classification of anxiety disorders. *Acta Psychiat.* 30, 169–109.

Wall, M., Tuchman, M. and Mielke, D. (1985). Panic attacks and temporal lobe seizures associated with a right temporal lobe arteriovenous malformation: case report. *J. Clin. Psychiat.* 46, 143–145.

Wolkowitz, T. B., Hoehn, D. M. and Sachs, S. (1987). Panic patients with concomitant panic attacks enhanced activity, possible clues to the neurobiology of anxiety states. *Biol. Psychiat.* 145, 1051–1055.

Wittchen, H. V. The epidemiology of anxiety disorder: rates, risks and familial transmission. *Psychiat. Res.* 22 (Suppl.) 3, 93–114.

World Health Organization. (1987). *Manual of the International Statistical Classification of Diseases, Injuries and Causes of Death (ICD-9).* WHO, Geneva.

The Clinical Relevance of Kindling
Edited by T. G. Bolwig and M. R. Trimble
© 1989 John Wiley & Sons Ltd

17

Kindling, drug holidays and disorders of movement

R. Fog & H. Pakkenberg*

*St Hans Hospital, Laboratory of Psychopharmacology, St Hans Hospital, DK-4000 Roskilde and *Hvidovre Hospital, Department of Neurology, DK-2650 Hvidovre, Denmark*

INTRODUCTION

Drug-induced dyskinesias have been subdivided as follows (Lees, 1985):

(1) neuroleptic-induced dyskinesias
   (a) acute dyskinesias
   (b) akathisia
   (c) tardive dyskinesias
(2) psychomotor stimulant-induced dyskinesias
   (a) pundning
   (b) chorea
   (c) tics
(3) L-dopa-induced dyskinesias
   (a) chorea-athetosis
   (b) dystonia
   (c) myoclonus
   (d) tics.

Among the neuroleptic-induced side-effects, tardive dyskinesia represents the most serious clinical problem, and the present paper will mainly deal with this syndrome. The approximate incidence of tardive dyskinesia in routine practice is 10–20%, and there is a predisposition among elderly patients (Lees, 1985). The symptoms (involuntary repetitive movements of the tongue, mouth and facial muscles, sometimes accompanied by limb and truncal chorea-athetosis) may occur during or following cessation of prolonged neuroleptic treatment, and may persist (Casey, 1984). The symptoms are accentuated by termination of medication, and also by repeated pauses (drug holidays) in the medication. A kindling model for the development of tardive dyskinesia has, therefore, been established (Glenthøj, Hemmingsen and Bolwig, 1988).

TARDIVE DYSKINESIA AND DRUG HOLIDAYS

In a recent comprehensive review with extensive references (Glenthøj, Hemmingsen and Bolwig, 1988), the kindling hypothesis for tardive dyskinesia has been discussed. Animal models have been developed, and rodents in long-term neuroleptic treatment have been shown to develop oral movements (for example vacuous chewing) with close resemblance to tardive dyskinesia. The movements tend to increase after discontinuation of neuroleptic treatment and are more often seen in older animals (Waddington et al., 1985). A few examples of animal and human studies will throw some light on the topic.

Sant and Ellison (1984) administered haloperidol to rats over 17 weeks in a drug holiday/no holiday regime. The duration of oral movements increased more rapidly in the animals having drug holidays.

Intermittent haloperidol treatment during 10 weeks in guinea pigs (Koller, 1984) caused an increase in the behavioural response to apomorphine, and also an increase of spiroperidol binding in the corpus striatum to the same degree as continuous haloperidol treatment.

Murugaiah et al. (1985) gave continuous or discontinuous trifluoperazine and flupenthixol to rats over a period of 12 months. The effect upon apomorphine-induced stereotyped behaviour was inconsistent with trifluoperazine, whereas an enhancing effect was seen after flupenthixol. No differences were found between the effect of continuous and discontinuous treatments. Ligand binding studies suggested that the overall change in striatal receptor function was not affected by the use of a discontinuous drug regime.

Glenthøj (personal communication) is now investigating abnormal oral movements in rats induced by continuous or discontinuous long-term haloperidol treatment in a kindling model (Clemmensen and Hemmingsen, 1984; Barry et al., 1987). She reports an increase of abnormal mouthing from the first week of treatment, and the dyskinesias induced by discontinuous treatment have the longest duration. She therefore suggests that discontinuous neuroleptic treatment may be correlated with irreversible tardive dyskinesias, and continuous treatment with reversible dyskinesias.

In a study of 57 hospitalized chronic psychiatric patients, Branchey and Branchey (1984) examined the patterns of psychotropic drug use and tardive dyskinesia. They found a correlation between the frequency of drug-free episodes and tardive dyskinesia. Other risk factors were increasing age and time since first neuroleptic intake.

Gerlach et al. (1986) conducted a video-controlled study of the effect of different neuroleptics in tardive dyskinesia. The effect of consecutive drug-free periods on withdrawal tardive dyskinesia was a significant increase in abnormal movements.

Thus it seems reasonable to suggest a relation between drug holidays and tardive dyskinesias.

OTHER DISORDERS OF MOVEMENT

Prolonged neuroleptic treatment may give rise to other forms of movement disorders than tardive dyskinesia. We have described three cases of tardive Tourette syndrome (Fog et al., 1982), and other authors have found similar cases with a symptomatology of motor and verbal tics (for review, see Lees, 1985). Even if the symptoms normally are present for shorter periods only, and to some extent may be controlled voluntarily, the syndrome seems related to tardive dyskinesia: It is induced by long-term neuroleptic treatment; it often starts upon drug withdrawal; and the symptoms may be suppressed by an increased dose of the neuroleptic drug (Fog et al., 1982).

Neuroleptic treatment may also diminish other forms of hyperkinesia such as Huntington's chorea, L-dopa-induced hyperkinesias, and amphetamine-induced pundning (Fog and Pakkenberg, 1980a). In these syndromes, as well as in the dystonias (torticollis, Meige syndrome), the relationship to tardive dyskinesia is, however, less obvious.

DISCUSSION

The etiology and pathogenesis of tardive dyskinesia ia still unknown. Is it impossible to deduct information about the mechanisms from effective treatment strategies?

Drugs causing partial suppression of symptoms are dopamine receptor blockers (neuroleptics); dopamine storage blockers (tetrabenazine, reserpine); and dopamine synthesis inhibitors (methylparatyrosine) (Lees, 1985). Cholinergic, GABAergic, and serotonergic agents have only uncertain or negligible effects (Lees, 1985).

There is evidence for the involvement of neurotransmitter systems in kindling (Glenthøj, Hemmingsen and Bolwig, 1988), and especially dopaminergic mechanisms may be relevant for the pathogenesis of tardive dyskinesia, since all known neuroleptic drugs have an antidopaminergic effect (Fog and Regeur, 1986). The most established theory of tardive dyskinesia has been that of a dopamine receptor supersensitivity (Christensen, 1979; Casey *et al.*, 1985). Further studies with drugs acting selectively on D-1 and D-2 receptors may elucidate this theory (Hyttel *et al.*, 1985).

The involvement of dopamine in tardive dyskinesia seems obvious, but just the same could be said, however, of other psychiatric and neurological disorders such as parkinsonism, Huntington's chorea, Tourette syndrome, schizophrenia, and mania (Fog and Pakkenberg, 1980a; Fog, 1989). This may not be very surprising, since dopaminergic areas in the basal ganglia represent the output system for a large number of brain functions. Influencing dopamine seems, therefore, to be the safest way of obtaining an effect upon a whole range of neuropsychiatric diseases (Fog, 1989).

If the kindling phenomenon is involved in tardive dyskinesia after neuroleptic treatment, it may also be involved in L-dopa-induced hyperkinesias, since there is a progressive increase of these dyskinesias with time (Lees, 1985).

Glenthøj (personal communication) has suggested a toxic effect of neuroleptics, because she is able to identify abnormal oral movements in the first week of treatment in her kindling model. This observation is in good accordance with our own findings of a neurotoxic effect of neuroleptics (Fog and Pakkenberg, 1980b). Long-term treatment with perphenazine induced a loss of neurons in the striatum of rats of about 20%, whereas no cell loss was found in the cortex. Similar effects have been found with flupenthixol (Nielsen, 1977).

New data from investigators using another neurotoxic agent, MPTP (methyl-phenyl-tetrahydropyridine) may support the hypothesis of a toxic effect. In man MPTP produces a Parkinson-like syndrome. Given to mice (Pakkenberg *et al.*, 1988) MPTP induces an initial increase in uridine uptake in neurons in substantia nigra followed by a decrease during the following 9 weeks. This may be interpreted as a hyperreactive state of these neurons.

CONCLUSION

The different hypotheses of the pathogenesis of tardive dyskinesia (kindling; supersensitivity; neurotoxicity; hyperreactive neurons) may be unified in a theory that repeated doses of neuroleptic drugs exert kindling effects, which in long-term treatment change the neurons to hyperreactive cells sensitive to a neurotoxic influence. This is, however, speculation, and further investigations are needed to clarify possible interactions of the above-mentioned mechanisms.

REFERENCES

Barry, D. I., Kikvadze, I., Brundin, P., Bolwig, T. G., Björklund, A. and Lindvall, O. (1987). Grafted noradrenergic neurons suppress seizure development in kindling-induced epilepsy. *Proc. Nat. Acad. Sci.*, **84**, 8712–8715.

Branchey, M. and Branchey, L. (1984). Patterns of psychotropic drug use and tardive dyskinesia. *J. Clin. Psychopharmacol.*, **4**, 41–44.

Casey, D. E. (1984). Tardive dyskinesia: new research. *Psychopharmacol Bull.*, **20**, 376–379.

Casey, D. E., Chase, T. N., Christensen, A. V. and Gerlach, J. (eds) (1985). *Dyskinesia: Research and Treatment*. Springer, Berlin.

Christensen, A. V. (1979). *Adaption in Dopamine Neurons After Single and Repeated Administration of Neuroleptics*. H. Lundbeck, A/S.

Clemmensen, L. and Hemmingsen, R. (1984). Physical dependence on ethanol during multiple intoxication and withdrawal episodes in the rat. Evidence of a potentiation. *Acta Pharmacol. Toxicol.*, **55**, 345–350.

Fog, R. (1989) On the state of knowledge in neurobiological psychiatry. In: *Interaction Between Mental and Physical Illness* (eds R. Öhman *et al.*), pp. 71–73. Springer, Berlin.

Fog, R. and Pakkenberg, H. (1980a). Combination treatment of choreiform and dyskinetic syndromes with tetrabenazine and pimozide. In: *Tardive Dyskinesia. Research and Treatment* (eds W. E. Fann, R. C. Smith, J. M. Davis and E. F. Domino), pp. 507–510. Spectrum, New York.

Fog, R. and Pakkenberg, H. (1980b). Anatomical and metabolic changes after long and short-term treatment with perphenazine in rats. In: *Tardive Dyskinesia. Research and Treatment* (eds W. E. Fann, R. C. Smith, J. M. Davis and E. F. Domino), pp. 89–92. Spectrum, New York.

Fog, R. and Regeur, L. (1986). Neuropharmacology of tics. *Rev. Neurol. (Paris)*, **142**, 856–859.

Fog, R., Pakkenberg, H., Regeur, L. and Pakkenberg, B. (1982). 'Tardive' tourette syndrome in relation to long-term neuroleptic treatment of multiple tics. In: *Gilles de la Tourette Syndrome* (eds A. J. Friedhoff and T. N. Chase), pp. 419–421. Raven Press, New York.

Gerlach, J., Ahlfors, U. G., Amthor, K. F., Dencker, S. J., Gravem, A., Gunby, B., Hagert, U., Korsgaard, S., Lunding, L., Noring, U., Ojannen, K., Pitkonen, T., Povlsen, U. J., Rossel, T., Tolvanen, E. and Wæhrens, J. (1986). Effect of different neuroleptics in tardive dyskinesia and parkinsonism. *Psychopharmacology*, **90**, 423–429.

Glenthøj, B., Hemmingsen, R. and Bolwig, T. G. (1988). Kindling: a model for the development of tardive dyskinesia? *Behav. Neurol.*, **1**, 29–40.

Hyttel, J., Larsen, J.-J., Christensen, A. V. and Arnt, J. (1985). Receptor-binding profiles of neuroleptics. In: *Dyskinesia. Research and Treatment* (eds D. E. Casey, T. N. Chase, A. V. Christensen and J. Gerlach). Springer, Berlin.

Koller, W. C. (1984). Effects of intermittent haloperidol treatment on dopamine receptor sensitivity in guinea pigs. *Psychopharmacology*, **84**, 98–100.

Lees, A. J. (1985). *Tics and Related Disorders*. Churchill Livingstone, London.

Murugaiah, K., Theodorou, A., Clow, A., Jenner, P. and Marsden, C. D. (1985). Effects of discontinuous drug administration on the development of dopamine receptor supersensitivity during chronic trifluoperazine or cis-flupenthixol administration to rats. *Psychopharmacology*, **86**, 228–232.

Nielsen, E. B. (1977). Long-term behavioural and biochemical effects following prolonged treatment with a neuroleptic drug (flupenthixol) in rats. *Psychopharmacology*, **54**, 203–208.

Pakkenberg, H., Pakkenberg, B., Fog, R. and Eldrup, E. (1988). The effect on MPTP on uridine uptake in murine nerve cells. *Brain Res.*, **460**, 146–149.

Sant, W. W. and Ellison, G. (1984). Drug holidays alter onset of oral movements in rats following chronic haloperidol. *Biol. Psychiat.*, **19**, 95–99.
Waddington, J. L., Molloy, A. G., O'Boyle, K. M. and Youssef, H. A. (1985). Spontaneous and drug-induced dyskinesias in rodents in relation to ageing and long-term neuroleptic treatment: relationship to tardive dyskinesia. In: *Biological Psychiatry* (eds E. Shagass *et al.*), pp. 1151–1153. Elsevier, New York.

The Clinical Relevance of Kindling
Edited by T. G. Bolwig and M. R. Trimble
© 1989 John Wiley & Sons Ltd

Discussion — Session 6

KINDLING AND PANIC DISORDERS

R. Adamec Dr Rosenberg, I was intrigued with your theory about the development of panic disorder in children. I was wondering how much actual data there was on human children, or whether you were merely speculating. Also, what about genetic data?

R. Rosenberg Recently Isac Marks reviewed the genetic evidence for anxiety disorder, and I think that there is very strong evidence that anxiety disorders have a genetic predisposition. With respect to childhood data, there have been studies by Gittelman, who has shown that in some panic disorder patients, retrospectively, you have a higher reported frequency of separation anxiety and so on. But it is soft data, and there are no prospective studies in which children with separation anxiety have been followed up.

J. Boas Although, Dr Fog, you relate some movement disorders to a possible kindling phenomenon, isn't it possible that they represent a neural imbalance in the basal ganglia?

R. Fog Yes, of course. I have considered the theory of kindling as one which might lead to degeneration in the nervous system, and in that sense neuroleptics may also induce cell losses in the basal ganglia. If that could be called a kindling effect, I would accept kindling as model for tardive dyskinesia.

E. H. Reynolds Is it not true that in some examples of tardive dyskinesia, if you increase the dose of the drug, the dyskinesia may disappear?

R. Fog Yes, that is true.

E. H. Reynolds What does that tell us about the mechanism? Does that not undermine the kindling theories and all sorts of other theories?

R. Fog This question has been answered by the believers in a receptor supersensitivity model. If you have a supersensitive dopaminergic receptor, you increase the blockage so much that you overcome the supersensitivity.

J. Majkowski You suggested that kindling might be something which leads to deterioration of the brain. This is not necessarily so. Our discussion has been mostly limited, as far as kindling is concerned, to epileptogenesis, and of course this is a limitation of the kindling concept, which is much broader. I think it underlies processes which are much wider and can modify behaviour, can modify the reaction between environmental stimuli and what is ongoing due to the processes which were started by kindling in the brain. This might lead to psychoses and other phenomena.

R. Fog I think it is necessary for us to define in which sense we will use the word 'kindling': if it is in a narrow or a broad sense.

J. Majkowski I think that you use what kindling produces. There are two effects: one local, which relates to the epileptogenic question, and another one, which is much wider, distributed all over the brain. Wherever you put your electrodes, you will get changes in evoked potentials, which were not present before kindling. These changes last for a long time. With the epileptic focus, of course we are dealing with something which is abnormal, and this is what is abnormal: the spreading of epileptic discharges and spiking going to certain areas. When these are associated with incoming environmental information, the latter is distorted, and may lead to psychic phenomena.

GENERAL DISCUSSION

R. Adamec I'd like to start off with a clarification of the word 'kindling'. Kindling refers, in a scientific sense, to a very specifically operationally defined phenomenon. A lot of people find parallels, for example in the development of psychotic behaviour, with repeated episodes leading to intensification. In that sense, the word kindling is used, because it resembles the intensification of seizures with repetition. The only explanation in any of these analogies is that they seem to have similar temporal characteristics, i.e. development over time and intensification with repetition and a long-lasting after-effect. These points are often made when the word kindling is used. This does not mean, however, that kindling — in the sense of kindling as the development of epilepsy — is the mechanism for other phenomena which develop in a similar fashion.

No one knows how kindling works. There are lots of correlates, or effects of kindling, but none of them have been conclusively proven to be crucial for the epileptogenic event. There are lots of secondary effects of kindling, which are produced by repeated seizures, that may not be contributors to the epileptic event, but nevertheless may result in changed behaviour.

I think at this stage it is premature to say that since something resembles kindling, in an operational sense — that it is therefore a process which is analogous or directly similar to kindling as it is used to produce epilepsy in animals.

E. Sindrup We are back to the narrow concept.

R. Racine I would like to reinforce what Adamec has just said: kindling has been defined as an increase in epileptogenesis as a result of a repeated application of an epileptogenic agent. I think it should remain defined as such. I think that these discussions that we have had are good ones. It is useful looking for parallels, but I do think it is a mistake to call some of these other phenomena kindling. Another point I would like to make is this. Many of us who work on the kindling phenomenon are interested in the cellular mechanisms of kindling. We find kindling a useful mechanism, because it allows us a very tight control over the developing epileptogenesis. In consequence, we choose to focus on the evoked measure of kindling, because of the control that we have over it. On the other hand, if you are looking for parallels between kindling and clinical epilepsy, i.e. superficial similarities, then it probably is a mistake to try to compare the evoked measures with the spontaneous events that you see in the human. If you look at the spontaneous events as they develop in the kindled preparation, you will find many more similarities with the clinical condition.

Going back to Dr Fink's talk on ECT: it would be unfortunate, I think, if people left this conference believing that ECT had no lasting effects. It may have minimal lasting effects, and the benefits may outweigh the risks. But the evidence so far is that it does produce lasting effects, and the presence of the electrodes in our own study does not explain those effects. The presence of those electrodes is controlled in every kindling experiment that has ever been done.

M. R. Trimble One of the reasons that Tom Bolwig and I thought this meeting should be convened is because of these difficulties that have arisen with the word 'kindling'. It has become already almost a part of popular clinical phraseology. What you have said restricts the term 'kindling' to epileptogenesis, and that is vital, because if you restrict kindling in that way (and I accept that may be one way to view it), a consequence is, as Dr Reynolds noted, that kindling has little relevance for developed clinical epilepsy. So you have a phenomenon, whose criteria is epileptogenesis, that has little relevance to the clinical setting. It has very limited value. However, I believe that it is a much more exciting concept than that. That it permeates other aspects of behaviour, other than a motor seizure and that it reflects a more widespread biological phenomenon. So, when we try to look at other states, for example panic disorder or tardive dyskinesia, I think that what one is saying is that if you remove the issue of epileptogenesis, but merely say that within the central nervous system mechanisms exist whereby sub-threshold stimuli can provoke effects that are qualitatively different from their added quantities, then you have a very interesting biological phenomenon. Kindling then becomes useful in looking at a whole range of phenomena.

R. Racine I think that kindling is an excellent model of clinical epilepsy. Again, if you look at the spontaneous epilepsy that develops with kindling, it looks very much like that described here for certain types of clinical epilepsy. So I disagree with you on that score. If you do what you were proposing, i.e. opening up the term, then it will become as useful as the term 'plasticity' which is not very useful. It loses its value as a term.

E. H. Reynolds I am not sure what kindling has to do with clinical epilepsy. I discussed what I call the Gower's phenomenon of the process of epilepsy, and I was careful not to call it kindling, which I do accept as an animal experimental model which might be very relevant to the development of the first seizure. But I do not know how the first seizure develops clinically, so kindling may be an excellent model for the initiation of epilepsy rather than for the perpetuation of it.

I think one thing that has come out of this meeting relates to the longitudinal view of the illness. Kindling has made us focus our attention on looking at illness in a longitudinal way, and looking at all the processes that make up the evolution of an illness into a chronic state. Of course there are parallels with kindling, but it does not mean they are the same things. In the Gower's phenomenon if a seizure leaves a mark on the nervous system, it does not have to be the same mark as occurs in kindling. And what's going on in ECT? Perhaps that has more in common with the Gower's phenomenon, but for ECT to be effective it has to be spaced out, and each one of the stimulations has some effect.

Let us try to agree what the word kindling means, and not be bogged down in interminable discussions that have gone on for centuries, for example about what is epilepsy. Michael Trimble and I have been down that road in a book recently published with the title *What is Epilepsy?* For the clinician, epilepsy is recurrent seizures, but once you say epilespy is a discharge of a hyperexcitable collection of neurons, then this opens up a Pandora's box, and a sneeze becomes healthy epilepsy. That's why there has been so much confusion in classifying both epilepsy and seizures! So let us try and agree on what kindling is, and I am quite prepared to stick to the original definitions of kindling as brought out by the experimental physiologists.

But there is one other point: one must be intrigued, as Post and I are, that we can both pursue our own interests, he in manic-depressive illness and me in epilepsy, and find that we are pursuing rather similar phenomena and theories about accelerating disease processes. That does not mean it is kindling, but there is something at work in these different disease processes. There are events, stimuli, leaving marks on the nervous system, things are never the same again, after you have had a convulsion, and that is a very intriguing observation. This is dynamic neurology (not dynamic psychiatry), and it raises practical issues about treatment: how early you should treat, and with what. Post's questions about using different drugs at different stages of manic-depressive illness is very relevant to other diseases, including epilepsy.

R. Post I would like to agree as well with Racine's definition and keep the kindling concept for that which has a seizure endpoint. I called that which was not associated with a seizure endpoint something else, sensitization or whatever. We are talking about phenomena that have some general properties of exacerbating over time: things get worse with repeated institution of the same process, and in one case, the case that we can call kindling, that leads to an epileptogenic process.

J. C. Ballenger For me it comes down to three terms. The first is the operationally defined kindling. After that everything else is an analogy, and we are trying to find words for that analogy. I write 'kindling-like', putting both words in quotes, even when describing paradigms that have convulsions as the final pathway, like the alcohol analogy, because it is truly just analogy. For the third, Post has suggested sensitization.

R. Adamec I think the word 'kindling-like' is probably very valuable, so that people are aware, when using the term, that it is an analogy.

M. R. Trimble Stevens, a number of years ago, described an experiment in which she placed stimulating wires into the ventral tegmental areas of cats. She carried out what I understand was a kindling paradigm, and yet she did not provoke seizures; but she produced marked behavioural changes. Now, was that a kindling experiment or not? Seizures were not produced, but the method was precisely the same as that which you are describing for amygdaloid kindled seizures.

R. Adamec When you kindle an animal, you produce seizure discharges which involve high frequency synchronous bursting of cells. This high frequency activation spreads to other areas, including ventral tegmental area and substantia nigra. What Stevens did was by-pass the necessary, what seem to be frequent, seizures to get to the point of high frequency and intense driving of the ventral tegmental and substantia nigra areas. That does happen in rats, but it takes many, many seizures. She may have been circumventing all of that, in doing to one particular part of the brain what repeated seizures do after a while in kindling. I would almost agree that she was doing something similar to what happens in kindling. It was not kindling in the epileptogenic sense, because she did not create epilepsy in her cats; but she did affect a particular circuit similar to what would happen during kindling to that circuit. I think I do that in my cats. I do something that requires seizure discharges, but it is very restricted, and I think these restricted phenomena are what are most behaviourally relevant. I also think repeated seizures can induce them, but it is not kindling in the strict sense. However, it is produced by repeated seizure activation. I call it partial kindling in my cats, because I am not driving them to motor convulsions.

R. Racine If kindling were defined in terms of the stimulation applied, rather than the events that are triggered, then you would have to call long-term potentiation kindling. I think most people would agree that it is not.

E. H. Reynolds I do not like the term 'kindling-like'. It smacks of 'epilepsy-like' and 'epileptiform' and 'epileptic equivalent' and 'masked epilepsy'. Either it is kindling, or it is not!

M. Dam Having been through all the different clinical syndromes and trying to think of kindling, I thought that infantile spasms and febrile seizures, if they started in a specific age group, have some similarity to kindling. It is easier to kindle animals in a specific age group. The same is the case with the Lennox-Gastaut syndrome. If the patients were young, they would develop severe epilepsy; if they got the syndrome later on, it was not so dangerous. The other group where you might suspect kindling is epilepsy with alcoholism. There we see patients coming in, first with abstinence seizures and after a short time we see them return more and more frequently with spontaneous seizures. We can treat them, and if we treat them early with carbamazepine, we will easily control their seizures.

T. G. Bolwig I have been convinced from what I've heard, that kindling should be reserved to kindling as it is now operationally defined. But what do we call the 'kindling-like' phenomena that are so intriguing in the clinical world today? I like sensitization.

Index

Note: Abbreviations used in sub-entries:

AD   Afterdischarge
CAR   Conditional avoidance reflex
CRF   Corticotropin releasing factor
CS   Conditioning stimulus
ECS   Electro-convulsive shock

ECT   Electro-convulsive therapy
EP   Evoked potential
GABA   Gamma-aminobutyric acid
LTP   Long-term potentiation
NMDA   *N*-Methyl-D-aspartate

For entries pertaining to Kindling, and not listed under this keyword, please see individual relevant subject headings.

Absence seizures, 73
  antieptileptic drug activity, 64
  overshooting inhibitory activity in, 64
  rat kindling as model, 65
Acetazolamide, 58, 61
Acetylcholine, agonists, kindling
  induced by, 35, 36
AD, *see* Afterdischarge
Addictive behaviour and kindling, 5–8,
  231–251
  see also Cocaine; Ethanol intoxication
  and withdrawal
Adrenocorticotrophic hormone
  (ACTH), 164, 171
Advance motor conditioned reflex
  (AMCR), 95
Affective illness, 2–3, 203
  animal model, 209
  in epilepsy, 8, 186
  factors influencing development, 209
  see also Manic-depressive illness
Afterdischarge (AD)
  associated with complex partial
  seizure, 93
  before motor convulsions, 20

  CAR latency, effect on, 94
  duration, effects on memory retrieval,
  93
  EEG patterns and effect on CAR
  performance, 94–98, 99
  in kindling phenomenon, 15–16, 19
  neocortical and limbic, 19
Aggression, 147–148
Agoraphobia, 265, 270
Alcoholism, 2, 5–7, 137–144
  see also Ethanol intoxication and
  withdrawal
Alprazolam, 266
Alumina focus model, 18
Amphetamines, 7–8, 210, 245, 260
Amygdala, 182
  behavioural biasing function, 127
  emotional behaviour, role in, 182, 266
  in ethanol withdrawal seizures, 6, 143
  facilitatory effect on defense
  behaviour in cats, 127
  glucose metabolism in, 142
  in hippocampal kindling, 80–81
  importance in kindling/epilepsy,
  80–81

Amygdala (*cont.*)
  individual differences in feline
    defensiveness, 128–129
  lesions, cocaine-induced behavioural
    sensitization block, 212
  noradrenergic denervation,
    kindling facilitation, 76, 77, 80,
    81
  reinnervation and hippocampal
    kindling suppression, 81
Amygdala kindling, 1, 15
  6-OHDA facilitation of, 76, 80
  anatomical and chemical specificity,
    43–46
  antiepileptic drugs suppression of, 55,
    56, 58, 60, 62–65, 144, 203,
    214–215, 221
  carbachol, 35, 36–37, 45, 46
  carbamazepine action, possible
    mechanisms, 226
  cross-sensitization with lidocaine
    kindling, 212, 246
  ECT antagonism, 203, 204, 261
  enkephalin-induced, 213–214
  ethanol intoxication and withdrawal
    relation, 6, 142, 143, 144, 148
  excitatory neurotransmitters role,
    38–39
  feline defensiveness, 127, 128
  focal response, then generalization,
    19–20
  long-term potentiation (LTP)
    similarity, 47, 70, 89
  neocortical tissue grafting, 78–79
  partial, feline behavioural changes,
    129–130
  rate and sensitivity, 1, 15, 18, 80, 142,
    187
  see also Kindling phenomenon;
    Limbic kindling
Amygdaloid-kindled seizures,
  antiepileptics effects on, 55, 57, 59,
    60–63, 65–66, 214, 215, 221
  comparative effects, 64–65
  see also individual drugs
Anaesthetics, local, *see* Cocaine;
  Lidocaine
Anatomical specificity of kindling
  circuits, 43–46
Animal model,
  affective illness, 209

anxiety and behavioural changes, 17,
    126–130, 266
  see also Anxiety; Cat
  complex partial seizures (CPS), 65,
    126
  ethanol intoxication and withdrawal,
    6, 139–144, 234, 235, 238, 244
  see also Amygdala kindling;
    Kindling phenomenon; Rat
Anti-absence drugs, 64, 65
Anticonvulsants,
  in alcohol withdrawal syndrome,
    242–244
  antimanic activity, 202–203, 204, 214,
    215, 221
  conditioned tolerance, 221, 223
  ECT as, 202, 204, 206
  kindling and, 72–73
  in manic-depressive illness, efficacy,
    202–203, 204, 210
  neocortical and limbic ADs response,
    19
  post-traumatic epilepsy, effect on, 72
  see also Antiepileptic drugs;
    Carbamazepine; *other specific
    drugs*
Antidepressants, 204–205
  ECT efficacy as, 204, 205
  in manic-depressive illness, 218, 219
  in panic disorder, 266, 267, 269
Antiepileptic drugs,
  anti-absence components, 64, 65
  epilepsy prognosis after withdrawal,
    168–169
  ethanol withdrawal, effect on, 144
  kindled seizures, effects on, 56–62,
    65–66, 144
  kindling and, 55–66, 213–214
  hypothesis on activity, 64–65
  kindling evolution, effects on, 56–62,
    62–65
  in newly diagnosed epilepsy, results,
    153
  see also Anticonvulsants; *individual
    drugs*
Antimania agents, 225
  ECT as, 203, 204, 205
Anxiety, 117–131, 123
  animal model, 126, 131
  cat, effects of seizures, 125, 126, 127
  in children, 265, 268

defensive behaviour in cats as model,
    126, 131
factors contributing to, in epilepsy,
    123, 125, 263
innate mechanisms, 266, 267, 268
limbic epilepsy and, 121, 123, 125,
    179, 263
local anaesthetics effect, 249, 261
neurobiology models of, 123, 125,
    266–267
see also Panic attacks; Panic disorder
Anxious personality, 118, 131
    premorbid, 125, 131
Area tempesta, 70
Aspartate, chemical kindling with, 39
Astrocyte activation,
    in kindling, 24–25, 27, 69
    in status epilepticus, 24–27, 28
Astrocyte hypertrophy, 24–25, 27, 69,
    70
Audiogenic seizures, 142
Auditory hallucinosis, 138, 143
Aura,
    fear, 119, 184
    limbic, 118–123, 120, 124, 125, 184
    questionnaire, 120
    subjective, 192
Automatisms, 85
Avoidance behaviour, 265, 268, 270

Baboons, antiepileptic agents and
    kindling, 56, 65, 66
Barbiturate anaesthesia, for ECT, 199,
    201
Basal ganglia, neural imbalance and
    movement disorders, 281
Basket cell activating systems, 75
Bear–Fedio questionnaire, 9, 118, 184
    modified, 119
Beck Depression Inventory (BDI), 121,
    122, 243
Behavioural changes,
    alcohol withdrawal, similarities with
        kindling, 6, 238, 240–241
    CRF-induced seizures, 213
    defensive, 17, 126–130, 147
    dopamine system kindling, 186–187
    interictal, in cats, 17, 125, 126–131,
        147
    in kindling, 16–17, 18, 89, 103–109,
        186–187, 240

possible mechanisms, 130
in temporal lobe lesions, see Temporal
    lobe epilepsy
in tetanus toxin model, 107
ventral tegmental area stimulation,
    285–286
Behavioural disorders, in epilepsy,
    177–180, 180, 240–241
    kindling as mechanism?, 185–187
    see also Psychopathology
Behavioural effects, convulsive therapy,
    198–199
Behavioural sensitization, 3, 260, 285,
    286
    affective illness relationship, 3, 4,
        214–216, 224
    cocaine-induced, see Cocaine-induced
        behavioural sensitization
    dopaminergic mechanisms, 210, 211,
        212, 245, 249
    pharmacological kindling comparison,
        7, 209–210, 247, 260
Behavioural therapy, 114, 270
Behavioural traits, personality
    behaviour inventory (PBI), 118
Benign familial neonatal convulsions,
    163, 171
Benign focal epilepsy, 165
Benzodiazepine receptor (BZR), 41,
    127, 128, 267
    agonists, feline defensive response
        reduced, 128
    antagonists, 41, 130
    in enhanced feline defensiveness,
        130–131
    inverse agonist, 41, 128
Benzodiazepines, 55
    amygdaloid-kindled seizures, effect,
        62, 241, 244
    anxiety reduction, 128, 266, 267
    in ethanol withdrawal reaction, 144,
        241, 242–244
    in manic-depressive illness, 218, 219
    in panic disorder, 267
    see also Diazepam
Betacarboline, 41
Bias, defensive, 127, 131
Bicuculline kindling, of cortex, 41, 42,
    45
Bio-feedback, 114
Brain maturation and schizophrenia, 5

Brain stem nuclei, in alarm and anxiety, 267, 268

CA1 and CA2–3 neurons, in kindling, 47, 49
CA3 hippocampal cells,
  loss in epilepsy, 104
  possible function, 109
  in tetanus toxin model, 107, 108–109
Calcium, 48, 103
Calmodulin kinase, 47
CAR, see Conditional avoidance reflex (CAR)
Carbachol kindling, of amygdala, 35, 36–38, 43, 45, 46
Carbamazepine, 55, 56, 57–59
  absence-type seizures precipitated by, 64, 65
  action against tonic–clonic seizures, 64
  in alcohol withdrawal syndrome, 242–244
  amydala kindling evolution, effect, 3, 56, 64–65, 192, 210, 214, 215, 221, 241, 247
  amygdaloid-kindled seizures, effect, 58, 59, 192, 214, 215, 221, 241–242, 247
  anitconvulsant and psychotropic effects, possible mechanisms, 226
  cocaine-induced seizures, 248
  contingent inefficacy and tolerance, 221, 223, 224, 225
  lidocaine-induced seizures block, 214, 215, 227, 247–248
  in manic-depressive illness, 3, 202, 210, 219, 221, 226
    contingent tolerance, 221, 223, 225
    mechanism, 226
    rapid-cycling, 218, 219
  segmental neuronal inhibition increase, 65
Carbamylcholine, 35, 36
Cat,
  anxiety, effects of seizures on, 126, 127
  anxiety disorder model, 127, 129–130, 131
  defensive behaviour, 17, 126, 127–130, 286

  defensive personality trait, 127, 128–129
    amygdala mediation, 127, 128, 128–129
    benzodiazepine receptor (BZR) function, 128, 130–131
  kindled seizure suppression by antiepileptics, 56, 66
  kindling in, tonic–clonic seizure model, 65
  personality, 127–130
    individual differences in behaviour, 128
    individual differences in limbic function, 128–129
    ontogeny, 129
    partial limbic kindling effect, 17, 127, 129–130, 286
Catecholamines and kindling, 41, 76–77
  cocaine effect on, 7, 211, 245, 246, 249
  depletion, kindling rate increase, 76, 77, 79, 81
Cell damage,
  after kindling, absence, 23, 24, 69, 104
  duration of status epilepticus, relation, 24–25
  in epilepsy, 104
Cellular changes associated with kindling, 46–49
Central tegmental area, kindling, 9
Cerbral ventricles, enlarged, in schizophrenia, 4
Cerebral blood flow (CBF), 4, 138, 269
Cerebral glucose metabolism, 6, 43, 64, 142, 185
Chemical kindling, 35–49, 76, 197
  agonists and antagonists, summary, 39
  comparison with electrical kindling seizures, 43, 214
  criteria for, 38
  excitatory neurotransmitters agonists, 38–40
  failures, 39
  inhibitory neurotransmitters antagonists, 41–42
  metabolic anatomy of seizures, 43–44
  muscarinic kindling, 36–38
  see also individual agents;
    Pharmacological kindling

Chemical specificity of kindling circuits, 46
Children,
  anxiety in and panic disorder, development, 265, 268, 270, 281
  epilepsy, 163–166, 168, 178
Clinical Institute Withdrawal Assessment for Alcohol (CIWA-A), 242–243
Clinic Interview Schedule, 178
Clobazam, 58, 62
Clonazepam, 58, 62
Clonic convulsion, in kindling, 16, 19
  see also Tonic–clonic seizures
Clonidine,
  cocaine-induced sensitization, block, 225
  reduced anxiety levels, 266–267
Cocaine, 3, 7–8, 210, 245
  affective changes, 7, 210, 245
  catecholamines, effect on, 7, 211, 245, 246, 249
  conditioned effects with, 211–212, 224–225, 249–250
  dysphoric effects, 249, 261
  euphorogenic effects (addiction), kindling not associated, 247, 249
  in kindling experiments, 41, 210
  local anaesthetic effects, kindling-like, 246, 248–249, 250
  as psychomotor stimulant, 7, 211, 245, 246
  self-administration, 245, 249
  tolerance to, and addiction, 210, 247
Cocaine-induced behavioural sensitization, 210–212, 224–225, 245–250, 260
  blocking of, 212, 225, 227, 247
  conditioning in, 3, 211–212, 224–225, 248, 249–250
  cross-sensitization, 211, 245
  dopaminergic mechanisms, 7, 210, 211, 212, 245, 249
  pharmacological kindling vs, 7, 209–210, 247
  phases, 248
Cocaine-induced panic attacks, 213, 249, 260–261
Cocaine-induced seizures, 210, 247–248
  mortality, 248
  spontaneous, absence, 261

Collaterals, sprouting, 24
Complex partial seizures, 167
  afterdischarge (AD) associated, 93
  alcoholism and kindling link, 7, 241
  behavioural changes, 167, 241
  mirror focus, 8, 21, 36
  model, 65, 126
  poor response to therapy and prognosis, 168, 184
  see also Partial seizures; Temporal lobe epilepsy
Conditional avoidance reflex (CAR), afterdischarge (AD), effect on, 93, 94
  effects of EEG patterns of afterdischarges (ADs), 94–98, 99
  latency, effects of, 94, 98
  memory retrieval and hippocampal kindling, 92
Conditioned emotional response (CER), panic disorder development, 268
Conditioned tolerance, carbamazepine, 221, 223, 225
Conditioning, 89, 114
  in cocaine-induced behavioural sensitization, 211–212, 224, 248, 249–250
  of kindling, 91–92
  kindling relation, 89
  in manic-depressive illness episode activation, 216, 224
Conditioning stimulus (CS),
  kindling retarded, 91–92
  presentation and CAR, 91, 92, 93, 95, 96, 97
Contingent inefficacy, 220–224, 225
  definition, 221
Contingent tolerance, 220–224, 225
  definition, 221
Convulsions, neonatal, 163, 171
Convulsive therapy, 195–206
  behavioural effects, 198–199
  kindling implications for, 196
  pharmacological, 198
  see also Electro-convulsive therapy
Corticotropin releasing factor (CRF), 211
  intrathecal administration, seizures, 213

Cross-sensitization,
  amphetamine and cocaine-induced
    behavioural sensitization, 211, 245
  intoxication–withdrawal episodes and
    electrical kindling, 6, 141, 143, 148,
    241
  lidocaine-induced seizures, 212, 246

Defensive behaviour in cats, 17,
  126–130, 266
  see also Cat, defensive personality
    trait
Defensive disposition in humans, 128
Delirium tremens (DTs), 5, 6, 137, 138,
  234
  rating scale, 138, 236, 237
Dementia paralytica, 198
Dementia praecox, see Schizophrenia
Demoralization hypothesis, 265
Dentate gyrus, 47–48
  kindling, neuronal and synaptic
    excitability changes, 47–48, 108
  possible function, 109
  reduction in excitability in tetanus
    toxin model, 107–108
2-Deoxyglucose, 6, 43
Depersonalization, 263, 269
Depression, 123
  limbic epilepsy and, 121, 179
  panic disorder relation, 265
  partial seizures and, 167
  see also Manic-depressive illness
Diagnostic and Statistical Manual of
  Mental Disorders (DSM-III, 1987),
  192, 263–264
Diazepam,
  in alcohol withdrawal syndrome, 241
  amygdaloid-kindled seizures, effect
    on, 62, 214, 215, 241
  amygdaloid-kindling evolution, effect
    on, 58, 214, 215
  cocaine-induced sensitization block,
    225
  see also Benzodiazepines
5,7-Dihyroxytryptamine, 77–78
Diphenylhydantoin, 72
'Doom anxiety', 249, 261
L-Dopa-induced dyskinesia, 275, 278
Dopamine, 5
  central depletion, effect on kindling,
    76

hyperactivity, in schizophrenia, 4, 5
  increase after kindling, 9
  postulated role in cocaine addiction,
    249
  receptor supersensitivity, 187, 277,
    282
  in tardive dyskinesia, 277–278
Dopaminergic mechanisms, 277
  behavioural sensitization (cocaine-
    induced), 7, 210, 211, 212, 245, 249
Dopaminergic neurone, 4
  transplantation, 82
Dopamine system kindling, seizures and
  behavioural changes, 186–187
DRL-20 task, 107
Drug abuse, see Cocaine
Drug holidays, 221, 276
Dyskinesia, drug-induced, 275–277

Ego-functioning, adaptive level, 10
Elderly, epileptic seizures in, 167–168
Electrical kindling, 15–17, 197, 212–214
  as anti-kindling agent, 205
  characteristics, 10, 15–17, 18–20
  comparison with chemical kindling,
    43, 214
  phases, 213
  see also Amygdala kindling; Kindling
    phenomenon; Limbic kindling
Electro-convulsive shock (ECS), 196,
  203
  lasting change in brain function, 259
Electro-convulsive therapy (ECT),
  anaesthesia for, 199, 201
  antagonism for kindled seizures, 3,
    202, 203, 204, 261
  as anticonvulsant, 202, 204, 206
  antidepressant efficacy, theory, 204,
    205
  clinical efficacy, kindling as model, 22,
    196–197, 202–204
  currents used in, 199, 200, 201
  direct brain stimulation and, 200–201
  epileptic psychosis, effect on, 203
  kindling comparison, 22, 200, 204,
    259–261, 284
    differences between, 22, 198,
      200–202, 259, 260
    similarities with, 198–200
    summary, 200
  kindling not valid as model, 204–205

lasting effect on brain function, 259, 283
mania, effect on, 3, 203, 204–205
number of inductions, 202
potentiation of inhibitory process by, 204
psychotherapeutic agents with, effect, 196
seizures, 198–199, 204
  duration and thresholds, 199, 201–202
spontaneous (tardive) seizures after, 22, 196, 199–200
therapeutic benefits, 205, 259, 283
tricyclic antidepressant drugs (TCA) comparison, 204–205
Electroencephalography (EEG),
afterdischarge (AD) patterns, 94–98, 99
non-convulsive component of withdrawal reactions, 148, 233, 238
Emotional behaviour, limbic system in, 182, 266
Emotional changes,
  in kindled animals, 105
  partial kindling of cat, 131
Emotional liability, temporal lobe focus associated, 167
Emotional problems, in epilepsy, 9–10
  see also Psychopathology
Endopiriform nucleus, 70
Endorphins, 40
Enkephalins, 40, 213–214
Entorhinal cortex kindling, 47, 48
Environmental context, cocaine-induced behavioural sensitization, 3, 211, 212, 248
Environmental stimulation, effects on kindling, 91
Epilepsy, 8–10, 149, 150, 284
  acute and chronic models, 18, 105
  antagonism with psychosis, 198, 203
  anxiety relationship, 121, 123, 125, 179, 263
  benign focal, 165
  'burst' pattern of seizures, 183
  case ascertainment difficulties, 161
  causes, 103, 150
  cell damage, 104
  chemical kindling relevance to, 36

chronic,
  development, 153, 154–155, 170, 183–184, 284
  evolution, 153
  kindling phenomenon as model of, 17, 18
  model, 18, 105
  prevention by early treatment, 157
classification, 181, 182
continuous pattern of seizures, 183
damping mechanisms reducing excitability, 109
destruction of structures involved in kindling, 36
drug refractoriness, 221
as dynamic process, 21, 149, 154–155, 156–157, 172, 191
in elderly, 167–168
GABA neurones in, 103
Gowers' Phenomenon relation, 150, 156, 157, 284
incidence after febrile seizures, 163
intermittent pattern of seizures, 183
juvenile myoclonic, 166, 172
kindling as different phenomenon, 21, 157–158, 284
kindling as model for, 2, 8–9, 17–20, 21, 22, 69, 104, 157–158, 284
development of first seizure, 158, 284
problems with, 81
kindling similarity, spontaneous seizures, 18–19, 157, 259–260, 283
learning relation, 88, 114, 158
limbic, see Limbic epilepsy
loss of inhibitory synapses, neurones in, 75, 103
manic depressive illness similarities, 158, 285
memory relation, 88, 158
monotherapy, 153, 154, 172
  failure, 170
natural history (untreated), 150–153, 162–163, 183
occipital focus, 165
personality changes, see Personality
possible transplantation therapy, 75, 78, 81–82, 83, 113
prevalence rate, 170, 178
prognosis, 103, 149, 161–172, 183–187
  after drug withdrawal, 168–169

Epilepsy, prognosis (*cont.*)
    age of onset effect, 163–165, 169,
        171
    duration of epilepsy, 155, 167, 170,
        171
    epileptic syndromes, 163–166,
        171–172
    factors, 168, 171, 172, 183, 184
    general aspects, 169–170
    individual seizure duration, 168,
        171
    influence of early treatment, 155,
        156–157, 172, 191, 221
    newly-diagnosed, 153, 154, 155, 183
    of single seizure, 103–104, 157,
        161–162, 183
    temporal lobe, 179–180
    *see also individual epileptic
        syndromes*
    psychomotor, 181, 182
    psychopathology, *see*
        Psychopathology in epilepsy
    psychosis link, 8–9, 184–185, 186,
        202–204
    remission, 153, 154, 155, 156, 169,
        170, 183
    seizure patterns, 183
    seizures, resistance to, after
        convulsion, 156
    'severe', concept of, 154
    spontaneous regeneration of
        neurones, 75, 78
    terminology, 180–181
    therapy, 191
        early, importance of correct drug,
            169, 192, 221
        effect on prognosis, 164, 166, 167,
            168–169
        newly-diagnosed, 153, 154–155, 156
        poor compliance, 155, 156
        poor outcome in chronic patients, 153,
            157, 221
Epileptic personality, 117–118, 147, 167,
    178, 179
Epileptogenesis, secondary, 8, 21, 36, 89
Ethanol, effects, 5, 233
Ethanol intoxication and withdrawal,
    5–7, 137–144, 231–245, 250
    altered CNS and behaviour during
        withdrawal, 6, 233, 238, 240–241
    animal models, 6, 139–144, 234, 235,
        238, 244
    behavioural and EEG similarities with
        kindling, 7, 238–241
    carbamazepine and oxazepam
        comparison, 242–244
    cerebral glucose metabolism and, 6,
        142
    clinical signs, 5, 138–139, 143, 232,
        236, 240
    convulsive component, cumulative
        effects, 140–141, 142, 234–237,
        239, 286
    detoxication episodes, withdrawal
        seizure predisposition, 6, 137, 238,
        239
    duration of alcohol, symptom severity
        relation, 236, 239
    intoxication, role in CNS dysfunction,
        143
    kindling analogy, stages, 6, 232, 250
    as kindling stimulus, evidence,
        233–234
    limbic structure hyperexcitability in,
        6, 233–234
    medications affecting kindling
        interaction, 233, 241–244, 250
    non-convulsive component,
        EEG changes, 148, 233, 238
        influence of duration of
            intoxication, 139–140
        kindling not found with, 140, 142,
            148
    physical signs, 138, 236
    predictions based on kindling model,
        233–245
    progression of severity with time,
        evidence, 234–237
    progression in stages in unidirectional
        manner, 233, 237
    psychotic signs, 138–139, 240
    regular use of alcohol vs binge
        drinking, 234, 239, 261
    susceptibility to relapse after, 245
    temporal lobe epilepsy relation, 7, 241
    two-component hypothesis, 142–143,
        148
    see also Delirium tremens (DTs)
Ethanol withdrawal seizures, 5, 6, 137,
    138, 140–141, 238–240, 286

cross-sensitization with kindled
seizures, 6, 141, 143, 148, 241
epilepsy kindled by?, 148
intensification after ECS, 196
kindled seizures similarities, 6, 141,
143, 148, 238
Ethosuximide, 60, 65
amygdaloid-kindled seizures and
kindling evolution, 58, 60, 61
Evoked potentials (EP),
enhancement in kindled animals, 46,
89
habituation of, 114
sensory-specific, changes during
kindling, 89
Excitotoxic effects, neurotransmitter
agonists, 39, 40

Fear, 118, 263
auras, 119, 184
in panic attacks, 263, 269
Febrile seizures, 163–164, 171, 286
Fetal neurones, grafting, see
Intracerebral grafting of fetal
neurones
FG-7142, 128
Flupenthixol, 276
Focal epilepsy, see Limbic epilepsy;
Partial seizures; Temporal lobe
epilepsy
Focal seizures, 105, 106
in kindling, 1, 19–20, 88
Folic acid, 158
'Forced normalization', 203
Forebrain, catecholamine depletion with
6-OHDA, 76, 77
Frontal lobe epilepsy, 182
Functional psychoses, see Manic-
depressive illness; Schizophrenia

Gamma-aminobutyric acid (GABA), 76
antagonists, kindling by, 35, 41, 42
folic acid block, 158
increase in ECT, 204
potentiators, kindling inhibition, 41,
45
receptors, desensitization in
epileptogenesis, 103
Gamma-aminobutyric acid (GABA)-
ergic circuits, recurrent, 47

Gamma-aminobutyric acid (GABA)-
ergic neurones, transplantation, 81
'Generalization', of response, 19–20
Generalized epilepsy, 43, 166, 171, 200
prognosis, 166, 169
psychopathology, reduced
susceptibility to, 179–180
Generalized seizures in kindling, 19–20,
88
Genetic predisposition,
anxious depression in epileptics, 123,
125
panic disorder, 265, 268, 281
Glia cells, 198
paucity in schizophrenia, 198
Glial fibrillary acidic protein (GFAP),
24
Gliosis, 25, 27, 69, 70
development of epilepsy, relation, 71
Glucose metabolism, cerebral, 6, 43,
142, 185
in absence seizures, 64
Glutamate and kindling, 39
antagonist, 40
'Gowers' Phenomenon, The', 150,
157–158, 163, 284
see also Kindling phenomenon
Grand mal epilepsy, 166, 171
in convulsive therapy, 200

Habituation, 40
of evoked potentials, 114
Hallucinations, 4, 138, 143, 192
Hallucinosis, withdrawal, 138, 143
Haloperidol, 276
Head trauma, 71
Hippocampal kindling, 1, 18, 22, 80
grafting of neocortical tissue, 79
grafting of noradrenergic neurons,
79–81, 113
interictal spiking, memory retrieval
and, 92
interictal spiking blocked by CS, 91
memory retrieval, effect on, 92
rate, 1, 18, 22
Hippocampal self-stimulation, 91
Hippocampus, 182
CA3 cells, 104, 107, 108–109
changes, tetanus toxin model and,
107–108
ventral (VH), 128, 129, 130

Hopkins symptoms checklist (SCL-90),
    243, 244
Humans, kindling in, 20–22, 187,
    200–201, 260
6-Hydroxydopamine (6-OHDA), 76
    effect on kindling rate, 76, 77, 79
    noradrenergic neurone grafting and
        hippocampal kindling, 79–80
Hyperactivity, 209
Hyper-reactivity, in tetanus toxin
    model, 105
Hypometabolism, 185, 226
Hypothalamo-pituitary hormones, 119
Hypothalamus, medial, feline
    defensiveness and, 126, 127, 128, 129

Immortalization oncogenes, 82
Infantile spasms (West's syndrome),
    164, 165, 171, 286
Inhibitory post-synaptic potentials, 64,
    72
Inhibitory seizures, 64
Interictal spikes in kindling, 1, 16, 91,
    92
    see also Spontaneous seizures
Intracerebral grafting of fetal neurones,
    75, 77–81, 113
    problems with, 81
    see also Transplantation of neurones

Jacksonian seizures, 180, 181
Juvenile myoclonic epilepsy, 166, 172

Kainic acid (KA), 23, 24, 126
    astrocyte activation, 24, 26, 28, 104
Kindling-induced sprouting, 24
'Kindling-like' process, 6, 263, 271,
    282–283, 285, 286
    functional psychoses, 3, 5, 224, 285
Kindling phenomenon, 1, 15–31, 56,
    69–72, 209
    anatomical substrates and structural
        changes, 22–27, 88, 197
    behavioural response, see Behavioural
        changes
    brain damage evidence, 197
    characteristics, 15–20, 88, 137, 197
    chemical, see Chemical kindling
    conditioning of, 91–92
    cortical vs subcortical sites, 19
    definition and concept, 10, 15, 75,
        195, 197, 212, 263, 282–286

broad, 197, 263, 271, 282, 284
    epileptogenesis, 10, 15, 17, 157,
        197, 212, 263, 282, 283
    three terms for, 285
difficulty in extrapolating to humans,
    205, 259
electrical, see Electrical kindling
evoked vs spontaneous events, 15–16,
    18–19, 197, 286
    see also Spontaneous seizures
focal vs generalized response, 19–20,
    88
future directions and research, 29, 31
Gowers' Phenomenon and, 150,
    157–158, 163, 284
histological measures, gross, 23, 24,
    69, 104
in humans, 20–22, 187, 200–201, 260
hyperexcitability of CNS in, 47–48,
    137
inhibition, 41, 45, 64
mechanisms, 27, 29, 48–49, 75, 88,
    158, 283
permanence of, 16, 104, 197, 259, 263
pharmacological, see Pharmacological
    kindling
phases, 213, 225
rate, 6-OHDA administration, 76
rate and regional sensitivity, 1, 15, 18,
    22, 80, 142, 187
responses with/without motor
    convulsion, 20
species susceptibility, 195
spontaneous events, see Spontaneous
    seizures
5-stage scale, 16
transfer, see Transfer of kindling
uses if broadly defined, 284
    see also individual related subjects

Lactate-induced panic attacks, 266, 269,
    270
Learning,
    CA3 region function, 109
    changes in tetanus toxin model, 107
    disturbance in temporal lobe lesions,
        115
    epilepsy relation, 88, 114, 115, 158
    interference by kindling, 91–92
    kindling as model, 88–92, 158
    memory and, 87, 88, 91

panic disorder development and, 268, 270
Lennox–Gastaut's syndrome, 164, 165, 171, 286
Lidocaine, 'doom anxiety', 249, 261
Lidocaine-induced seizures, 41, 212, 246, 261
  CRF release, block by carbamazepine, 214, 215, 227, 247–248
Limbic auras, 118–123, 120, 124, 125, 184
  psychopathology prediction, 125
Limbic disturbances,
  kindling-like process, 125
  vulnerability to response to social stress, 117, 123, 125, 187
Limbic epilepsy, 180–183
  defensive personality trait in cat and, 127
  identification, 182–183
  prognosis, 183–184, 184, 185
  psychopathology associated, 118–123, 119, 131, 184–185
    nature of, 120–123
  as specific form of epilepsy, 184, 185, 187
  terminology and classification, 180–182
  treatment difficulties, 184, 185
  see also Temporal lobe epilepsy
Limbic excitability,
  in alcohol withdrawal syndrome, 231, 233–234
  carbamazepine action, 226
  cat personality, defensive behaviour and, 127–128, 129
Limbic function, interictal changes in animal models, 125
Limbic hyperfunction, 118, 126–131
Limbic kindling, 1, 15, 16, 17, 179, 185
  impact on animal behaviour, 126–131, 186–187
  induced by CRF, 213
  interictal spikes, 16
  model of temporal lobe epilepsy, 17, 20, 186–187
  partial, effect on cat personality, 127, 129–130, 131
  rate, 1, 15, 16, 18, 22
  reduced noradrenergic inhibition, 77

response to and characteristics, 19, 20, 185–187
  spontaneous remission, 187
  in tetanus toxin model, 107
  see also Amygdala kindling; Kindling phenomenon
Limbic system,
  cocaine effect on, 7, 246
  in psychopathology development in epilepsy, 8, 10, 119, 179, 183, 184–185
  stress diathesis model and, 3, 213
  vulnerability to epileptogenic conditions, 123, 125, 187
Lithium, effect on behavioural sensitization and kindling, 247
Lithium carbonate, in manic-depressive illness, 218, 219
Locus coeruleus,
  6-OHDA facilitation of kindling, 76, 77
  kindling development suppression, 77
  panic disorder and, 266, 269
  role in alarm, 266, 267–268
Long-term potentiation (LTP),
  blocking, 104
  defensive behaviour in cat, 127, 147
  dependent on NMDA receptors, 104, 130
  kindling comparison, 46–47, 70, 89, 147, 286
  learning and memory requiring, 89, 104
  limbic kindling producing, 130
  not necessary for kindling occurrence, 70–71, 147

Manic-depressive illness, 2–3, 209–227
  anticonvulsant efficacy, 3, 202–203, 204, 210
    see also Carbamazepine
  behavioural sensitization to psychomotor stimulants relation, 3, 214–216, 224
  conditioning effect in episode activation, 3, 216, 224
  contingent inefficacy and contingent tolerance, 220–224, 225
  course of, 3, 214–215, 216, 217, 224
  ECT in, 3, 203, 204, 205
  epilepsy similarities, 158, 285

Manic-depressive illness (*cont.*)
  kindling-like process, 3, 202–203
  as learning phenomenon, 158, 224
  pharmacological kindling
    relationship, 3, 216, 218–220, 224,
    226
  psychopharmacological intervention,
    dual effects, 224
  psychotherapy response as function of
    stage, 220, 225
  rapid cycling, carbamazepine
    response, 218, 219
  response to lesser inducing stimuli,
    mechanism, 3, 158, 216, 218, 224
  therapeutic agents effectiveness,
    function of stage, 191, 218–220,
    225, 285
Medial hypothalamus (MH), feline
    defensiveness, 126, 127, 128, 129
Memory, 88
  changes in tetanus toxin model, 107
  consolidation,
    interference by kindling, 91–92
    kindled epileptogenesis similarities,
      88–91
  drugs facilitating and convulsions, 104
  effect of electrical stimulation on, 92
  epilepsy and, 87, 88, 109, 158
  habit, 220
  kindling relation, 87–100, 103–109,
    158
  learning and, 87, 88, 109
  long-term potentiation (LTP) in, 89,
    104
  multiple systems, 87, 220
  representational, 220
  retrieval,
    afterdischarge (AD) duration effect
      on, 93
    EEG patterns of afterdischarges
      (ADs), effect, 94–98, 99
    epileptic discharges/seizures relation,
      92
  interictal hippocampal spiking and, 92
Mental handicap, 168, 180
Metabolic activity in kindling, 6, 43–44,
    142
Metabolic rates, during synaptic
    inhibition, 64, 72
N-Methyl-D-aspartate (NMDA)
    receptor, *see* NMDA receptors

Minnesota Multiphasic Personality
    Inventory, 9, 184
Mirror foci, 8, 21, 36, 89
MK-801, 40
Monoamine oxidase inhibitors
    (MAOIs), 218, 219, 267
Mood lability, 126
Movement disorders, 277, 281
MPTP (methyl-phenyl-
    tetrahydropyridine), 278
Muscarinic agonists, 35, 36–38
Muscarinic blockers, 37
Muscarinic kindling, 35, 36–38
Muscarinic receptors and kindling
    induction, 37
Myoclonic seizures, 64, 65, 73

Neocortical epilepsy, 20
Neocortically-kindled seizures,
    suppression by antiepileptic drugs, 19,
      58, 62, 63
    tonic response, 19, 20
Neocortical tissue, grafting and
    amygdaloid kindling, 78–79
Neonatal convulsions, 163, 171
Nerve growth factor, 79
Neural cell lines, 82
Neuroleptic drugs, 2, 224–225
    cocaine-induced behavioural
      sensitization, effect on, 225, 248
    discontinuous and tardive dyskinesia,
      276–277
    neurotoxic effects, 278, 281
    schizophrenia pathogenesis and, 4, 5
    timing of treatment with, effect of,
      225
Neuroleptic-induced dyskinesia, 275,
    276–277
Neuronal activity, excessive in
    epileptogenesis, 98, 103
Neuronal excitability, increase in
    kindling, 29, 48–49, 89, 137
Neuronal plasticity, 88, 89
Neurophysiological mechanisms,
    seizures, 29, 47–48, 75, 89, 98, 103,
    158
Neurosis, epileptic, 184
Neurosyphilis, 198
Neuroticism, 118, 131
Neurotransmitters and kindling, 75–83,
    113–115, 277

excitatory, agonists inducing kindling,
    35, 38–40
inhibitory, antagonists inducing
    kindling, 41–42
NMDA receptors, 38–39
    activation, in epileptogenesis, 103
    antagonist, learning impairment, 104
    blockers, and electrical kindling
        block, 40
    in kindling, 38–39, 40, 47–48
    -linked ionic channels, 29, 48, 103
    LTP dependent on, 104, 130
Noradrenaline,
    central depletion and kindling, 76
    inhibitory to amygdaloid kindling, 9,
        76
Noradrenergic neurones,
    denervation, kindling facilitation by,
        76, 77, 79, 81
    grafting, 82, 83, 113
        to amygdala/pyriform cortex, 81
        hippocampal kindling, 79–81, 113
        seizure suppression, 269
    in locus coeruleus, in panic disorder,
        266, 269
Nucleus accumbens lesions, 212, 245

Olfactory bulb kindling, serotoninergic
    neurone grafting, 77–78
Oxazepam, in alcohol withdrawal
    syndrome, 242–244
Oxcarbazepine, 55, 57, 192
    kindling evolution, effect on, 55, 57,
        64–65

Panic attacks, 264
    cocaine-induced, 213, 249, 260–261
    lactate-induced, 266, 269, 270
Panic disorder,
    appearance of kindling phenomenon,
        249, 269
    biology of, 266
    depression and, 265
    development, in children, 265, 268
    diagnostic criteria, 264
    epidemiology and genetics, 265, 268,
        281
    kindling and, 249, 263, 267–270,
        281–282
    natural history, 265, 269

repetitive subthreshold stimuli and
    intervals, 267–268
stable duration of kindling
    phenomenon, 269–270
treatment, 266, 267, 269, 270
Paranoid psychosis, 210
Partial kindling of cat, 16–17, 129–130,
    131, 286
    in amygdala, 130
    effect on personality, 127, 129–130
    in ventral hippocampus, 129–130
Partial seizures, 150
    fear in, 263
    prognosis, 167, 169, 171, 191
    progression to generalization, 191
    psychopathology associated, 147, 167,
        179–180, 184, 241
    secondary generalized seizure
        frequency, 167, 171
    see also Complex partial seizures;
        Temporal lobe epilepsy
Penicillin/hippocampal slice model, 18
Pentylenetetrazol, 104, 198, 199, 201
Personality,
    changes, 117, 123, 125, 130, 131,
        147–148
        in animals, 125, 127, 129, 130, 131
        in epilepsy, 9, 123, 125, 131, 241
    epileptic, 117–118, 147, 167, 178, 179
    see also Cat, personality
Personality Behaviour Inventory (PBI),
    118, 119, 184
    modified (PBI-2), 119–120
Petit mal, 156
    pyknoleptic, 165–166, 172
Petit-mal seizures, 72, 73
Pharmacological kindling, 3, 7, 210,
    212–214
    behavioural sensitizations vs, 7,
        209–210, 247, 260
    manic-depressive episodes
        relationship, 3, 216, 218–220, 224,
        226
    phases, 213, 216, 225
Phenobarbital, 55, 59–60
    absences provoked by, 73
    amygdaloid-kindled seizures, effect
        on, 60
    amygdaloid-kindling evolution, effect
        on, 58, 59, 60, 63
    post-traumatic epilepsy and, 71–72

Phenytoin, 55, 56–57
  absence-type seizures precipitated by,
    64, 65
  action against tonic–clonic seizures, 64
  amygdaloid-kindled seizures, effect
    on, 57, 59, 214, 215
  amygdaloid kindling evolution, effect
    on, 55, 56–57, 64–65, 214, 215
  depression and, 123
  hypothesis on effects on kindling,
    64–65
  segmental neuronal inhibition
    increase, 65
Photosensitivity, prognosis, 166
Picrotoxin, 41
Post-synaptic potentials,
  excitatory, 48
  inhibitory, 64, 72
Post-traumatic epilepsy, 71, 72
Potassium, 49, 69
Prefrontal cortex, dorsolateral, in
  schizophrenia, 4, 5
Procaine, 246, 249
Psychomotor stimulants, 7–8, 210, 214,
  215, 245
  see also Cocaine
Psychopathology,
  in ethanol withdrawal, 137–144,
    240–241
  prevalence rates, 178
Psychopathology in epilepsy, 8–9, 9,
  117–118
  argument against kindling as
    mechanism, 187
  development, hypotheses, 8, 10,
    177–188
  due to secondary consequences?, 177,
    185
  epileptic personality and, 117–118,
    147, 167, 178, 179
  improvement over time, 187
  kindling as mechanism?, 179,
    185–187, 202–204
  limbic epilepsy, limbic auras, and,
    118–123, 147
  nature of, seizure association, 120–123
  overrepresentation?, 177–178
  partial seizures association, 167, 241
  percent epileptics classified as,
    120–121, 147–148, 178

temporal lobe, association, 9, 115,
    119, 167, 179–180, 182–183,
    184–185, 203
  temporal lobe vs generalized, 179–180
  vulnerability and limbic disturbances,
    123–126, 187
  see also Anxiety; entries beginning
    Behavioural
Psychosis, antagonism between epilepsy
  and, 198, 203
Psychosis, epileptic, 8–9, 184–185, 186
  ECT efficacy, kindling as model for,
    202–204
Psychotherapy, in manic-depressive
  illness, 220, 225
Psychopathology, neurotic and
  psychotic, 184
Psychomotor epilepsy, 181, 182
Pyknoleptic petit mal, 165–166, 172
Pyriform cortex, 1, 18, 70
  cell changes after kindling, 29
  in chronic epileptogenic condition, 18
  gliosis, in status epilepticus, 25, 28
  in hippocampal kindling, 80
  in induction of status epilepticus,
    23–24
  kindling rate, 1, 15, 18, 22, 80
  spontaneous events in, 22, 24

Radial arm maze, 107, 109
Raphe cells, transplantation, 78
Rat,
  amygdaloid-kindled seizures, human
    seizure comparison, 66
  antiepileptics, effect on kindling
    evolution, 56, 57, 63–65, 247
  difficulty in extrapolating kindling
    evidence, 205
  model for absence/myoclonic-type
    seizures, 65
Receptor supersensitivity, 187, 277, 282
Recurrent inhibition, 47, 129, 130
Reserpine, 76
Rhesus monkeys, 65
RO-15-1788, 41, 128, 130–131
Rolandic epilepsy, 172

Schizoid–paranoid personalities, 167
Schizophrenia, 4–5, 192
  antagonism with seizures, 198, 203
  temporal lobe involvement, 193

Schizophrenia-like psychosis, in
    epilepsy, 8, 193
Secondary foci, *see* Mirror foci
Seizure threshold, 199, 201
    fall in kindling, 201
    rise in ECT, 199, 201–202
Sensitization, 3, 260, 285, 286
    see also Behavioural sensitization
Sensory–limbic hyperconnection, 118,
    131
Serotonergic disturbance in panic
    attacks, 267
Serotonin, inhibitory effect on epileptic
    activity, 77
Serotoninergic neurones, grafting, 77–78
Social stress, response, *see* Stress,
    psychosocial
Spielberger Trait Anxiety Scale, 121,
    122, 125, 243
Spike-wave complexes, 64, 65, 72
Spontaneous seizures, 103, 284
    cell damage absence, 104
    in electro-convulsive therapy (ECT),
    199–200
    in kindling, 16, 18–19, 22, 103, 157,
    197, 212, 259–260, 283, 284
    lidocaine-induced, 212
    neurophysiology, 103
    see also Ethanol withdrawal seizures
Standard response criterion, kindling, 16
State-Trail Inventory (Spielberger), 121,
    122, 125, 243
Status epilepticus,
    astrocyte activation, 24–27, 28
    cell damage, 104
    relevance of models to kindling,
    23–24, 24–27, 28
Sterotypy, 209
Stratum radiatum–stratum moleculare,
    of hippocampus, 48
Stress diathesis model, 3
Stress, psychosocial, 260
    cocaine as model, 211, 212
    epileptic psychopathology and, 117,
    123, 125
    response to psychotherapy, 220
    seizures induced by, after kindling,
    214
    sensitization increase and, 260
    triggering manic-depressive illness, 3,
    214–215, 220, 224

Stress-related peptide, inducing
    behavioural changes, 213
Suicide-oncogenes, 82
Suitably spaced successive seizures
    (SSSS), 158
Suitably spaced successive subclinical
    stimuli (SSSSS), 157
Superkindling, 187
Synaptic mechanism, in kindling, 46,
    47–48, 70, 89

Tardive dyskinesia, 2, 5, 275, 276–277
    disappearance with increasing drug
    dosage, 281–282
    dopamine involvement, 277–278
    kindling hypothesis for, 276–277, 278
    pathogenesis hypotheses, 278, 281
Tardive seizures during ECT, 199–200
Temporal lobe, sensitivity to
    epileptogenesis, 21
Temporal lobe abnormality, in
    schizophrenia, 193
Temporal lobe epilepsy,
    alcoholism relationship, 7, 241
    anticonvulsants for, 203
    behavioural syndrome associated,
    115, 117–118
    classification, 182
    consequences, learning changes, 115
    focus of seizure in medial temporal
    lobe, 171, 179, 180
    gross structural damage absent, 185
    kindling as model of, 17, 105
    onset of seizures and
    psychopathology, time between, 186
    panic disorder similarities, 269
    prognosis, 179–180
    psychopathology, 9, 115, 119, 167, 203
    limbic structures in, 182–183, 185
    psychopathology susceptibility, 179,
    180, 203
    seizure frequency and psychosis
    relation, 186
    terminology, development of,
    180–181
    see also Limbic epilepsy
Tetanus toxin-induced epilepsy model,
    104, 105–109
    long-term effects, 107–109
Thalamus, stimulation, 22

Tolerance,
   cocaine, 210, 247
   conditioned, carbamazepine, 221,
      223, 225
Tonic–clonic seizure,
   anti-absence drugs effect, 65
   kindling model for, 65, 66
   memory retrieval, effect on, 93
   in natural history of epilepsy, 150, 162
   resistance to partial seizures after, 156
Tourette syndrome, 277
Transfer of kindling, 35, 36, 45, 79, 88,
      89
   chemical specificity, 46
   failure, 45
   influence of neocortical tissue grafts,
      79
   partial, 46
Transplantation of neurones, 75, 77–81,
      113
   dopaminergic, 82
   ethical aspects, 82
   growth of, 113
   neural cell lines, establishment, 82
   noradrenergic, 79–81, 82, 83, 113, 269
   serotoninergic to olfactory bulb, 78
Transplantation therapy, in epilepsy,
      81–82, 83

Tricyclic antidepressant drugs (TCA),
   ECS comparisons, 204–205
   in manic-depressive illness, 218, 219
   in panic disorder, 266, 267, 269
Trifluoperazine, 276
Trigeminal neuralgia, 221, 225
Trimethadione, effect on amygdaloid-
   kindled seizures, 61

Uncinate gyrus, 181

Valproate, 60, 65
   amygdaloid-kindled seizures, effect
      on, 60, 61
   amygdaloid-kindling evolution, effect
      on, 58
Ventral hippocampus (VH),
   enhanced feline defensiveness, 17,
      128, 129–130
   partial kindling, 16–17, 129–130
Ventral tegmental area stimulation,
      285–286

West's syndrome, 164, 165, 171
Withdrawal seizures, see Ethanol
   withdrawal seizures

Yohimbine, 266–267